Ischemic Stroke

Ischemic Stroke

Diagnosis and Treatment

Edited by **Sheryl Martin-Schild,
Hen Hallevi, and Andrew Barreto**

Rutgers University Press

New Brunswick, Camden, and Newark, New Jersey, and London

Library of Congress Cataloging-in-Publication Data

Names: Martin-Schild, Sheryl, editor. | Hallevi, Hen, editor. | Barreto,
    Andrew, editor.
Title: Ischemic stroke : diagnosis and treatment / edited by Sheryl
    Martin-Schild, Hen Hallevi, and Andrew Barreto.
Other titles: Ischemic stroke (Martin-Schild)
Description: New Brunswick : Rutgers University Press, 2018. | Includes
    bibliographical references and index.
Identifiers: LCCN 2018030027| ISBN 9780813592572 (pbk.) |
    ISBN 9780813592589 | ISBN 9780813592596 | ISBN 9780813592602
Subjects: | MESH: Stroke—therapy | Stroke—diagnosis | Brain
    Ischemia—therapy | Brain Ischemia—diagnosis
Classification: LCC RC388.5 | NLM WL 356 | DDC 616.8/1—dc23
LC record available at https://lccn.loc.gov/2018030027

A British Cataloging-in-Publication record for this book is available from
the British Library.

www.rutgersuniversitypress.org

Manufactured in the United States of America

CONTENTS

CONTRIBUTORS

Andrew Barreto, MD MS
Associate Professor of Neurology
Stroke Division, Department
  of Neurology
University of Texas Health Science
  Center at Houston
Houston, TX

Liliana Cohen, MD
Jersey City Medical Center
Jersey City, NJ

Michael G. Fara, MD
Department of Neurology
NYU Langone Health
New York, NY

Christopher Favilla, MD
Assistant Professor of Neurology
University of Pennsylvania
Philadelphia, PA

Rahul Garg, MD
Department of Radiology
Rutgers Robert Wood Johnson
  Medical School
New Brunswick, NJ

Toby I. Gropen, MD, FAHA
James H. Halsey Jr., MD
  Endowed Professor and Chief,
Division of Cerebrovascular
  Disease
Department of Neurology
Director, Comprehensive
  Neurovascular and Stroke Center
The University of Alabama at
  Birmingham
Birmingham, AL

Hen Hallevi, MD
Director, Neurology Department
  A (Stroke)
Tel-Aviv Sourasky Medical Center
Tel Aviv, Israel

**Nneka Ifejika, MD, MPH,
FAAPMR, FAHA**
Stroke Section Chief
Associate Professor of Physical
  Medicine and Rehabilitation
Associate Professor of Neurology
  and Neurotherapeutics
University of Texas Southwestern
Dallas, Texas

Koto Ishida, MD
Medical Director of Stroke
Department of Neurology
NYU Langone Health
New York, NY

Lester Y. Leung, MD, MSc
Director, Comprehensive Stroke
    Center
Director, Stroke and Young Adults
    Program
Tufts Medical Center
Boston, MA

Ava L. Liberman, MD
Assistant Professor of Neurology
Albert Einstein College
    of Medicine
Montefiore Medical CenterBronx,
    NY

Kira Long, MD
Tulane University Department
    of Surgery
Tulane Medical School
University of Chicago
Chicago, IL

**Sheryl Martin-Schild, MD, PhD,
FANA, FAHA**
Stroke Medical Director
    for Louisiana Emergency
    Response Network (LERN)
Medical Director of Neurology
    & Stroke—Touro Infirmary
Medical Director of Neurology—
    New Orleans East Hospital
Co-Director of the Stroke
    Program—Our Lady of the Lake
President & CEO—Dr. Brain, Inc.
New Orleans, LA

James S. McKinney, MD
Medical Director of NHRMC
    Stroke Program
New Hanover Regional Medical
    Center
Wilmington, NC

Deviyani Mehta, MD
Assistant Professor of
    Neurology
Department of Neurology
Rutgers Robert Wood Johnson
    Medical School
New Brunswick, NJ

Steven R. Messé, MD
Associate Professor of Neurology
University of Pennsylvania
Philadelphia, PA

**Michael T. Mullen, MD,
MSCE**
Assistant Professor
University of Pennsylvania
Department of Neurology
Philadelphia, PA

Vikas Patel, MD
Vascular Neurology Fellow
Rutgers New Jersey Medical
    School
Parlin, NJ

Christopher Renner, MD
Vascular Neurology Fellow
University of Pennsylvania
Philadelphia, PA

Igor Rybinnik, MD
Assistant Professor of Neurology
Rutgers Robert Wood Johnson
    Medical School
New Brunswick, NJ

Amardeep Saluja, MD, FHRS
Director, Clinical Cardiac
    Electrophysiology Laboratory
Robert Wood Johnson University
    Hospital
New Brunswick, NJ

Albert D. Sam II, MD, MS, MMM, FACS
The Vascular Experts/Southern CT
  Vascular Center
Director, Middlesex Hospital Limb
  Preservation Program
Middletown, Connecticut

Rajbeer Singh Sangha, MD
Fellow of Neurocritical Care
Northwestern Memorial Hospital
Chicago, IL

Steven M. Schonfeld, MD
Clinical Professor of Radiology
Chief, Division of Neuroradiology
Robert Wood Johnson Medical School
New Brunswick, NJ

Magdy Selim, MD, PhD
Professor of Neurology
Harvard Medical School
Chief, Division of Stroke &
  Cerebrovascular Disease
Department of Neurology
Beth Israel Deaconess Medical Center
Boston, MA

Christina Mijalski Sells, MD, MPH
Clinical Assistant Professor,
  Neurology & Neurological Sciences
Telestroke Program Medical Director
Stanford University Medical Center
Stanford Stroke Center
Palo Alto, CA

James E. Siegler, MD
Vascular Neurology Fellow
University of Pennsylvania
Philadelphia, PA

Joseph Tarsia, MD
Assistant Professor of Neurology
University of Queensland,Ochsner
  Clinical School
Department of Vascular Neurology,
  Ochsner Neuroscience Institute
New Orleans, LA

Monica Verduzco-Gutierrez, MD
Assistant Professor of Physical
  Medicine and Rehabilitation
Vice Chair of Compliance, Quality
  and Patient Safety
McGovern Medical School at
  UTHealth
Medical Director of Brain Injury
  and Stroke Programs
TIRR/Memorial Hermann
Houston, TX

Linda C. Wendell, MD
Assistant Professor, Division of
  Neurocritical Care
Departments of Neurology and
  Neurosurgery and Section
  of Medical Education
Vice Chair of Education of Neurology
Director—Clinical Neurosciences
  Clerkship (Neurology),
  Sub-Internship in Neurology, and
  Advanced Elective in Neurology
The Warren Alpert School of
  Medicine at Brown University
Providence, RI

Ashlie White, MD
Department of Surgery
Tulane Medical School
New Orleans, LA

Frank Wilklow, MD
Interventional Cardiologist
Touro Infirmary
New Orleans, LA

Ischemic Stroke

Emergent Evaluation of the Suspected Stroke Patient

Lester Y. Leung and Andrew Barreto

TIME IS BRAIN

Acute stroke is a treatable medical emergency, and time is a critical determinant of permanent disability and death. For every minute the human brain is starved of oxygen and nutrients in acute ischemic stroke, 1.9 million neurons are lost.[1] In acute intracerebral hemorrhage, patients can rapidly decompensate secondary to expansion of the hematoma, leading to obstructive hydrocephalus or brain herniation. Early recognition and treatment of both ischemic stroke and intracerebral hemorrhage can significantly reduce stroke severity and improve chances of achieving functional independence and, in an increasing number of cases, a return to baseline neurologic function.

While there are many efforts to bring patients with acute stroke to stroke centers during early, intervenable stages of their illnesses, there are few organized programs for medical providers to improve the detection and management of acute stroke in the inpatient and outpatient settings. Therefore, non-neurologists (including primary care physicians, hospitalists, intensivists, cardiologists, surgeons, anesthesiologists, and others) must remain vigilant in detecting symptoms of stroke early and develop clinical skills to optimize the management of acute stroke during the first few critical minutes and hours while calling for guidance from vascular neurology specialists.

THE STROKE CHAIN OF SURVIVAL

To organize care systems around rapid triage, evaluation, and treatment of acute stroke, the American Heart Association/American Stroke Association developed the *stroke chain of survival*.[2]

Detection

Most individuals with acute stroke develop their neurologic symptoms and deficits in the community setting. Because many strokes result in impaired awareness or communication, neurologic deficits must be recognized by family members, friends, co-workers, and bystanders. Unfortunately, public awareness of stroke symptoms is poor, with only modest improvements gained through several public health campaigns to improve awareness of stroke warning signs; risk factors; and time-limited, emergent treatments.[3–11]

However, clinicians are better equipped with background knowledge on stroke presentations and the emergent nature of the condition as well as with better familiarity with healthcare systems. Both inpatient and outpatient clinicians have opportunities to identify and triage patients with acute stroke symptoms in a healthcare setting with resources that can be mobilized to initiate the stroke evaluation or quickly transfer the patient to a stroke center. (Stroke symptoms and signs will be discussed in greater detail in Chapter 2.)

Dispatch

In the community, the initial contact between a patient or family member and the healthcare system ideally proceeds through a telephone call to emergency medical services (EMS): dialing 9-1-1. (Some individuals subscribe to remote activation of EMS through wearable devices.) The 9-1-1 operator attempts to obtain a few historical details to triage the urgency of the call; in some cases, a specialized EMS team that includes stroke experts available via video-conference telemedicine can be dispatched to evaluate the patient.[12] Upon arriving on the scene, the EMS team quickly assesses the patient with the basic ABCs of resuscitation; proceeds with a brief, stroke-oriented clinical assessment; and then prepares the patient for transportation to the nearest hospital. Ideally, if the stroke is recognized by EMS personnel, the patient may actually bypass the nearest hospital and instead be taken to a certified primary or comprehensive stroke center.[13] (The examination of the stroke patient is described in Chapter 2.)

For clinicians in outpatient and inpatient settings, the dispatch process is more heterogeneous. In clinic and outpatient procedure settings (even those connected to a hospital), the fastest method of patient transfer is usually through activation of EMS; however, the clinician can begin the initial clinical examination and obtain key historical details to convey to EMS. (Exceptions occur with procedural services such as cardiology that have inpatient services and beds where the patient can be quickly admitted and medically stabilized.) When a patient is admitted to a hospital without vascular neurology specialists, the inpatient clinician should call for emergent consultation with the hospitalist's on-call neurologist or through telestroke services. When a patient is admitted to a hospital with a stroke service, a stroke activation or stroke code can be called to mobilize the neurology team for rapid assessment. (The key historical details that must be obtained by the clinician are described later in this chapter.)

Delivery

EMS is tasked with rapidly transporting patients to stroke centers that are capable of providing intravenous fibrinolytic therapy (IV tissue plasminogen activator, or IV tPA) for acute ischemic stroke. Outcomes are better for these patients.[14] Additionally, some patients may benefit from intra-arterial therapies (mechanical thrombectomy), which are usually performed by appropriately trained vascular neurologists, interventional radiologists, or neurosurgeons. Other surgical treatments such as decompressive hemicraniectomies for large hemispheric strokes and hemicraniectomies and ventriculostomies for intracerebral hemorrhages are provided by neurosurgical specialists. Ideally, a city's or region's EMS services may be organized to routinely bring patients with possible acute stroke to these centers and provide prehospital notification. This expedites the mobilization of the stroke team and other ancillary services and permits faster treatment. For example, the stroke team meets the patient at the door and escorts her directly to the CT scanner, which has already been cleared and prepared for stroke neuroimaging.

During this phase, EMS providers and other clinicians use prehospital stroke scales to estimate stroke severity. Several scores have been developed, including the Los Angeles Prehospital Stroke Screen (LAPSS), a shortened version called the Los Angeles Motor Score (LAMS), and the Cincinnati Prehospital Stroke Scale (CPSS).[15–17] Of these, LAMS and CPSS have been validated to help predict the presence of persistent large-vessel occlusions (LVOs) with high severity scores.[18,19] Accordingly, these scores may help triage patients to centers that can deliver optimal, expedient care. In some regions, stroke centers that provide intra-arterial therapies (comprehensive stroke centers, CSCs) are within relatively close proximity to centers that only provide intravenous therapies (primary stroke centers, PSCs). Some PSCs lack additional capabilities, including emergent angiographic studies (CT angiography or MR angiography), MR imaging, or intensive care unit (ICU)–level care. In light of clinical trials demonstrating the efficacy of combined intravenous fibrinolysis and intra-arterial therapy for ischemic strokes due to LVO, early identification of patients with persistent LVO can help EMS providers direct patients to centers that can provide both therapies in a timely manner without delay in diagnosis, transport, or mobilization of specialized teams. In other situations, eligible patients may need to receive intravenous fibrinolysis at a PSC before rapid transport (e.g., via helicopter) to a CSC for subsequent intra-arterial therapy.

For the clinician evaluating a patient with acute stroke, arranging transportation to the next stage of care is vital. While EMS ground transport between a clinic and an adjacent hospital is straightforward, some patients may need to be transported by helicopter to the nearest stroke center. In some cases, transportation may occur after the non-neurologist clinician has assessed the patient, obtained requisite imaging and laboratory data, confirmed the absence of contraindications, and proceeded with treatment with IV tPA. If an in-hospital stroke activation is called, the clinician may need to arrange for hospital transport services to bring the patient to the CT scanner or assist the stroke team in transporting the patient.

Door

If the EMS services were able to provide prehospital notification of a patient's arrival, the stroke team can be present when the patient enters the doors of the emergency department. The emergency medicine team is tasked with rapidly assessing the patient within 10 minutes of the patient's arrival. During this phase, EMS communicates the initial historical details and findings from a prehospital stroke screening assessment.

The non-neurologist clinician evaluating a patient with possible acute stroke must provide essential details of the patient's history and examination to expedite the evaluation and treatment of the patient. When EMS, an on-call neurologist, or the stroke team arrives, a brief assessment should be presented:

> The patient is a 65-year-old woman with an acute onset of aphasia and right face and arm weakness in the setting of atrial fibrillation, not on anticoagulation. She was last seen normal 30 minutes ago by the physical therapists.

Some stroke centers have developed pathways through which patients with suspected stroke may be delivered from EMS directly to the CT scanner, dramatically reducing treatment times (i.e., "door-to-needle" time).[20] Point-of-care laboratory testing is often implemented to quickly assess blood glucose, coagulation studies, and renal function. If a patient is eligible for fibrinolysis after head CT images are acquired, tPA can be drawn from a medication repository in the scanner room and administered while the patient is still in the CT scanner. Often, once renal function has been assessed, the patient then undergoes CT angiography to assess for critical stenosis and occlusions of the extracranial and intracranial blood vessels.

Data

In the emergency department, a few key data are quickly acquired in order to assist the decision-making process regarding intravenous fibrinolytic and intra-arterial therapies and to exclude common stroke mimics. While several laboratory tests, cardiac telemetry and electrocardiography, and vital signs are obtained, the most essential data required before the administration of IV tPA are as follows:

1. The National Institutes of Health Stroke Scales (NIHSS), a brief standardized examination quantifying the patient's neurologic deficits.
2. Blood pressure, as the patient's systolic blood pressure should be below 185 and diastolic blood pressure should be below 110 prior to administration of IV tPA.
3. Glucose measurement, generally obtained as a point-of-care fingerstick blood draw to exclude severe hypoglycemia and hyperglycemia (common stroke mimics).
4. A noncontrast head CT to exclude intracranial hemorrhage. (Imaging is discussed in greater detail in Chapter 4.)
5. Coagulation studies (prothrombin time/international normalized ratio, partial thromboplastin time [PT/INR, PTT]) if the patient is known to be taking anticoagulants.

The non-neurologist clinician can obtain several of these data prior to arrival of EMS, the on-call neurologist, or the stroke team; an updated set of vital signs and glucose measurement are readily available in most clinics and on inpatient wards, and the NIHSS is an easy assessment tool to learn. While awaiting the arrival of EMS or the neurologist, an order can be placed for a STAT noncontrast head CT for the acute stroke evaluation.

With these data, the assessment is richer and can expedite treatment even further:

The patient is a 65-year-old woman with an acute onset of aphasia and right face and arm weakness in the setting of atrial fibrillation, not on anticoagulation. She was last seen normal 30 minutes ago by the physical therapists. Her NIHSS is 6. Her blood pressure is 170/80, and her glucose is 105. I have ordered a STAT head CT and called Radiology; they are ready for us.

Decision

The initial decision focuses on the administration of IV tPA for possible acute ischemic stroke. In most cases, decision support provided by vascular neurologists maximizes the chances of administering IV tPA appropriately while minimizing the risk of harm (i.e., hemorrhagic complications) through inadequate patient selection. In emergency departments without neurology or vascular neurology support, emergency medicine clinicians typically follow strict protocols and assess a comprehensive list of contraindications to the administration of IV tPA. If these contraindications are not present, then IV tPA can be administered as an emergent treatment. If the patient is unable to communicate and no family or medical provider is available to corroborate a medical history, then the clinician must use her clinical judgment regarding whether or not to proceed with fibrinolytic therapy. Verbal consent is generally obtained when possible, but it is not essential in order to proceed with this proven therapy undertaken to reduce permanent disability. The American Heart Association (AHA)/American Stroke Association (ASA) provides guidelines regarding the administration of IV tPA and a list of suggested contraindications.[21] At the time of this publication, IV tPA is approved for the treatment of acute ischemic stroke within 3 hours of the onset of symptoms, and the AHA/ASA also recommends its administration between 3 and 4.5 hours after the onset of symptoms for eligible patients with a few additional contraindications. IV tPA has been demonstrated repeatedly to reduce disability and improve the chances of achieving functional independence. (Fibrinolytic therapy is discussed in greater detail in Chapter 6). Visual aids to help with the decision analysis and discussions with patients and family members have previously been published and effectively illustrate the benefit and risk of IV tPA.[22]

Importantly, intravenous fibrinolysis for patients presenting to emergency departments with most stroke mimics is safe.[23–26] In the absence of strict contraindications, treatment with intravenous fibrinolysis is commonly the safest and best option for most patients with possible acute ischemic stroke. The situation may be more complicated for patients admitted to the hospital with other medical conditions. However, the administration of IV tPA for patients with acute stroke while admitted to the hospital is a common practice.[27]

Selected ischemic stroke patients achieve additional benefit from intra-arterial therapy. This therapy, also known as thrombectomy, applies to patients with acute ischemic stroke due to large artery occlusions of the intracranial vasculature (and sometimes, tandem occlusions in the extracranial arteries) for which combination therapy with IV tPA and intra-arterial therapy is more effective than IV tPA alone. The 2018 AHA/ASA guidelines for the management of acute ischemic stroke now recommend thrombectomy for selected patients who have proximal (terminal internal carotid and middle cerebral artery) occlusions and in which thrombectomy can be started within 6 hours of symptom onset.[21] For select patients with favorable pretreatment neuroimaging indicating a slow progression to brain infarction, endovascular therapy can be considered within 24 hours of symptom onset. While some patients with strict contraindications to systemic fibrinolytics may undergo intra-arterial therapy, these catheter-based treatments have not been demonstrated to be a suitable replacement for IV tPA in the majority of cases of acute ischemic stroke. (Endovascular therapy is discussed in greater detail in Chapter 7.)

For patients with acute intracerebral hemorrhage, additional data are obtained to determine the cause and treatable exacerbating factors that may predispose to hematoma expansion. These include uncontrolled hypertension, coagulopathies (often induced by anticoagulant medications), and vascular malformations (e.g., aneurysms, arteriovenous malformations).

Drug

If the decision is made to proceed with IV tPA, the medication is administered as a weight-based dose with 10% of the dose injected over 1 minute and the remaining 90% infused over 1 hour (maximum dose of 90 mg). During this time, additional laboratory and clinical data may be obtained; some of these data may actually prompt the cessation of the infusion if a contraindication to fibrinolysis is discovered (e.g., an elevated INR, a low platelet count, etc.). The patient is closely monitored during the course of the infusion for early complications of IV tPA, including intracranial hemorrhage and orolingual angioedema.

If patients are found to have intracerebral hemorrhage, the major tenets of care focus on rapidly identifying and attenuating the impact of factors that expand hemorrhages and worsen outcomes.[28] This typically involves monitoring and treatment of high blood pressure, reversal of coagulopathies (often pharmacologic), and identification and treatment of arterial vascular malformations (such as ruptured aneurysms and arteriovenous malformations). Most hemorrhages are associated with hypertension, and treatment of high blood pressure to a systolic blood pressure goal of less than 140 has been demonstrated to be safe and possibly beneficial.[29] This is particularly important for patients who present early in the course of hemorrhage or have imaging signs that predict hematoma expansion (and, thus, the increase in volume of the intracranial mass, increased intracranial pressure, development of hydrocephalus, and damage to surrounding structures).[30]

Disposition

After the administration of IV tPA in an emergency department, patients with acute ischemic stroke are typically admitted to a specialized stroke unit (in some cases, an intermediate care unit on the neurology floor or an intensive care unit). If the patient is eligible for intra-arterial therapy, she may be transferred to the angiography suite for endovascular treatment prior to admission to the stroke unit or intensive care unit.

For the non–neurologist clinician evaluating and treating a patient with possible acute stroke, the disposition decision may be complex. For outpatient clinicians, all patients with acute stroke symptoms should be transported to the closest stroke center, regardless of eligibility for acute recanalization therapies: the risk of stroke recurrence, neurologic deterioration, and complications of stroke are high in the first few days after stroke. For clinicians in community hospitals without a stroke service, some minor strokes and transient ischemic attacks may be managed with the assistance of a neurology consultation, as long as careful attention is given to the numerous possible post-stroke complications and the core tenets of post-stroke care, including appropriate secondary prevention and rehabilitation (i.e., the AHA/ASA's Get With the Guidelines program for the standardization of inpatient stroke care). Patients with more severe or complicated presentations of stroke may warrant transfer to a comprehensive stroke center that can provide care guided by a vascular neurology specialist, neurosurgical treatments, cardiovascular and hematology consultation, and neurocritical care management. (Critical care management is described in Chapter 8.) Patients undergoing IV tPA or intra-arterial therapies should be admitted to a stroke unit with appropriately trained nursing staff and telemetry whenever possible to provide the appropriate monitoring and response to complications of treatment.

ESSENTIALS FOR IN-HOSPITAL STROKES

Clinicians in all fields can use a few basic tools to establish:

1. The possibility of eligibility for acute, time-limited treatments for stroke.
2. The likelihood of acute stroke as the underlying cause of a patient's symptoms and signs.
3. The necessity of emergent neurology consultation.

The first essential detail is the last seen normal (LSN) time: this is the start time for the time window during which acute recanalization therapies for acute ischemic stroke can be administered, including intravenous fibrinolysis and intra-arterial therapy. In order to proceed with acute stroke treatments, an LSN time must be established to as high a degree of certainty as possible. The nature of this time is dependent on the clinical scenario: if the patient cannot communicate, the LSN time is the time when she was last seen by another person at her neurologic baseline. If the patient awoke with neurologic deficits, the LSN time is the time when she went to sleep. In some cases, a patient may have a witnessed onset of neurologic deficits, which represents the LSN time. If the patient can communicate, the LSN time is when she experienced the onset of her neurologic deficits (unless she awoke with those deficits, whereupon the LSN time is, again, the time when she went to sleep). In some cases, symptoms may occur and then completely resolve. If the symptoms recur, the time of recurrence (after confirmed full resolution of symptoms and deficits) is the LSN time.

In many cases of in-hospital stroke, the LSN time is the last time a patient was evaluated by a nurse for a routine assessment, underwent a vital signs check from a nursing assistant, or before a patient undergoes anesthesia for a procedure. Unfortunately, many ischemic strokes occur while a patient is sleeping, so new neurologic deficits discovered at the time of morning rounds do not always warrant an emergent Neurology evaluation but may still require early initiation of post-stroke therapies. At other times, stroke symptoms and signs are detected very early during a physical therapy evaluation or when a nurse returns to the patient's bedside to administer a medication. It is imperative that concerns brought forward by ancillary staff about a change in neurologic status are taken seriously and addressed promptly.

Second, not all sudden-onset neurologic symptoms are due to acute stroke. The syndromic definition of *acute ischemic stroke* is an acute onset of focal neurologic deficits referable to a vascular territory in the setting of cerebrovascular risk factors. Acute intracerebral hemorrhage follows similar patterns, but the neurologic syndrome does not need to be restricted to a vascular territory. The more features of the syndromic definition a patient's presentation matches, the more likely the patient's deficits are due to stroke. (Stroke symptoms and signs are described in Chapter 2.)

Finally, does neurology need to be emergently consulted? If a patient has an established LSN time placing her within a time window for intravenous fibrinolysis and/or intra-arterial therapy, then the answer is yes. In stroke centers, emergent evaluations by vascular neurology specialists and neurologists can be accomplished at the bedside through in-person examinations or through telemedicine technologies. While these services are being mobilized, it is essential for the primary physician to initiate preliminary supportive care measures. Outside the time window for these treatments, early consultation is still advisable as there are numerous complications that can follow acute stroke, including cerebral edema, brain herniation, infections, seizures, cardiac arrhythmias, myocardial infarction, cardiopulmonary arrest, and death.

IN-HOSPITAL STROKE SCENARIOS

Strokes commonly occur in the setting of concurrent illnesses, and these may present with acute symptoms during a patient's hospitalization for another medical condition. The following are common scenarios encountered by vascular neurology specialists organized by consulting service:

1. Cardiology
   a. After cardiac catheterization, either immediately after awakening from anesthesia or in the first few days after the procedure
   b. After atrial fibrillation ablation
   c. During or immediately after endovascular replacement of aortic or mitral valves
   d. After patent foramen ovale or atrial septal defect closure
   e. After treatment of cardiogenic shock or arrhythmia electrocardioversion
   f. During medical or surgical treatment for infective endocarditis
   g. With patients receiving multiple antithrombotics for treatment of concurrent cardiovascular conditions (e.g., coronary artery disease, atrial fibrillation, mechanical valve replacement, etc.)
2. Cardiothoracic surgery
   a. After coronary artery graft bypass surgery
   b. After open valvular repair or replacement
3. Vascular surgery
   a. After carotid endarterectomy
   b. After open or endovascular aortic dissection repair
4. Neurosurgery
   a. After coiling or stenting of intracranial aneurysms
   b. After coiling of arteriovenous malformations
   c. After temporal lobectomy for the treatment of epilepsy
5. Gastroenterology
   a. Following cessation of antiplatelet or anticoagulant therapy in preparation for endoscopy
6. Obstetrics
   a. Around the time of delivery and puerperium
7. Medical intensive care unit
   a. During treatment for infective meningitis
   b. During treatment of septic or anaphylactic shock

c. During treatment for patients with liver failure complicated by coagulopathies

Acute stroke is a common, critical, treatable illness encountered by clinicians in a variety of scenarios and practice environments. Understanding the essential steps to initiate care, the stages of stroke diagnostic and treatment pathways, and the roles and responsibilities of clinicians encountering patients with stroke is as essential as recognizing the signs and symptoms of neurologic dysfunction due to stroke. These initial steps are crucial to improving the outcomes of patients with stroke through early recognition, mobilization, and treatment.

References

1. Saver JL. Time is brain—quantified. *Stroke*. 2006;37:263–266.
2. Jauch EC, Cucchiara B, Adeoye O, et al. 2010 American Heart Association Guidelines for Cardiopulmonary Resuscitation and Emergency Cardiovascular Care Science. Part 11: Adult Stroke. *Circulation*. 2010;122:S818–828.
3. Greenlund KJ, Neff LJ, Zheng ZJ, et al. Low public recognition of major stroke symptoms. *Am J Prev Med*. 2003;25(4):315–319.
4. Kleindorfer DO, Miller R, Moomaw CJ, et al. Designing a message for public education regarding stroke: does FAST capture enough stroke? *Stroke*. 2007;38(10):2864–2868.
5. Kleindorfer DO, Khoury K, Broderick JP, et al. Temporal trends in public awareness of stroke: warning signs, risk factors, and treatment. *Stroke*. 2009;40(7):2502–2506.
6. Kleindorfer DO, Lindsell CJ, Moomaw CJ, et al. Which stroke symptoms prompt a 911 call? A population-based study. *Am J Emerg Med*. 2010;28(5):607–612.
7. Lecouturier J, Murtagh MJ, Thomson RG, et al. Response to symptoms of in the UK: a systematic review. *BMC Health Serv Res*. 2010;10:157.
8. Robinson TG, Reid A, Haunton VJ, et al. The face arm speech test: does it encourage rapid recognition of important stroke warning symptoms? *Emerg Med J*. 2013;30(6):467–471.
9. Lundelin K, Graciani A, Garcia-Puig J, et al. Knowledge of stroke warning symptoms and intended action in response to stroke in Spain: a nationwide population-based study. *Cerebrovasc Dis*. 2012;34(2):161–168.
10. Rasura M, Baldereschi M, Di Carlo A, et al. Effectiveness of public stroke educational interventions: a review. *Eur J Neurol*. 2014;21(1):11–20.
11. Yang J, Zheng M, Cheng S, et al. Knowledge of stroke symptoms and treatment among community residents in Western Urban China. *J Stroke Cerebrovasc Dis*. 2014;23(5):1216–1224.
12. Rajan S, Baraniuk S, Parker S, et al. Implementing a mobile stroke unit program in the United States: why, how, and how much? *JAMA Neurol*. 2015;72(2):229–234.
13. Brandler ES, Sharma M, Sinert RH, et al. Prehospital stroke scales in urban environments: a systematic review. *Neurology*. 2014;82(24):2241–2249.
14. de la Ossa NP, Sanchez-Ojanguren J, Palomeras E, et al. Influence of the stroke code activation source on the outcome of acute ischemic stroke patients. *Neurology*. 2008;70(15):1238–1243.
15. Kidwell CS, Starkman S, Eckstein M, et al. Identifying stroke in the field. Prospective validation of the Los Angeles prehospital stroke screen (LAPSS). *Stroke*. 2000;31(1):71–76.

16. Llanes JN, Kidwell CS, Starkman S, et al. The Los Angeles Motor Scale (LAMS): a new measure to characterize stroke severity in the field. *Prehosp Emerg Care*. 2004;8(1):46–50.

17. Kothari RU, Panciolo A, Liu T, et al. Cincinnati Prehospital Stroke Scale: reproducibility and validity. *Ann Emerg Med*. 1999;33(4):373–378.

18. Nazliel B, Starkamn S, Liebeskind DS, et al. A brief prehospital stroke severity scale identifies ischemic stroke patients harboring persisting large arterial occlusions. *Stroke*. 2008;39:2264–2267.

19. Katz BS, McMullan JT, Sucharew H, et al. Design and validation of a prehospital scale to predict stroke severity: Cincinnati Prehospital Stroke Severity Scale. *Stroke*. 2015;46:1508–1512.

20. Meretoja A, Strbian D, Mustanoja S, et al. Reducing in-hospital delay to 20 minutes in stroke thrombolysis. *Neurology*. 2012;79:306–313.

21. Powers WJ, Rabinstein AA, Ackerson T, et al. 2018 guidelines for the early management of patients with acute ischemic stroke: a guideline for healthcare professionals from the American Heart Association/American Stroke Association. *Stroke*. 2018;49:e46–e110.

22. Saver JL, Gornbein J, Starkman S. Graphic reanalysis of the two NINDS-tPA trials confirms substantial treatment benefit. *Stroke*. 2010;41:2381–2390.

23. Chernyshev Y, Martin-Schild S, Albright KC, et al. Safety of tPA in stroke mimics and neuroimaging-negative cerebral ischemia. *Neurology*. 2010;74(17):1340–1345.

24. Giraldo EA, Khalid A, Zand R. Safety of intravenous thrombolysis within 4.5 h of symptom onset in patients with negative post-treatment stroke imaging for cerebral infarction. *Neurocrit Care*. 2011;15(1):76–79.

25. Zinkstok SM, Engelter ST, Gensicke H, et al. Safety of thrombolysis in stroke mimics: results from a multicenter cohort study. *Stroke*. 2013;44(4):1080–1084.

26. Tsivgoulis G, Zand R, Katsanos AH, et al. Safety of intravenous fibrinolysis in stroke mimics: prospective 5-year study and comprehensive meta-analysis. *Stroke*. 2015;46:1281–1287 [epub ahead of print, Mar 19]

27. Emiru T, Adil MM, Suri MF, et al. Thrombolytic treatment for in-hospital ischemic strokes in United States. *J Vasc Interv Neurol*. 2014;7(5):28–34.

28. Hemphill III JC, Greenberg SM, Anderson CS, et al. Guidelines for the management of spontaneous intracerebral hemorrhage. *Stroke*. 2015;46:2032–2060.

29. Anderson CS, Heeley E, Huang Y, et al. Rapid blood-pressure lowering in patients with acute intracerebral hemorrhage. *N Engl J Med*. 2013;368:2355–2365.

30. Wada R, Aviv RI, Fox AJ, et al. CT angiography "spot sign" predicts hematoma expansion in intracerebral hemorrhage. *Stroke*. 2007;38:1257–1262.

Clinical Signs and Symptoms of Stroke   2

Christopher Renner and Deviyani Mehta

In the realm of neurology, when a patient's presenting deficits are "sudden" in onset and "focal," all neurologists would agree that *stroke* is at the top of the differential. The two broad categories of stroke are *ischemic* and *hemorrhagic*. Ischemic stroke is caused by occlusion of one or more blood vessels in the brain for sufficient time to cause cerebral infarction. When these occlusions are temporary, resulting in complete resolution of symptoms *and* no evidence of infarction on brain imaging, the term *transient ischemic attack* (TIA) is used instead. Various stroke syndromes result, depending upon the location of the occlusion. Recognition of the particular signs and symptoms of the various stroke syndromes can help to localize the infarct as well as the occluded vessel and, therefore, the volume of infarcted brain tissue. The more common stroke syndromes will be described in this chapter.

MCA SYNDROME

Known to supply the largest portion of the cerebral hemisphere, the middle cerebral artery (MCA) and its branches are some of the most common sites of occlusion and infarct. Broadly speaking, the main cortical areas supplied by the MCA include the lateral frontal and lateral temporal cortices, the parietal cortex, and the insula and operculum.[1] Deeper structures supplied by the MCA include most of the anterior and posterior limbs of internal capsule, the basal ganglia, extreme capsule, putamen, claustrum, globus pallidus, substantia innominate of Reichert, as well as the body and posterior head of caudate nucleus.[2-4] A complete MCA distribution infarct will produce contralateral hemiplegia, hemianesthesia,

13

hemianopia, ipsilateral gaze preference, global aphasia (dominant hemisphere), and contralateral hemineglect.

The MCA is supplied by the internal carotid artery (ICA) and divides to form a superior division and an inferior division. These cortical branches supply the lateral portion of the cerebral hemisphere. Proximal to this bifurcation, multiple deep penetrating, or lenticulostriate branches, exit and supply subcortical structures. These include the internal capsule, lentiform nucleus (putamen and pallidum), and body of caudate nucleus. When a blockage occurs in the portion of MCA proximal to its first division, termed the M1 segment or middle cerebral stem, an MCA stem occlusion syndrome results. While distal occlusion of the stem will not affect the deep penetrating vessels (as they originate from the stem), proximal or total occlusion will result in a combination of cortical and deep branch deficits, as outlined in Table 2.1.

The superior division supplies the frontal lobe and rolandic regions, while the inferior division supplies the temporal, parietal, and lateral occipital lobes.[5] Superior division occlusions result in a Broca's (expressive or motor) aphasia when the dominant hemisphere is affected.[6] Also seen is a hemiparesis mainly

TABLE 2.1 MCA syndromes

	Left hemisphere	Right hemisphere
Superior division	• Right face and arm weakness	• Left face and arm weakness
	• Right face and arm sensory deficit	• Left face and arm sensory deficits
	• Broca's (nonfluent) aphasia	• Left hemineglect
Inferior division	• Wernicke's (fluent) aphasia	• Profound left hemineglect
	• Right visual field cut	• Left visual field cut
	• Right face and arm sensory deficit	• Left face and arm weakness (mild)
	• Confusion	• Right gaze preference
	• Mild right-sided weakness (at the onset)	
Deep penetrating branches	• Right pure motor hemiparesis	• Left pure motor hemiparesis
MCA stem (combination of the above)	• Right hemiplegia	• Left hemiplegia
	• Right hemianesthesia	• Left hemianesthesia
	• Global aphasia	• Profound left hemineglect
	• Right homonymous hemianopia	• Left homonymous hemianopia
	• Left gaze preference	• Right gaze preference

involving the contralateral face and arm because the leg is more so affected in anterior cerebral artery (ACA) occlusions. Inferior division occlusions produce a Wernicke's (receptive or sensory) aphasia when the dominant hemisphere is affected.[6] A contralateral hemianopia is also seen; however, hemiparesis, gaze deviations, and sensory disturbances are not typical of inferior division occlusions. Inferior division strokes are vulnerable to misdiagnosis because they often lack these obvious focal deficits.

In addition to these proximal MCA syndromes, smaller infarcts can occur within isolated territories due to blockage of higher-order (smaller, distal) branches to produce more focal deficits. When small infarcts occur due to isolated blockage of a small penetrating branch, the infarct that results is termed *lacuna* (pl. *lacunas* or *lacunae*).[6]

ACA SYNDROME

The ACA supplies a large portion of the medial surface of the frontal lobe, including a portion of the anterior corpus callosum. Whereas occlusions of the MCA affect mainly the contralateral face and arm, occlusions of the ACA have greater impact on the contralateral lower extremity due to infarction of the paracentral lobule. Special attention should be paid to the distal leg muscles due to the fact that proximal muscle representation receives input from MCA collaterals as well.[7,8] However, the pattern may include "grip sparing" and face-sparing hemiparesis. A comprehensive set of exam findings—including distal paresis (flaccid initially then spastic over days to weeks), the presence of Babinski's sign, loss of two-point discrimination, impaired proprioception, and incontinence due to loss of the voluntary micturition center—may therefore assist in localizing the lesion to the ACA territory (Table 2.2). Variations in anatomy do, however, occur and have the potential to mislead the practitioner. For instance, if the initial segments of both ACAs (i.e., the A1 segments) arise from one side, occlusion of the ACA can result in the type of paraparesis usually seen in spinal cord infarcts.[9,10] Careful sensory exam can help to localize the lesion, as this ACA anomaly should not produce the sensory deficit seen in spinal cord infarcts.

One of the ACA's deep branches, termed the *recurrent artery of Heubner*, depending on relative development, supplies the head of the caudate in conjunction with lenticulostriate branches from the MCA. Therefore, an ACA territory stroke can look like a classic lacunar infarct. As Heubner's artery supplies the anterior limb and genu of the internal capsule, its involvement can cause contralateral face and arm weakness as well.[11] An ACA territory stroke in the dominant hemisphere can also produce a transcortical motor aphasia, recognized by

TABLE 2.2 ACA syndrome

Left hemisphere	Right hemisphere
• Right leg weakness	• Left leg weakness
• Right leg sensory deficit	• Left leg sensory deficit
• Transcortical aphasia	• Left hemineglect
• Behavioral changes	• Behavioral changes
• Grasp reflex	• Grasp reflex

impaired fluency, but with intact comprehension and *intact* repetition. This type of aphasia is commonly seen with ACA-MCA watershed infarcts because the location impairs proper functioning of Broca's area but spares peri-sylvian connections from posterior to anterior language areas, allowing for repetition. When an ACA occlusion impacts the medial prefrontal cortex of the dominant hemisphere as well as the anterior corpus callosum, the patient may display semiautomatic movements of the contralateral arm. This has been termed *alien hand syndrome* because the patient loses voluntary control of the arm, and the limb has a "mind of its own."[12] Along with the cingulate gyrus, lesions affecting the supplementary motor area can also present with an affect of indifference, apathy, and detachment with "limited responsiveness to the environment" not attributed to paralysis or coma.[13] The term *abulia* or *akinetic mutism* is used to describe a person in this emotionally flattened state. These individuals are awake and alert, and they display appropriate, albeit muted, responses to stimuli; however, their spontaneous verbal communication is significantly reduced. Special attention should be paid to these patients because they will often not ask for food when hungry and can be incontinent.[14]

PCA SYNDROME

The posterior cerebral artery (PCA) arises from the terminal bifurcation of the basilar artery in 70% of cases.[15] In some individuals, however, one or both PCAs originate from the ipsilateral ICA via a large posterior communicating artery. These individuals are said to have a "fetal PCA" because it retains embryologic origin from the ICA. This variant of cerebrovascular anatomy can allow for PCA syndromes to result from *anterior* circulation occlusions (specifically in the ICA) or anterior circulation emboli.[16] The PCA supplies the midbrain and thalamus via its small *thalamoperforating* branches. It supplies the posterior thalamus, lateral geniculate body, and choroid plexus via medial and lateral posterior

TABLE 2.3 PCA syndrome

Left hemisphere	Right hemisphere
• Right homonymous hemianopia • Alexia without agraphia (with mass effect on the corpus callosum)	• Left homonymous hemianopia

choroidal arteries. Finally, the PCA divides posteriorly to form the calcarine artery and anteriorly to form the anterior and posterior inferior temporal arteries to supply the ventral temporal and occipital lobes.[17]

Occlusion of the PCA stem can result in contralateral hemiplegia, hemianesthesia, hemianopia, Horner's syndrome, and contralateral hyperhidrosis. When the thalamogeniculate branch of the PCA becomes occluded, the Déjerine-Roussy syndrome may result, which involves rapidly improving hemiparesis with choreic movements and ataxia, as well as hyperesthesia with later paroxysmal pain on the hyperesthetic side.[18] It is important to note that, while the thalamus is supplied by the posterior cerebral artery, infarction to this structure can also produce motor deficits as a consequence of its location near the internal capsule. When the infarct lies on the edge of the thalamus, ischemia can occur within the adjacent internal capsule. These *thalamocapsular* infarcts can therefore cause motor deficits that mimic MCA distribution infarcts (Table 2.3).

The PCA supplies the lower portions of the visual radiations throughout their entire course. Infarctions of the lateral geniculate body, temporal or occipital lobe, or calcarine cortex will produce visual disturbances, including homonymous hemianopia and amblyopia.[19] As the primary visual pathway is strictly unilateral, improvement in vision after infarction along the visual pathways is not common. Spontaneous improvement in vision is expected within the first 2 weeks to 2 months of recovery. Any remaining deficit after 6 months is usually permanent.[20–22] In one retrospective study, 40% of 263 patients with homonymous hemianopia (not limited to stroke as etiology) showed improvement, with the probability of improvement decreasing steadily after injury and reaching <10% by 6 months. However, that 40% figure may be falsely low due to the occurrence of spontaneous recovery in many patients prior to initial visual field testing.[22] Other studies report spontaneous improvement in 50% to 60% of patients within the first month, limited improvement after 3 months, and virtually no improvement after 6 months.[23] Lastly, with damage to the ventral temporo-occipital region, patients may present with a phenomenon called *prosopagnosia*, which is an inability to recognize familiar faces.[24]

Vertebrobasilar

The two vertebral arteries merge to form the basilar artery. Occlusion of the basilar artery can produce unilateral paresthesia, hemiplegia (and/or quadriplegia), speech disturbance, anisocoria, gaze palsy, or coma. Patients may be seen to have decerebrate posturing along with myoclonic jerks. The possibility of crossed signs is typical for a lesion in this territory and can present as ipsilateral lower motor neuron facial paresis and dysesthesia along with contralateral limb hemiparesis and hemidysesthesia.[25] Truncal ataxia is also seen with lesions in this territory along with vertical nystagmus—a sign that a central lesion exists. Moreover, eye abnormalities such as *ocular bobbing* can occur with infarction to the pontine base. Internuclear opthalmoplegia (INO) can result from damage to the medial longitudinal fasciculus (MLF), where adduction is impaired for the ipsilateral eye and there is associated nystagmus of the abducting eye. Furthermore, rhythmic jerking of the soft palate and pharyngopalatine arch, termed *palatal myoclonus*, may indicate a lesion within the Guillain-Mollaret triangle, which comprises the red nucleus, the dentate nucleus of the cerebellum, and the inferior olivary nucleus along with their connections.[26] Finally, the locked-in syndrome is seen with basilar artery occlusion resulting in extensive destruction to the pontine base. The patient is paralyzed and unable to speak, but he can move his eyes vertically and raise his eyebrows.

Occlusion of the paramedian arteries can cause damage to the midbrain, producing a third nerve palsy along with other symptoms dictated by the particular involvement of adjacent structures. Weber syndrome is caused by infarction of the ventral midbrain and causes damage to cranial nerve III and the corticospinal tract, resulting in ipsilateral oculomotor palsy and contralateral hemiparesis. Infarction of the tegmentum of the midbrain can cause damage to the third cranial nerve, red nucleus, and superior cerebellar peduncles, causing Claude syndrome. This is characterized by ipsilateral oculomotor palsy with contralateral hemiataxia. Infarction of the ventral and tegmental midbrain results in damage to cranial nerve III, corticospinal tracts, red nucleus, substantia nigra, and superior cerebellar peduncle, causing Benedikt syndrome. This syndrome is characterized by ipsilateral oculomotor palsy, contralateral hemiparesis, contralateral hemiataxia, and involuntary movements such as hemiathetosis or hemichorea.[27]

When an occlusion occurs at the distal basilar artery, appropriately termed *top of the basilar artery occlusion*, bilateral infarction of paramedian midbrain, medial thalamus, occipital lobes, and medial temporal lobes occurs.[28] This can produce sudden onset of somnolence or loss of consciousness due to ischemia of the reticular activating system within the medial mesencephalon and diencephalon. Damage to the rostral interstitial MLF (riMLF), the interstitial nucleus of Cajal, and posterior commissures results in vertical (upward and/or downward) gaze palsy with preservation of vertical vestibulo-ocular reflex.[29] Additionally, deficits in convergence, pupillary reactivity, and eyelid movement are seen due to damage to the medial midbrain tegmentum, diencephalon, or rostral brainstem. Infarction of the rostral brainstem can also cause hallucinations, termed *peduncular hallucinosis*, that are usually visual involving objects, colors, and scenes.[30] Moreover, abnormal spontaneous movements such as hemiballism and hemichorea can result from damage to the subthalamic nucleus.[31] While these are some of the more common signs of the top of the basilar artery syndrome, its clinical presentation can vary depending upon the areas affected by the infarction.

Lateral Medullary Syndrome

The lateral medullary syndrome, as its name implies, results from an infarct to a portion of the lateral medulla. Known also as Wallenberg syndrome, this condition most commonly results from thrombosis to lateral medullary branches of the vertebral artery; however, due to variable origin of medullary perforating vessels, occlusions to the posterior inferior cerebellar artery (PICA) can also result in this syndrome. The brainstem structures affected produce the clinical features shown in Table 2.4.[25]

TABLE 2.4 Lateral medullary syndrome

Clinical features	Brainstem structures affected
• Contralateral loss of pain and temperature over body	• Spinothalamic tract
• Ipsilateral pain, burning, and paresthesia over face	• 5th cranial nerve nucleus and tract
• Ipsilateral Horner syndrome	• Descending sympathetic tract
• Vomiting, vertigo, nystagmus, oscillopsia	• Vestibular nuclei
• Hoarseness, dysphagia, hiccough, diminished gag reflex	• 9th and 10th cranial nerve tracts
• Loss of taste	• Nucleus and tractus solitarius
• Vertical diplopia, tilting vision	• Utricular nucleus
• Ipsilateral ataxia of limbs and lateropulsion	• Olivocerebellar, spinocerebellar, restiform body, inferior cerebellum

It is important to note that not all of these signs and symptoms need to be present to suspect a lateral medullary infarct. Patients may present with various combinations of the clinical features listed.

Cerebellar

The rostral half of the cerebellar hemispheres and dentate nucleus are supplied by the superior cerebellar artery (SCA).[32] The classic SCA territory infarction involves loss of pain and temperature sensation of the contralateral face, arm, leg, and trunk, as well as ipsilateral limb ataxia, ipsilateral Horner's syndrome, and contralateral fourth cranial nerve palsy.[33,34] The middle cerebellar peduncle and the flocculus are supplied by the anterior inferior cerebellar artery (AICA).[35] Patients with infarction of these structures will present with vertigo, vomiting, tinnitus, hearing loss, dysarthria, ipsilateral facial palsy, trigeminal sensory loss, Horner's syndrome, ipsilateral limb dysmetria, and contralateral pain and temperature sensory loss of limbs and trunk. In fact, this is the only stroke syndrome that presents with unilateral hearing loss. To be clear, the hearing loss is actually not caused by the stroke itself but rather by occlusion of the labyrinthine artery (vascular supply to the cochlea), which is a branch of the AICA. Occlusions to the posterior inferior cerebellar artery (PICA) can present with vertigo, headache, vomiting, dysarthria, gait and trunk ataxia, ipsilateral axial lateroplusion, nystagmus, ipsilateral limb dysmetria, and impairment of consciousness in some patients.[34] These patients often have difficulty standing upright or walking in a straight line (Table 2.5).

TABLE 2.5 Cerebellar stroke syndromes

SCA	AICA	PICA
• Ipsilateral limb ataxia	• Vertigo	• Vertigo
• Ipsilateral Horner's syndrome	• Vomiting	• Headache
• Contralateral loss of pain and temperature sensation in the face, arm, leg, and trunk	• Tinnitus	• Vomiting
	• Hearing loss	• Ipsilateral limb dysmetria
• Contralateral fourth cranial nerve palsy	• Dysarthria	• Ipsilateral axial lateropulsion
	• Horner's syndrome	• Nystagumus
	• Ipsilateral limb dysmetria	• Wallenberg syndrome (dorsolateralmedullary)
	• Contralateral loss of pain and temperature sensation of limbs and trunk	
	• Ipsilateral facial palsy	
	• Trigeminal sensory loss	

COMMONLY MISSED STROKE PRESENTATIONS

The term *stroke chameleon* has been used to describe syndromes that are initially thought to be caused by a non-stroke disease process but ultimately are discovered to be due to an acute infarct.[36] Cerebellar stroke syndromes in particular can be difficult to recognize at initial presentation. Patients presenting with vague complaints of vomiting, dizziness, and headache are often seen by internists and gastroenterologists before the neurologist is called to evaluate them. For instance, vomiting, vertigo, occipital headache, neck pain, and ataxia are often seen with an inferior cerebellar stroke caused by PICA occlusion. It can also be challenging to distinguish delirium or "confusion" from aphasia. The former is often caused by metabolic disorders, which can be usually diagnosed with routine blood tests and a "nonfocal" physical exam. In addition, *wrist drop* is often prematurely attributed to radial nerve palsy, with subsequent MRI revealing a small infarct involving a precentral knob in the precentral gyrus.[37] Moreover, stroke, in general, should be placed high in the differential for patients who present with unexplained acute hypertension. A premature diagnosis of hypertensive urgency may delay emergent treatment in patients who are actually hypertensive due to acute stroke. A hyperacute MRI of the brain can distinguish stroke from stroke mimics; however, it is often not feasible to obtain in most stroke centers when time is of the essence. Therefore, it is important for emergency physicians and general practitioners to consider stroke in the differential for these classically nonfocal symptoms that occur suddenly so that emergent treatment can be administered if warranted.

References

1. Gibo H, Carver CP, Rhoton AL, et al. Microsurgical anatomy of the middle cerebral artery. *J Neurosurg.* 1981;54:151–169.
2. Abbie AA. The morphology of the fore-brain arteries, with special reference to the evolution of the basal ganglia. *J Anat.* 1934;68:433–470.
3. Shellshear JC. A contribution to our knowledge of the arterial supply of the cerebral cortex in man. *Brain.* 1927;50:236.
4. Grotta, JC, Albers GW, Broderick JP, et al, eds. *Stroke: Pathophysiology, Diagnosis, and Management.* 6e. Philadelphia, PA: Elsevier; 2016:362.
5. Ibid., 363.
6. Ibid., 367–369.
7. Penfield W, Jasper H. *Epilepsy and the Functional Anatomy of the Human Brain.* Boston: Little, Brown; 1954.
8. Grotta, JC, Albers GW, Broderick JP, et al, eds. *Stroke: Pathophysiology, Diagnosis, and Management.* 6e. Philadelphia, PA: Elsevier; 2016:351.
9. Perlmutter D, Rhoton AL. Microsurgical anatomy of the anterior cerebral-anterior communicating-recurrent artery complex. *J Neurosurg.* 1976;45:259.

10. Perlmutter D, Rhoton AL. Microsurgical anatomy of the distal anterior cerebral artery. *J Neurosurg.* 1978;49:204.

11. Critchley M. The anterior cerebral artery and its syndromes. *Brain.* 1930;53:120.

12. Feinberg TE, Schindler RJ, Flanagan NG, et al. Two alien hand syndromes. *Neurology.* 1992;42:19.

13. Segarra JM. Cerebral vascular disease and behavior. I: the syndrome of the mesencephalic artery (basilar artery bifurcation). *Arch Neurol.* 1970;22:408.

14. Laplane D, Degos JD, Baulac M, Gray F. Bilateral infarction of the anterior cingulate gyri and of the fornices: report of a case. *J Neurol Sci.* 1981;51(2):289–300.

15. Cereda C, Carrera E. Posterior cerebral artery territory infarctions. *Front Neurol Neurosci.* 2012;30:128–131.

16. Pessin MS, Kwan ES, Scott RM, et al. Occipital infarction with hemianopsia from carotid occlusive disease. *Stroke.* 1989;20(3):409–411.

17. Erdem A, Yasargil G, Roth P. Microsurgical anatomy of the hippocampal arteries. *J Neurosurg.* 1993;79:256–265.

18. Bogousslavsky J, Regli F, Uske A. Thalamic infarcts: clinical syndromes, etiology, and prognosis. *Neurology.* 1988;38(6):837–848.

19. Kumral E, Bayulkem G, Atac C, et al. Spectrum of superficial posterior cerebral artery territory infarcts. *Eur J Neurol.* 2004; 11(4):237–246.

20. Goodwin D. Homonymous hemianopia: challenges and solutions. *Clin Ophthalmol.* 2014;8:1919–1927.

21. Zhang X, Kedar S, Lynn MJ, et al. Homonymous hemianopias: clinical-anatomic correlations in 904 cases. *Neurology.* 2006;66;906–910.

22. Zhang X, Kedar S, Lynn MJ, et al. Natural history of homonymous hemianopia. *Neurology.* 2006;66:901–905.

23. Das A, Huxlin KR. New approaches to visual rehabilitation for cortical blindness: outcomes and putative mechanisms. *Neuroscientist.* 2010;16:374–387.

24. Meadows JC. The anatomical basis of prosopagnosia. *J Neurol Neurosurg Psychiatry.* 1974;37(5):489–501.

25. Kim JS. Pure lateral medullary infarction: clinical-radiological correlation of 130 acute, consecutive patients. *Brain.* 2003;126(8):1864–1872.

26. Lapresle J, Hamida MB. The dentato-olivary pathway. Somatotopic relationship between the dentate nucleus and the contralateral inferior olive. *Arch Neurol.* 1970;22(2):135–143.

27. Ruchalski K, Hathout GM. A medley of midbrain maladies: a brief review of midbrain anatomy and syndromology for radiologists. *Radiol Res Pract.* 2012;2012:258524.

28. Caplan LR. "Top of the basilar" syndrome. *Neurology.* 1980;30(1):72–79.

29. Buttner-Ennever JA, Buttner U, Cohen B, et al. Vertical glaze paralysis and the rostral interstitial nucleus of the medial longitudinal fasciculus. *Brain.* 1982;105(1):125–149.

30. Benke T. Peduncular hallucinosis: a syndrome of impaired reality monitoring. *J Neurol.* 2006;253(12):1561–1571.

31. Martin JP. Hemichorea resulting from a local lesion of the brain (the syndrome of the body of Luys). *Brain.* 1927;50:637–642.

32. Hardy DG, Peace DA, Rhoton AL Jr. Microsurgical anatomy of the superior cerebellar artery. *Neurosurgery.* 1980;6(1):10–28.

33. Mills CK. Preliminary note on a new symptom complex due to lesion of the cerebellum and crebello-rubro-thalamic system, the main symptoms being ataxia of the upper and lower extremities of one side, and the other side deafness, paralysis of emotional expression in the face, and loss of the senses of pain, heat, and cold over the entire half of the body. *J Nerv Ment Dis.* 1912;39:73–76.

34. Kase CS, Norrving B, Levine SR, et al. Cerebellar infarction. Clinical and anatomic observations in 66 cases. *Stroke*. 1993;24(1):76–83.

35. Kumral E, Kisabay A, Atac C. Lesion patterns and etiology of ischemia in the anterior inferior cerebellar artery territory involvement: a clinical—diffusion weighted—MRI study. *Eur J Neurol*. 2006;13(4):395–401.

36. Dupre CM, Libman R, Dupre SI, et al. Stroke chameleons. *J Stroke Cerebrovasc Dis*. 2014;23:374–378.

37. Tahir H, Daruwalla V, Meisel J, Kodsi SE. Pseudoradial nerve palsy caused by acute ischemic stroke. *J Investig Med High Impact Case Rep*. 2016;4(3):2324709616658310.

Mechanisms of Ischemic Stroke 3

Michael G. Fara and Koto Ishida

INTRODUCTION

Ischemic stroke occurs when regional blood flow to the central nervous system is limited due to blockage or narrowing of the involved vasculature. Multiple stroke subtypes exist that are distinct in risk factor profile, pathologic mechanism, management, and prognosis. The emergent therapeutic management of acute ischemic stroke is largely independent of subtype. However, determination of stroke etiology is essential in providing optimal long-term care because both chronic management and secondary stroke prevention vary considerably depending on the specific mechanism.

Several classification systems have been proposed for distinguishing subtypes of ischemic stroke on the basis of underlying mechanism. The most influential of these is the TOAST (Trial of Org 10172 in Acute Stroke Treatment) classification,[1] which divides ischemic strokes into five major mechanistic categories: large-artery atherosclerosis, cardioembolism, small-vessel occlusion, stroke of other determined etiology, and stroke of undetermined etiology (see Figure 3.1). Originally published in 1993, the TOAST classification has since been modified to allow for advances in imaging techniques and stroke epidemiology. This has yielded the Stop Stroke Study TOAST (SSS-TOAST) system,[2] the Causative Classification of Stroke (CCS) system,[3] and others. These differ from TOAST primarily in allowing the weighing of evidence to assign a likelihood that the classification of any given stroke is correct, while still maintaining the five basic TOAST categories. There are alternative classification schemes that subtype

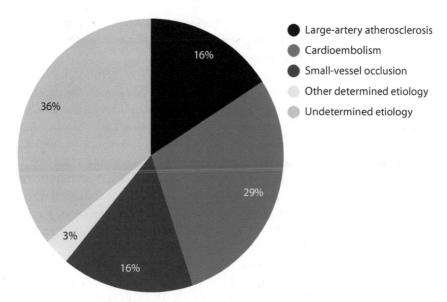

FIGURE 3.1 Relative incidence of stroke subtypes by TOAST criteria

Source: Data from Reference 17.

strokes into different categories altogether, but TOAST and its variants remain the most widely used in stroke research, and we largely follow the TOAST classification in organizing this review.

LARGE-VESSEL ATHEROSCLEROSIS

Considerable variation exists in the literature regarding what qualifies as "large vessel" for the purpose of classification of ischemic stroke subtype.[4] Some researchers use a size cutoff, considering any vessel with a diameter of at least 1.5 mm as large.[5] Others appeal to anatomical landmarks—for example, limiting this distinction to only the extracranial portions of the major arteries of the neck.[6] Still others consider any artery with an individual name as large arteries, including segments and branches of the middle cerebral artery (MCA), anterior and posterior choroidal arteries, and even the recurrent artery of Heubner. In clinical practice, this large-vessel classification definitively includes the common and internal carotid arteries, as well as the vertebral arteries. Often, the basilar and the proximal segments of the three major cerebral arteries (anterior, middle, and posterior) are also included. Though it may seem counterintuitive, the aortic arch and its major branches, while clearly of wide diameter, are typically not considered large vessels in this mechanistic context because their role in the pathogenesis of ischemic stroke is usually as a source of embolism rather than atherosclerotic occlusion.

Large-vessel atherosclerotic stroke requires evidence of significant atherosclerosis in a large vessel supplying the territory correlating with the patient's clinical symptoms. Having evidence of occlusion of a large artery is not enough to determine large-vessel atherosclerosis because the vessel may be occluded by an embolus of undetermined source. The TOAST classification and its descendants count atherosclerosis as significant if it leads to a greater than 50% stenosis of the vessel. However, some investigators favor using measurement of overall atherosclerotic plaque burden rather than degree of vessel stenosis when assessing for large-vessel atherosclerotic causes of stroke, proposing a total plaque area of at least 1.19 cm^2 as the critical threshold.[7] For intracranial disease, 70% stenosis is often used as the cutoff rather than 50%.[8]

The development of atherosclerosis is an inflammatory process that typically takes years to decades to evolve. It begins with the accumulation of lipoprotein particles within the intima of an artery, which leads to a cytokine-mediated recruitment of inflammatory cells. These cells include macrophages, which engulf the lipoprotein particles, forming foam cells. An inflammatory cascade then ensues, leading to destruction of the extracellular matrix within the intima, proliferation of endovascular smooth muscle cells, and development of fibrosis. The result is a fibrous, lipid-laden plaque, or atheroma, protruding from within the arterial intima.[9]

This long, indolent process of plaque formation in a large vessel can result in acute ischemic stroke via one of two major mechanisms. Most commonly, a thrombus detaches from the atheromatous site and is swept distally in the bloodstream until it lodges as the vessel narrows, occluding flow and causing ischemia to the regions of brain supplied by that vessel and its distal branches (artery-to-artery embolism).[10] The thrombus itself typically forms at the site of atheroma in one of two ways. Sometimes a defect develops in the fibrous cap of the atheroma, exposing the lipid core to the circulating blood. This lipid core is extremely thrombogenic, and its exposure drives rapid platelet aggregation and subsequent thrombus formation. This mechanism of thrombus formation is termed *plaque rupture*. Alternatively, thrombus can form without a distinct disruption of the fibrous cap via a mechanism called *plaque erosion*. While this mechanism is not well understood, it also involves aggregation of platelets on the surface of the atheroma but without any distinct structural defect in the atheroma's fibrous cap.[11] In either case, the primary role of platelet activation in thrombus formation explains the success of platelet inhibitors in reducing the risk of stroke in patients with atherosclerotic disease.[12]

An alternative mechanism of large-vessel atherosclerotic stroke is by complete or partial vessel occlusion, either by the atheroma itself or by overlying thrombus that forms in situ but does not dislodge. Complete occlusion of a large artery can cause devastating infarction of the entire region supplied by the parent artery and its distal branches. Alternatively, complete occlusion can be relatively asymptomatic if collateral circulation is sufficiently well developed; in these cases, subsequent stroke in the territory of the occluded artery is either limited or doesn't occur.[13] More worrisome is the high risk for first or recurrent stroke in patients with incomplete occlusion of a large vessel, classified as severe or critical stenosis. As the vessel lumen narrows, blood flow distal to the occlusion decreases given a fixed arterial pressure (a consequence of Poiseuille's law). If flow decreases enough, ischemia develops, usually in the "watershed" territories perfused by the most distal portions of the major cerebral arteries. Patients suffering a stroke due to a critically stenosed large vessel frequently report a prodrome of stuttering, transient symptoms prior to the infarction itself, presumably a result of transient episodes of relative systemic hypotension. It is important to recognize such a prodrome of symptomatic stenosis, both because stroke can be temporarily averted by raising the systemic blood pressure and because if the stenosis is in the common or internal carotid artery then surgical or endovascular intervention has been shown to be beneficial as will be reviewed in Chapter 12.[14] For symptomatic, critical intracranial stenosis, a condition with up to 15% recurrence rate at 1 year if treated with aspirin alone,[15] aggressive medical management with dual antiplatelet therapy is usually indicated as will be further examined in Chapter 13.[8]

CARDIOEMBOLIC DISEASE

Epidemiological studies have repeatedly shown cardioembolism to be the most common mechanism of ischemic stroke in adults, with one population-based study finding cardioembolism to be the cause of 27% of all ischemic strokes and 42% of those whose cause was known.[16] Furthermore, patients with cardioembolic stroke as a group have the poorest long-term survival relative to those with ischemic stroke due to other mechanisms. In one study, the 5-year mortality rate of patients with cardioembolic stroke was 80%, twice that of patients with stroke due to large-vessel atherosclerosis after adjusting for age, sex, cardiac comorbidity, and stroke severity.[17]

In cardioembolic stroke, a proximal thrombus, either intracardiac or other proximal source (e.g., the aortic arch) distally embolizes until it occludes a cerebral artery, causing ischemia or, ultimately, infarction. Many of the conditions that have been shown to carry a high risk of causing stroke (greater than 2% annually) are discussed below.

By far the most common cause of cardioembolism in patients with ischemic stroke is atrial fibrillation, accounting for 45% of all cardioembolic strokes in one stroke registry.[18] In an analysis of vascular risk factors, the Framingham study found stroke incidence to be five times higher in patients with non-valvular atrial fibrillation compared with healthy controls.[19] Given recent evidence showing that many patients with cryptogenic stroke probably have occult paroxysmal atrial fibrillation (to be discussed), these figures likely underestimate the proportion of strokes due to atrial fibrillation.

Impaired atrial contractility in fibrillation leads to impaired flow and pooling of blood in the left atrium, particularly in the left atrial appendage, which is the site of thrombus formation in approximately 90% of patients with non-valvular atrial fibrillation. Echocardiographic studies have shown that blood flow across the left atrial appendage is significantly reduced in atrial fibrillation, and that this decrease in flow correlates with thrombus formation.[20] In contrast to arterial atheromatous plaque rupture, there is no significant endothelial disruption involved in left atrial thrombus formation in patients with atrial fibrillation, at least initially.[21] Instead, thrombogenesis appears to be primarily a result of hemostasis, although there is increasing evidence that various systemic prothrombotic factors may also play a pivotal role.[22]

Ischemic stroke due to atrial fibrillation occurs when an atrial thrombus is dislodged and travels through the arterial system, occluding a distal vessel. Often, the thrombus degrades as it travels, leading to smaller thrombi being swept into multiple branches of the cerebral vasculature. This phenomenon accounts for the fact that radiographic or clinical evidence of simultaneous strokes in different vascular territories is associated with a cardioembolic source of the strokes. It is important to recognize that distal embolization of thrombus can occur at any time, even if the heart has returned to normal sinus rhythm. Early studies reported substantial risk of cerebral embolization at the time of electrical cardioversion, with one study reporting an incidence of 7% within 72 hours of cardioversion for patients not treated with anticoagulation.[23] Surprisingly, there may be a similarly high risk even during spontaneous conversion from atrial fibrillation to normal sinus rhythm. Additionally, while the risk of stroke seems low in patients who have been in atrial fibrillation of only very brief duration, thrombi can develop surprisingly quickly. In one study, 14% of patients with new atrial fibrillation (either continuous or paroxysmal) lasting less than 3 days had a left atrial thrombus seen on transesophageal echocardiography.[24] These observations play an important role in guiding primary and secondary stroke prevention for patients with atrial fibrillation.

Valvular heart disease, even without accompanying atrial fibrillation, is another important source of cardioembolic stroke. The risk is highest in patients with rheumatic mitral valve disease,[25] with natural history studies finding an approximate 10% incidence of embolic stroke.[26,27] Early rheumatic heart disease frequently leads to mitral regurgitation, where turbulent retrograde flow during ventricular systole causes both damage to the atrial endothelium and pooling of blood, providing a mechanism for atrial thrombogenesis. Later in the course of the disease, mitral stenosis typically develops. Decreased forward flow across the mitral valve again leads to pooling of blood in the atrium, promoting thrombogenesis; the chronic increase in left atrial pressure ultimately leads to structural dilatation, which itself may cause atrial fibrillation. This provides an additional mechanism for thrombus formation as described earlier, although notably in atrial fibrillation due to valvular disease, the majority of thrombi form outside of the left atrial appendage.[28]

The significance of other valvular lesions for the development of cardioembolic stroke is less clear. Calcification of the aortic valve, with or without accompanying aortic stenosis, is not itself a risk factor for ischemic stroke and does not, in isolation, warrant antiplatelet or anticoagulation therapy for primary stroke prophylaxis.[29] In rare cases, however, it can provide a unique mechanism for stroke because a piece of calcium can break off and embolize distally, usually in the context of surgical or endovascular manipulation.[30] Calcification of the mitral annulus has been associated with increased incidence of ischemic stroke. Much of this risk has been attributed to increased risk of atrial fibrillation and endocarditis rather than an independent mechanism. However, autopsy and echocardiographic studies have demonstrated thrombus at or near sites of annulus calcification, suggesting a primary role in thrombogenesis.[31] Mitral valve prolapse, once thought to subserve an independent mechanism for cardioembolic stroke, does not, in fact, appear to do so, although it may lead to severe mitral regurgitation over time, with subsequent thrombus formation and potential embolization.[32]

Infectious endocarditis carries a huge risk for ischemic stroke, with an incidence as high as 23% in one study.[33] Infected valvular vegetations are friable, particularly early in the course of disease due to elevated inflammatory response, and are thus prone to rupture, causing embolic stroke. The risk of stroke decreases dramatically with prompt initiation of appropriate treatment. In one large prospective cohort study, 15% of patients with infective endocarditis suffered a stroke, but only one-fifth of these occurred after 1 week of effective antibiotic therapy.[34] Non-infectious or "marantic" endocarditis also carries a significant risk for ischemic stroke, although the prothrombotic state that leads to noninfectious endocarditis itself confers a risk, and the mechanism of ischemia in such patients is not always cardioembolic (to be discussed).

Left-sided heart structure and function is impaired after acute myocardial infarction (MI) and in patients with cardiomyopathy, so it is unsurprising that patients with these conditions are at increased risk of stroke. Approximately 1% of patients with an acute MI will develop an ischemic stroke within 28 days, with half of these occurring within the first 5 days.[35] Once again, the phenomena of impaired forward blood flow and stasis as well as atrial dilatation leading to endothelial disruption combine to increase risk of left atrial thrombus formation and subsequent embolization. Additionally, both MI and chronic cardiomyopathy can lead to left ventricular thrombus formation, providing another potential source of embolic stroke. Ischemic cardiomyopathy as a result of MI compounds the risk of stroke, with one large trial showing that patients with a left ventricular ejection fraction less than 28% had almost twice the risk of stroke compared with those with an ejection fraction greater than 40% over the course of 5 years following an acute MI.[36]

The role of atheromatous plaque in the ascending aorta or aortic arch as a source of cerebral embolism is controversial. One case-control study using transesophageal echocardiography investigated 250 consecutive patients admitted with ischemic stroke, and found arch plaques thicker than 4 mm in 36 of them, compared with 5 in the control group. This resulted in an odds ratio of greater than 9 for ischemic stroke in patients with atherosclerotic arch plaque diameter >4 mm after adjusting for other vascular risk factors ($p < 0.001$).[37] However, a subsequent longitudinal, population-based study did not find any association between aortic arch atherosclerosis and stroke incidence.[38] Nevertheless, there is increasing evidence that aortic arch atheromatous disease is an independent risk factor for stroke. A meta-analysis of prospective studies showed an odds ratio of 4 for ischemic stroke in patients with large atheromatous lesions, increasing to 12 for mobile lesions.[39] While the mechanism of stroke from aortic arch disease is not well understood, in addition to the more familiar embolization of in situ thrombus formation from plaque rupture, another possibility is direct embolization of the unstable, mobile plaque itself.

More rare causes of cardioembolic stroke, particularly in adults, include cardiac tumors. Atrial myxomas are the most common primary cardiac tumors in adults, with an annual incidence of 0.5 case per 100,000,[40] and they carry a significant risk of stroke if left untreated. Although large studies are lacking because of the relative rarity of the tumor, one retrospective case series of adults with atrial myxomas found that 11% had an ischemic stroke before the tumor was resected.[41] The mechanism of stroke from myxomas usually involves fragmentation and embolization of tumor tissue, although occasionally thrombus that forms on the primary myxoma can also embolize.[42] Papillary fibroelastomas of the cardiac valves are other benign tumors with a propensity to cause embolic stroke, again either from tumor fragment or from thrombus that has formed on the tumor surface.[43] These and other benign cardiac tumors are usually treated surgically. Malignant tumors of the heart, either primary or metastatic, can similarly lead to embolic stroke, although the role for surgery in these cases is unfortunately limited.[44]

Secondary prevention of stroke due to atrial fibrillation and other cardioembolic causes of stroke are covered in Chapters 10 and 11, respectively.

SMALL-VESSEL DISEASE

Chronic hypertension and diabetes mellitus have been well established as significant, independent risk factors for ischemic stroke. While these conditions are also risk factors for diffuse atherosclerotic disease and increase stroke risk via some of the mechanisms described earlier, ischemic strokes suffered by patients with isolated hypertension or diabetes often have a characteristic pattern seen either at autopsy or, more commonly today, on neuroimaging. This pattern of lacunar infarction involves small (less than 15 mm) ischemic lesions of the basal ganglia, thalamus, pons, internal capsule, or deep cerebral white matter. There are characteristic clinical syndromes associated with lacunar strokes, and this association led to the *lacunar hypothesis* that these syndromes are predictive of the anatomical or radiographic pattern of lacunar infarction. Although C. Miller Fisher famously described more than 20 clinical syndromes associated with lacunar strokes,[45] the most common are pure motor hemiparesis, pure sensory syndrome, sensorimotor syndrome, dysarthria–clumsy hand, and ataxia–hemiparesis. In one prospective study, the presence of one of these clinical syndromes had a positive predictive value of 87% for detecting a radiographically lacunar infarct.[46]

Lacunar strokes are caused by occlusion of small, penetrating arteries that supply the deep subcortical structures. This occlusion may occur in different ways, and there is controversy about which mechanism predominates. One mechanism, associated predominantly with chronic hypertension and initially believed to be the major pathological contributor to lacunar infarction, is the process of lipohyalinosis. Early autopsy series demonstrated the presence of intracerebral microaneurysms in chronically hypertensive patients, increasing risk of endothelial rupture. This rupture leads to lipid and hyaline accumulation within the vessel wall, resulting in progressive concentric hypertrophy.[47] At some point, this hypertrophy progresses to the point of either critical "microstenosis," or complete vessel occlusion and subsequent infarction.

Microatheromatous disease is another proposed mechanism of small-vessel lacunar strokes. Similar to the process in the larger vessels, smaller cerebral vessels can accumulate lipid-laden plaque within their intima via a chronic inflammatory process, providing a nidus for occlusive thrombus formation and subsequent infarction. Alternatively, the microatheroma itself can grow sufficiently large to occlude the lumen of the vessel.[48] Although there are conflicting reports in the literature, there is some evidence suggesting that lacunar infarcts due to microatheromatous disease tend to be larger and more symptomatic, whereas infarcts due to lipohyalinosis tend to be small, multiple, and clinically silent.[49]

Atherosclerosis can also develop at the origins of the small vessels, where they branch off from the larger intracranial arteries. Termed *branch atheromatous disease*, this has been proposed to represent a distinct pathological entity.[50] Radiographically, branch disease should be suspected if the vascular territory of an entire penetrating artery is infarcted, and the resulting ischemic lesion is often larger than the 15-mm cutoff used to define lacunar infarction. Clinically, suspicion of branch atheromatous disease is important because, in contrast to lipohyalinosis, the predominant vascular risk factors are not hypertension but, rather, diabetes and hyperlipidemia.[51]

Another mechanism of lacunar infarction is microembolism, from either a large artery or cardiac source. Some authors argue that, while possible, embolic causes of lacunar infarction are rare.[52] Others disagree, with one study of consecutive lacunar infarctions finding that of the patients without either hypertension or diabetes, 32% had a possible carotid or cardiac source of embolism.[53] While the true incidence of microembolic lacunar stroke is unknown, its possibility demands that patients presenting with lacunar infarctions should never be assumed to have intrinsic small-vessel disease and should be thoroughly evaluated for other potential causes of their disease so that secondary stroke prevention can be optimized. Small-vessel disease is covered in more detail in Chapter 14.

OTHER MECHANISMS

Among cases of ischemic stroke whose etiology is known, the vast majority are due to either cardioembolism or large- or small-vessel disease—97% in one population-based study of adults with first stroke.[11] However, other less common sources of stroke exist, especially in younger patients or those lacking traditional vascular risk factors.

Hypercoagulability is one such mechanism and can be either acquired or inherited. Among the acquired causes of hypercoagulability, malignancy is most strongly associated with risk for ischemic stroke, with an incidence of 7.5% in one large autopsy series of cancer patients.[54] Other acquired hypercoagulable states known to increase risk of ischemic stroke include antiphospholipid antibody syndrome (RR 2.6 for women),[55] postpartum state (RR 8.7),[56] and estrogen-containing oral contraceptive use (RR 2.8).[57] Yet others include myelo-proliferative disorders, heparin-induced thrombocytopenia, and certain chemo-therapeutic agents.[58,59]

The relationship between inherited hypercoagulable states and ischemic arterial stroke is more controversial. Studies suggest an association between ischemic stroke and many of the inherited thrombophilias, including factor V Leiden,[60] the prothrombin gene mutation,[61] antithrombin III deficiency,[62] protein C deficiency,[63] and protein S deficiency.[64] However, for each of these conditions, there are also studies suggesting they confer no increased risk of stroke.[65] The most robust data linking hypercoagulability to stroke involves the prothrombotic role of homocysteine, with multiple prospective and retrospective studies demonstrating an association between high-serum homocysteine levels and increased risk of ischemic stroke.[66] Hyperhomocysteinemia can be acquired, for example by vitamin deficiencies, or it can be inherited via a polymorphism in the gene encoding methylenetetrahydrofolate reductase (MTHFR), an enzyme involved in homocysteine catabolism. There is growing evidence that MTHFR gene polymorphisms confer an increased risk of ischemic stroke.[67]

The discussion so far has been exclusively about ischemic stroke due to occlusion of an arterial vessel. Importantly, ischemic stroke can also occur if there is occlusion in the venous system, and there is no doubt in the literature that hypercoagulable states substantially increase the risk of venous infarction. For example, one case-control study showed a five-fold increase in relative risk for cerebral venous thrombosis in patients with the prothrombin gene mutation, while at the same time showing no difference in relative risk for arterial ischemic stroke or transient ischemic attack (TIA).[68]

Ischemic stroke from venous occlusion can occur if a thrombus forms anywhere in the cerebral venous system, including the internal jugular and other large veins of the neck, the cerebral venous sinuses, and the most proximal small cortical veins. When a thrombus occludes a vein, the vasculature proximal to the obstruction swells as venous pressure increases, and venous infarction occurs in approximately 50% of cases. While the exact mechanism of infarction in these cases is not fully understood, animal models and imaging studies show that increased venous pressure likely causes neuronal death via an interplay of reduced capillary perfusion pressure, increased cerebral blood volume, and parenchymal tissue edema.[69] Because of extensive venous collateral circulation, venous infarction tends to evolve slowly, and patients typically present with subacute progression of neurological deficits, in contrast to arterial ischemic stroke. Additionally, compared with arterial infarcts, venous infarcts are far more likely to present with headache, with an incidence of headache at presentation reported as around 90%.[70]

Among young adults whose mechanism of stroke is identified, arterial dissection is the most common.[71] Dissection occurs when a tear develops in the intimal wall of an artery and blood seeps through this tear, leading to a hematoma within the vessel wall. Stroke due to dissection is primarily a consequence of distal embolization of thrombus from the site of dissection. Rarely, hematoma expansion causes infarction due to occlusion of the vessel lumen itself.[72] As such, ischemic strokes can present days to weeks after the actual dissection.[73]

The reason non-aneurysmal dissections occur remains, in many cases, poorly understood. Obvious causes such as severe neck trauma or inadvertent disruption of an artery during neck surgery are sometimes manifest, but many patients present with dissections that appear to be more spontaneous. Extrinsic risk factors for dissection have been studied, and the risk of dissection appears to be increased with either acute infection[74] or trivial neck injury (e.g., minor vehicle accidents while seat-belted, roller-coaster rides, or chiropractic spinal manipulation).[75] However, these occurrences are commonplace, whereas cervical artery dissections are rare, implying that the patients who suffer dissection after one of these events may also have other underlying predisposing risk factors.

Patients with inherited connective tissue disorders, particularly Ehlers-Danlos syndrome, are at increased risk for spontaneous cervical artery dissection.[76] Although most patients with dissections do not have Ehlers-Danlos syndrome, in a study of skin biopsies of patients with dissection, 55% had structural connective tissue abnormalities, suggesting a substantial underlying contribution.[77] Additionally, hyperhomocysteinemia and MTHFR gene mutations have also been shown to be risk factors for cervical artery dissection,[78] suggesting a possible relationship between dissection and atherosclerotic disease.[79]

Atherosclerosis and dissection are just two of the many acquired vasculopathies that can affect cerebral arteries and lead to stroke. A whole array of toxic, rheumatologic, infectious, and other systemic processes can affect cerebral vasculature and cause stroke. Most of these systemic vasculopathies involve inflammation and necrosis of vessel walls, which can lead to vascular stenosis or occlusion. In these cases, the term *vasculitis* is used.[80] But noninflammatory vasculopathies can also lead to stroke. One important example is cerebral vasospasm, a severe and potentially fatal complication in many patients with aneurysmal subarachnoid hemorrhage. Although the mechanism is still unclear, subarachnoid blood can lead to severe cerebral vasoconstriction that is not responsive to vasodilators, resulting in secondary brain injury due to ischemic stroke.[81] Other causes of cerebral vasospasm that can lead to stroke include vasoactive toxins and medications, traumatic brain injury, and the reversible cerebral vasoconstriction syndrome.

A second important noninflammatory vasculopathy can be caused by radiation therapy to the head or neck. The exposure of vessels to radiation causes a progressive loss of their endothelium, leading to subsequent thrombus formation and stroke.[82] Although data are limited regarding the relative incidence of ischemic stroke in patients who have received prior radiation therapy, isolated studies indicate increase in stroke risk, thought due to accelerated atherosclerosis resulting from radiation-induced endothelial injury.[83]

Recreational drugs of abuse, particularly stimulants, are associated with increased risk of stroke. For example, one large cross-sectional study found that the incidence of ischemic stroke in cocaine users was twice that of the general population.[84] While there are case reports of cerebral vasculitis secondary to acute stimulant abuse, the mechanism of stroke in these patients likely has more to do with increased risk of hypertension and cardiac arrhythmias.[85]

Cerebral vasculitis leading to stroke is an uncommon but important finding in many of the systemic vasculitides. Those that most frequently affect the central nervous system are systemic lupus erythematosus (SLE), Sjögren syndrome, Takayasu disease, Kawasaki disease, and Behçet disease.[61] Although the neurological symptoms are more often nonfocal—including headache, encephalopathy, and seizure—patients with these diseases are also at increased risk of ischemic stroke. For example, one large cross-sectional study showed that the relative risk of stroke in patients with SLE was 1.5.[86] Mechanistically, however, stroke in SLE patients is far more likely to be due to cardioembolism or thrombosis than cerebral vasculitis.[87] In addition to treating the underlying rheumatological disorder, therefore, aggressive management of modifiable stroke risk factors is of paramount importance in these patients.

Vasculitis with subsequent ischemic stroke is a relatively common consequence of several central nervous system infections. Stroke is a frequent complication of bacterial meningitis, with one series reporting an incidence of 27%.[88] Angiography in patients with bacterial meningitis complicated by stroke often reveals abnormalities, ranging from stenosis and tortuosity of large intracranial vessels to focal hypervascularity of distal arterioles and capillaries. These vascular changes are likely multifactorial, including intravascular inflammatory changes, extravascular compression by purulent fluid, and cytokine-mediated dilation or constriction of vessels.[89]

HIV infection leading to immunodeficiency also increases risk for stroke. One large cohort study found that patients with poorly controlled HIV (defined by CD4 count <200 cells/μL) had a relative risk of 3.2 for ischemic stroke compared with HIV-negative controls, whereas patients with well-controlled HIV (CD4 count >500 cells/μL) had no increased risk.[90] There is a wide variety of stroke mechanisms in HIV patients, although a disproportionate number are due to vasculitis (13% in one series).[91] In many cases, this vasculitis is related to opportunistic infections, although primary HIV-associated vasculitides have also been described.[92]

Varicella zoster virus (VZV) is another important viral source of ischemic stroke. Although it is relatively rare in adults, VZV infection may account for up to a third of all arterial ischemic strokes in children.[93] Either primary infection (chickenpox) or reactivation (shingles) can cause a vasculitis of both the large and small intracranial vessels, leading to ischemic stroke. Other infectious syndromes that can cause stroke through cerebral vasculitis include Lyme disease, syphilis, tuberculosis, fungal infections, neurocysticercosis, and malaria.[94]

Many genetic syndromes have a high incidence of ischemic stroke. By far the most prevalent of these is sickle-cell disease, which is overall the most common cause of stroke in children. One study found sickle-cell disease to be the cause of 39% of ischemic strokes in children.[95] Additionally, almost a quarter of patients with sickle-cell disease will have a stroke before age 45, and children with sickle-cell disease are over 400 times more likely to suffer an ischemic stroke than their peers. Mechanistically, a range of proximal causes of ischemic stroke is found in patients with sickle-cell disease, including large-vessel critical stenosis, large- and medium-vessel occlusive thrombus, and artery-to-artery embolism. Sickled red cells bind tightly to vascular endothelium and cross-polymerize to form a red cell thrombus; damage to the endothelium from sickled cells leads to platelet activation and other prothrombotic events; and intravascular hemolysis likely also has a vasoactive effect, further contributing to vessel narrowing.[96]

Moyamoya disease is an inherited vasculopathy that frequently leads to both ischemic and hemorrhagic stroke. The term *moyamoya*, Japanese for "puff of smoke," refers to a characteristic angiographic appearance of a diffuse haze of tiny collateral vessels distal to stenotic internal carotid and proximal major cerebral arteries. Given the degree of stenosis of the large vessels, the network of collaterals in moyamoya is maximally dilated in order to maintain cerebral perfusion. Any insult that reduces cerebral blood flow, such as decreased systemic blood pressure due to dehydration or cerebral vasoconstriction due to hypocarbia, can lead to ischemia. As well as being an inherited disease, moyamoya vasculopathy can be acquired, in which case it is called moyamoya syndrome. Conditions that have been linked to moyamoya syndrome include radiotherapy to the head and neck, sickle-cell disease, Down syndrome, neurofibromatosis type 1, autoimmune thyroiditis, and others.[97]

Fabry disease, an X-linked recessive lysosomal storage disorder, is another inherited condition that can manifest with stroke. Before the advent of enzyme-replacement therapy, approximately 5% of patients with Fabry disease developed ischemic stroke, many as young adults. In almost half of these patients, Fabry disease was undiagnosed at the time of stroke.[98] A study of young adults with strokes of undetermined cause found that 1% of them had Fabry disease, making it an important source of otherwise cryptogenic stroke.[99] Fabry disease results in a vasculopathy of both the small and large intracranial vessels, with a predilection for the vertebrobasilar system. The mechanism of this vasculopathy is poorly understood.[100]

Several genetic syndromes include ischemic stroke as part of their pathognomonic characterization. Cerebral autosomal dominant arteriopathy with subcortical infarcts and leukoencephalopathy (CADASIL) is the most common inherited cause of stroke in adults. Mutations in the NOTCH3 gene expressing a smooth muscle transmembrane receptor cause an arteriopathy, leading to a characteristic progressive symptomatology of migraine with aura, subcortical ischemic strokes and TIAs, mood disturbances, apathy, and dementia.[101] An analogous autosomal recessive disorder, CARASIL, is caused by mutations in the HTRA1 gene and leads to a syndrome of ischemic strokes, premature baldness, dementia, and paroxysmal severe lower back pain.[102] Rarer inherited genetic syndromes leading to stroke include mitochondrial encephalopathy, lactic acidosis, and stroke-like episodes (MELAS); hereditary endotheliopathy with retinopathy, nephropathy, and stroke (HERNS); and various inborn errors in metabolism.[103]

CRYPTOGENIC STROKE

More than a third of ischemic strokes in adults are categorized as cryptogenic, in that they have no known etiology even after appropriate diagnostic investigation has been performed.[104] This is likely a heterogeneous group; however, many cryptogenic strokes appear to be due to occult cardioembolic events. Some evidence for this comes from two recent prospective trials investigating the use of long-term cardiac rhythm monitoring for patients with cryptogenic ischemic stroke or TIA. EMBRACE randomized patients to either 30 days of cardiac rhythm monitoring with an event-triggered loop recorder or 24 hours of continuous Holter monitoring. The rate of detection of atrial fibrillation was five times higher in the group receiving 30-day monitoring.[105] Similar results were seen in the CRYSTAL AF trial, which randomized patients to either an insertable cardiac monitor (ICM) or regular clinic visits with periodic electrocardiographic surveillance, and followed patients for at least 6 months. The rate of detection of atrial fibrillation was six times higher in the ICM group.[106]

Another source of occult cardioembolism in cryptogenic stroke is paradoxical embolism of a venous thrombus through a patent foramen ovale (PFO) or other atrial septal defect. While the prevalence of PFO in the general population is approximately 25%,[107] it is much higher in patients with stroke and higher still in patients with cryptogenic stroke. One case-control study found a 40% prevalence of PFO in patients with stroke compared with 10% in controls;[108] another reported a 48% prevalence in patients with cryptogenic stroke compared with 4% in those with stroke of determined cause.[109] These findings suggested that patients with PFO might be at risk for arterial stroke via venous thromboembolism crossing from the right to the left atrium. Prospective studies examining the risk of stroke recurrence in patients with PFO have failed to establish this, however. A recent meta-analysis of 14 prospective studies found that the risk of recurrent stroke or TIA in patients with PFO was no higher than in those without PFO.[110]

One possible explanation is that the majority of PFOs are not "functional." In theory, for paradoxical venous thromboembolism to occur, a PFO must be large enough for a clot to pass through, and the cardiac hemodynamics must be such that blood is shunted right-to-left through the PFO rather than the physiologic left-to-right shunting favored by the normal trans-atrial pressure gradient. However, large prospective studies and meta-analyses of patients with cryptogenic stroke have not found an association between either the degree of right-to-left shunting[111] or PFO size[91] and risk of recurrent stroke.

Some data suggest that PFO is pathologic in a subset of patients, and there have been risk stratification scores proposed to help identify this group. Most influential of these is the Risk of Paradoxical Embolism (RoPE) score, which predicts the likelihood of a cryptogenic stroke being due to a pathologic PFO based on the patient's age, conventional vascular risk factors, and stroke location.[112] For patients with pathologic PFOs, correction of the defect might be a promising strategy for stroke prevention, although compelling outcome data are lacking, and risk of recurrent stroke has been shown to be low in this group. Three major trials compared percutaneous device closure of PFOs with medical therapy for secondary stroke prevention. Despite some results from these trials suggesting a benefit to PFO closure, on intention-to-treat analysis, no significant benefit was found.[113] The most recent clinical trials are reviewed in Chapter 11.

While there is hope that the proportion of strokes that are cryptogenic will decrease as new mechanisms are discovered and as appropriate diagnostic tests are perfected, it will likely remain a substantial, highly heterogeneous category.

References

1. Adams HP Jr, Bendixen BH, Kappelle LJ, et al. Classification of subtype of acute ischemic stroke. Definitions for use in a multicenter clinical trial. TOAST. Trial of Org 10172 in Acute Stroke Treatment. *Stroke.* 1993;24:35–41.

2. Ay H, Furie KL, Singhal A, et al. An evidence-based causative classification system for acute ischemic stroke. *Ann Neurol.* 2005;58:688–697.

3. Ay H, Benner T, Arsava M, et al. A computerized algorithm for etiologic classification of ischemic stroke: The Causative Classification of Stroke system. *Stroke.* 2007;38: 2979–2984.

4. Aboyans V, Lacroix P, Criqui MH. Large and small vessels atherosclerosis: similarities and differences. *Prog Cardiovasc Dis.* 2007;50:112–125.

5. Reed DM, Resch JA, McLean C, et al. A prospective study of cerebral artery atherosclerosis. *Stroke.* 1998;19:820–825.

6. Wityk RJ, Lehman D, Klag M, et al. Race and sex differences in the distribution of cerebral atherosclerosis. *Stroke.* 1996;27:1974–1980.

7. Bogiatzi C, Wannarong T, McLeod AI, et al. SPARKLE (Subtypes of Ischaemic Stroke Classification System), incorporating measurement of carotid plaque burden: a new validated tool for the classification of ischemic stroke subtypes. *Neuroepidemiology.* 2014;42: 243–251.

8. Derdeyn CP, Chimowitz MI, Lynn MJ, et al. Aggressive medical treatment with or without stenting in high-risk patients with intracranial artery stenosis (SAMMPRIS): the final results of a randomised trial. *Lancet.* 2014;383:333–341.

9. Libby P. The vascular biology of atherosclerosis. In Bonow RO, Mann DL, Zipes DP, et al. *Braunwald's Heart Disease: A Textbook of Cardiovascular Medicine.* Philadelphia, PA: Saunders; 2012:897–913.

10. Grotta JC. Carotid stenosis. *N Engl J Med.* 2013;369:1143–1150.

11. Bentzon JF, Otsuka F, Virmani R, Falk E. Acute coronary syndromes compendium: mechanisms of plaque formation and rupture. *Circ Res.* 2014;114:1852–1866.

12. Antiplatelet Trialists' Collaboration. Collaborative overview of randomised trials of antiplatelet therapy: prevention of death, myocardial infarction, and stroke by prolonged antiplatelet therapy in various categories of patients. *Brit Med J.* 1994;308:81–106.

13. Powers WJ, Derdeyn CP, Fritsch SM, et al. Benign prognosis of never-symptomatic carotid occlusion. *Neurology.* 2000;54:878–882.

14. Rerkasem K, Rothwell PM. Carotid endarterectomy for symptomatic carotid stenosis. *Cochrane Database Syst Rev.* 2011 Apr 13;(4):CD001081.

15. Chimowitz MI, Lynn MJ, Howlett-Smith H, et al. Comparison of warfarin and aspirin for symptomatic intracranial arterial stenosis. *N Engl J Med.* 2005;352:1305–1316.

16. Kolominsky-Rabas PL, Weber M, Gefeller O, et al. Epidemiology of ischemic stroke subtypes according to TOAST criteria: incidence, recurrence, and long-term survival in ischemic stroke subtypes: A population-based study. *Stroke.* 2001;32:2735–2740.

17. Petty GW, Brown RD, Whisnant JP, et al. Ischemic stroke subtypes: A population-based study of functional outcome, survival, and recurrence. *Stroke.* 2000;31:1062–1068.

18. Cerebral Embolism Task Force. Cardiogenic brain embolism. *Arch Neurol.* 1986; 43:71–84.

19. Wolf PA, Abbott RD, Kannel WB. Atrial fibrillation as an independent risk factor for stroke: The Framingham Study. *Stroke.* 1991;22:983–988.

20. Pathophysiologic correlates of thromboembolism in nonvalvular atrial fibrillation: I. Reduced flow velocity in the left atrial appendage (the Stroke Prevention in Atrial Fibrillation [SPAF-III] study. *J Am Soc Echocardio.* 1999;12:1080–1087.

21. Hart RG, Halperin JL. Atrial fibrillation and stroke: Concepts and controversies. *Stroke.* 2001;32:803–808.

22. Watson T, Shantsila E, Lip GYH. Mechanisms of thrombogenesis in atrial fibrillation: Virchow's triad revisited. *Lancet.* 2009;373:155–166.

23. Weinberg DM, Mancini GBJ. Anticoagulation for cardioversion of atrial fibrillation. *Am J Cardiol.* 1989;63:745–746.

24. Stoddard MF, Dawkins PR, Prince CR, et al. Left atrial appendage thrombus is not uncommon in patients with acute atrial fibrillation and a recent embolic event: A transesophageal echocardiographics study. *J Am Coll Cardiol.* 1995;25:452–459.

25. Salem DN, Daudelin DH, Levine HJ, et al. Antithrombotic therapy in valvular heart disease. *Chest.* 2001;119:207–209S.

26. Wood P. An appreciation of mitral stenosis: Part I: clinical features. *Brit Med J.* 1954;1: 1051–1063.

27. Szekely P. Systemic embolism and anticoagulant prophylaxis in rheumatic heart disease. *Brit Med J.* 1964;1:1209–1212.

28. Mahajan R, Brooks AG, Sullivan T, et al. Importance of the underlying substrate in determining thrombus location in atrial fibrillation: Implications for left atrial appendage closure. *Heart.* 2012;98:1120–1126.

29. Boon A, Lodder J, Cheriex E, et al. Risk of stroke in a cohort of 815 patients with calcification of the aortic valve with or without stenosis. *Stroke.* 1996;27:847–851.

30. Walker BS, Shah LM, Osborn AG. Calcified cerebral emboli, a "do not miss" imaging diagnosis: 22 new cases and review of the literature. *Am J Neuroradiol.* 2014;35: 1515.

31. Murtagh B, Smalling RW. Cardioembolic stroke. *Curr Atherosd Rep.* 2006;8(4):310–316.

32. Gilon D, Buonanno FS, Joffe MM, et al. Lack of evidence of an association between mitral-valve prolapse and stroke in young patients. *N Engl J Med.* 1999;341:8–13.

33. Cabell CH, Pond KK, Peterson GE, et al. The risk of stroke and death in patients with aortic and mitral valve endocarditis. *Am Heart J.* 2001;142:75–80.

34. Dickerman SA, Abrutyn E, Barsic B, et al. The relationship between the initiation of antimicrobial therapy and the incidence of stroke in infective endocarditis: An analysis from the ICE Prospective Cohort Study (ICE-PCS). *Am Heart J.* 2007;154:1086–1094.

35. Mooe T, Eriksson P, Stegmayr B. Ischemic stroke after acute myocardial infarction: A population-based study. *Stroke.* 1997;28:762–7.

36. Loh E, Sutton MSJ, Wun CC, et al. Ventricular dysfunction and the risk of stroke after myocardial infarction. *N Engl J Med.* 1997;336:251–257.

37. Amarenco P, Cohen A, Tzourio C, et al. Atherosclerotic disease of the aortic arch and the risk of ischemic stroke. *N Engl J Med.* 1994;331:1474–1479.

38. Meissner I, Khandheria BK, Sheps SG, et al. Atherosclerosis of the aorta: Risk factor, risk marker, or innocent bystander? A prospective population-based transesophageal echocardiography study. *J Am Coll Cardiol.* 2004;44:1018–1024.

39. Macleod MR, Amarenco P, Davis SM, et al. Atheroma of the aortic arch: An important and poorly recognised factor in the aetiology of stroke. *Lancet Neurol.* 2004;3:408–414.

40. O'Rourke F, Dean N, Mouradian MS, et al. Atrial myxoma as a cause of stroke: Case report and discussion. *CMAJ.* 2003;169:1049–1051.

41. Lee VH, Connolly HM, Brown RD. Central nervous system manifestations of cardiac myxoma. *Arch Neurol.* 2007;64:1115–1120.

42. Goodwin JF. Diagnosis of left atrial myxoma. *Lancet.* 1963;281:464–468.

43. Gowda RM, Khan IA, Nair CK, et al. Cardiac papillary fibroelastoma: A comprehensive analysis of 725 cases. *Am Heart J.* 2003;146:404–410.

44. Butany J, Nair V, Naseemuddin A, et al. Cardiac tumors: Diagnosis and management. *Lancet Oncol.* 2005;6:219–228.

45. Fisher CM. The arterial lesions underlying lacunes. *Acta Neuropath.* 1969;12:1–15.

46. Gan R, Sacco RL, Kargman DE, et al. Testing the validity of the lacunar hypothesis: The Northern Manhattan Stroke Study experience. *Neurology.* 1997;48:1204–1211.

47. Russell RWR. How does blood-pressure cause stroke? *Lancet.* 1975;2:1283–1285.

48. Fisher CM. Capsular infarcts: The underlying vascular lesions. *Arch Neurol.* 1979;36: 65–73.

49. De Jong G, Kessels F, Lodder J. Two types of lacunar infarcts: Further evidence from a study on prognosis. *Stroke.* 2002;33:2072–2076.

50. Caplan LR. Intracranial branch atheromatous disease: A neglected, understudied, and underused concept. *Neurology.* 1989;39:1246–1250.

51. Nakase T, Yoshioka S, Sasaki M , et al. Clinical evaluation of lacunar infarction and branch atheromatous disease. *J Stroke Cerebrovasc Dis.* 2013;22:406–412.

52. Macdonald RL, Kowalczuk A, Johns L. Emboli enter penetrating arteries of monkey brain in relation to their size. *Stroke.* 1995;26:1247–1251.

53. Horowitz DR, Tuhrim S, Weinberger JM, et al. Mechanisms in lacunar infarction. *Stroke.* 1992;23:325–327.

54. Graus F, Rogers LR, Posner JB. Cerebrovascular complications in patients with cancer. *Medicine.* 1985;64:16–35.

55. Janardhan V, Wolf PA, Kase CS, et al. Anticardiolipin antibodies and risk of ischemic stroke and transient ischemic attack: The Framingham cohort and offspring study. *Stroke.* 2004;35:736–741.

56. Kittner SJ, Stern BJ, Feeser BR, et al. Pregnancy and the risk of stroke. *N Engl J Med.* 1996;335:768–774.

57. Gillum LA, Mamidipudi SK, Johnston SC. Ischemic stroke risk with oral contraceptives: A meta-analysis. *JAMA.* 2000;284:72–78.

58. Hiatt BK, Lentz SR. Prothrombotic states that predispose to stroke. *Curr Treat Options Neurol.* 2002;4:417–425.

59. Nachman RL, Silverstein R. Hypercoagulable states. *Ann Intern Med.* 1993;119:819–827.

60. Kenet G, Sadetzki S, Murad H, et al. Factor V Leiden and antiphospholipid antibodies are significant risk factors for ischemic stroke in children. *Stroke.* 2000;31:1283–1288.

61. De Stefano V, Chiusolo P, Paciaroni K, et al. Prothrombin G20210A mutant genotype is a risk factor for cerebrovascular ischemic disease in young patients. *Blood.* 1998;91(10): 3562–3565.

62. Martinez HR, Rangel-Guerra RA, Marfil LJ. Ischemic stroke due to deficiency of coagulation inhibitors. Report of 10 young adults. *Stroke.* 1993;24:19–25.

63. Camerlingo M, Finazzi G, Casto L, et al. Inherited protein C deficiency and non-hemorrhagic arterial stroke in young adults. *Neurology.* 1991;41:1371.

64. Sacco RL, Owen J, Mohr JP, et al. Free protein S deficiency: A possible association with cerebrovascular occlusion. *Stroke.* 1989;20:1657–1661.

65. Hankey GJ, Eikelboom JW, van Bockxmeer FM et al. Inherited thrombophilia in ischemic stroke and its pathogenic subtypes. *Stroke.* 2001;32:1793–1799.

66. Homocysteine Studies Collaboration. Homocysteine and risk of ischemic heart disease and stroke: A meta-analysis. *JAMA.* 2002;288:2015–2022.

67. Li P, Qin C. Methylenetetrahydrofolate reductase (MTHFR) gene polymorphisms and susceptibility to ischemic stroke: A meta-analysis. *Gene.* 2014;535:359–364.

68. Reuner KH, Ruf A, Grau A, et al. Prothrombin gene G20210(A) transition is a risk factor for cerebral venous thrombosis. *Stroke.* 1998;29:1765–1769.

69. Schaller B, Graf R. Cerebral venous infarction: The pathophysiological concept. *Cerebrovasc Dis.* 2004;18:179–188.
70. Stam J. Thrombosis of the cerebral veins and sinuses. *N Engl J Med.* 2005;352:1791–1798.
71. Kristensen B, Malm J, Carlberg B, et al. Epidemiology and etiology of ischemic stroke in young adults aged 18 to 44 years in northern Sweden. *Stroke.* 1997;28:1702–1709.
72. Benninger DH, Georgiadis D, Kremer C, et al. Mechanism of ischemic infarct in spontaneous carotid dissection. *Stroke.* 2004;35:482–485.
73. Biousse V, D'Anglejan-Chatillon J, Touboul P-J, et al. Time course of symptoms in extracranial carotid artery dissections: A series of 80 patients. *Stroke.* 1995;26:235–239.
74. Guillon B, Berthet K, Benslamia L, et al. Infection and the risk of spontaneous cervical artery dissection: A case-control study. *Stroke.* 2003;34:e79–e81.
75. Haldeman S, Kohlbeck F, McGregor M. Risk factors and precipitating neck movements causing vertebrobasilar artery dissection after cervical trauma and spinal manipulation. *Spine.* 1999;24:785–794.
76. Pepin M, Schwarze U, Superti-Furga A, et al. Clinical and genetic features of Ehlers-Danlos syndrome type IV, the vascular type. *N Engl J Med.* 2000;342:673–680.
77. Brandt T, Orberk E, Weber R, et al. Pathogenesis of cervical artery dissections. *Neurology.* 2001;57:24–30.
78. Pezzini A, Del Zotto E, Archetti S, et al. Plasma homocysteine concentration, C677T MTHFR genotype, and 844ins68bp CBS genotype in young adults with spontaneous cervical artery dissection and atherothrombotic stroke. *Stroke.* 2002;33:664–669.
79. Brandt T, Grond-Ginsbach C. Spontaneous cervical artery dissection: From risk factors toward pathogenesis. *Stroke.* 2002;33:657–658.
80. Ferro JM. Vasculitis of the central nervous system. *J Neurol.* 1998;245:766–776.
81. Crowley RW, Medel R, Dumont AS, et al. Angiographic vasospasm is strongly correlated with cerebral infarction after subarachnoid hemorrhage. *Stroke.* 2011;42:919–923.
82. Belka C, Budach W, Kortmann RD, et al. Radiation induced CNS toxicity: Molecular and cellular mechanisms. *British J Cancer.* 2001;85:1233–1239.
83. Dorresteijn LDA, Kappelle AC, Boogerd W, et al. Increased risk of ischemic stroke after radiotherapy on the neck in patients younger than 60 years. *J Clin Oncol.* 2002;20:282–288.
84. Westover AN, McBride S, Haley RW. Stroke in young adults who abuse amphetamines or cocaine: A population-based study of hospitalized patients. *JAMA Psychiatry.* 2007;64:495–502.
85. Treadwell SD, Robinson TG. Cocaine use and stroke. *Postgrad Med J.* 2007;83:389–394.
86. Krishnan E. Stroke subtypes among young patients with systemic lupus erythematosus. *Am J Med.* 2005;118:1415.e1-e7.
87. Futrell N, Millikan C. Frequency, etiology, and prevention of stroke in patients with systemic lupus erythematosus. *Stroke.* 1989;20:583–591.
88. Weststrate W, Hijdra A, de Gans J. Brain infarcts in adults with bacterial meningitis. *Lancet.* 1996;347:399.
89. Pfister H-W, Borasio GD, Dirnagl U, et al. Cerebrovascular complications of bacterial meningitis in adults. *Neurology.* 1992;42:1497–1504.
90. Marcus JL, Leyden WA, Chao CR, et al. HIV infection and incidence of ischemic stroke. *AIDS.* 2014;28:1911–1919.
91. Ortiz G, Koch S, Romano JG, et al. Mechanisms of stroke in HIV-infected patients. *Neurology.* 2007;68:1257–1261.
92. Chetty R. Vasculitides associated with HIV infection. *J Clin Pathol.* 2001;54:275–278.

93. Askalan R, Laughlin S, Mayank S, et al. Chickenpox and stroke in childhood: A study of frequency and causation. *Stroke.* 2001;32:1257–1262.

94. Ionita CC, Siddiqui AH, Levy EI, et al. Acute ischemic stroke and infections. *J Stroke Cerebrovasc Dis.* 2011;20:1–9.

95. Earley CJ, Kittner SJ, Feeser BR, et al. Stroke in children and sickle-cell disease. *Neurology.* 1998;51:169–176.

96. Switzer JA, Hess DC, Nichols FT, et al. Pathophysiology and treatment of stroke in sickle-cell disease: Present and future. *Lancet Neurol.* 2006;5:501–512.

97. Scott RM, Smith ER. Moyamoya disease and moyamoya syndrome. *N Engl J Med.* 2009;360:1226–1237.

98. Sims K, Politei J, Banikazemi M, et al. Stroke in Fabry disease frequently occurs before diagnosis and in the absence of other clinical events. *Stroke.* 2009;40:788–794.

99. Rolfs A, Böttcher T, Zschiesche M, et al. Prevalence of Fabry disease in patients with cryptogenic stroke: A prospective study. *Lancet.* 2005;366:1794–1796.

100. Moore DF, Kaneski CR, Askan H, et al. The cerebral vasculopathy of Fabry disease. *J Neurol Sci.* 2007;257:258–263.

101. Chabriat H, Joutel A, Dichgans M, et al. CADASIL. *Lancet Neurol.* 2009;8:643–653.

102. Fukutake T. Cerebral autosomal recessive arteriopathy with subcortical infarcts and leukoencephalopathy (CARASIL): From discovery to gene identification. *J Stroke Cerebrovasc Dis.* 2011;20:85–93.

103. Testai FD, Gorelick PB. Inherited metabolic disorders and stroke part 1: Fabry disease and mitochondrial myopathy, encephalopathy, lactic acidosis, and strokelike episodes. *Arch Neurol.* 2010;67:19–24.

104. Schulz UGR, Rothwell PM. Differences in vascular risk factors between etiological subtypes of ischemic stroke: Importance of population-based studies. *Stroke.* 2003;34:2050–2059.

105. Gladstone DJ, Spring M, Dorian P, et al. Atrial fibrillation in patients with cryptogenic stroke. N Engl J Med. 2014;370:2467–2477.

106. Sanna T, Diener H-C, Passman RS, et al. Cryptogenic stroke and underlying atrial fibrillation. *N Engl J Med.* 2014;370:2478–2486.

107. Hagen PT, Scholz DG, Edwards WD. Incidence and size of patent foramen ovale during the first 10 decades of life: An autopsy study of 965 normal hearts. *Mayo Clinic Proc.* 1984;59:17–20.

108. Lechat P, Mas JL, Lascault G, et al. Prevalence of patent foramen ovale in patients with stroke. *N Engl J Med.* 1988;318:1148–1152.

109. Di Tullio M, Sacco RL, Gopal A, et al. Patent foramen ovale as a risk factor for cryptogenic stroke. *Ann Intern Med.* 1992;117:461–465.

110. Katsanos AH, Spence JD, Bogiatzi C, et al. Recurrent stroke and patent foramen ovale: A systematic review and meta-analysis. *Stroke.* 2014;45:3352–3359.

111. Serena J, Marti-Fàbregas J, Santamarina E, et al. Recurrent stroke and massive right-to-left shunt: Results from the prospective Spanish multicenter (CODICIA) study. *Stroke.* 2008;39:3131–3136.

112. Kent DM, Ruthazer R, Weimar C, et al. An index to identify stroke-related vs incidental patent foramen ovale in cryptogenic stroke. *Neurology.* 2013;81:619–625.

113. Spencer FA, Lopes LC, Kennedy SA, et al. Systematic review of percutaneous closure versus medical therapy in patients with cryptogenic stroke and patent foramen ovale. *BMJ Open.* 2014;4:e004282.

Neuroimaging of Acute Stroke 4

Rahul Garg and Steven M. Schonfeld

In the last 20 years, we have seen significant developments in the screening, diagnosis, and treatment of ischemic and hemorrhagic stroke. These include advancements in CT and MRI technology; changes in stroke imaging algorithms; and novel treatment devices and techniques, such as intravenous tissue plasminogen activator (IV tPA), carotid artery stenting, intra-arterial therapy (IAT) of ischemic stroke, and endovascular embolization of vascular malformations. These innovative techniques have helped achieve reductions in the relative rate of stroke deaths compared to other cardiovascular deaths by 35.8% and the actual number of stroke deaths by 22.8% from 2001 to 2011.[1,2]

Many imaging modalities are available to the clinician and radiologist for evaluating a variety of focal neurologic deficits. The application of these modalities largely depends on the working diagnosis, the urgency of the clinical problem, the availability of the modality, and the comorbidities of the patient. Modalities such as CT and MRI are used as first-line imaging examinations and tend to provide useful diagnostic information.[3] However, CT angiography (CTA), CT venography (CTV), CT perfusion (CTP), MR angiography (MRA), MR venography (MRV), MR perfusion (MRP), and digital subtraction angiography (DSA) also play major roles when evaluating cerebrovascular disease.[1] In practice, the challenge for clinicians is to understand the multiple complex facets of these techniques, including which technique to implement and how to optimally implement it in the appropriate clinical setting. Many important factors must be considered, including time urgency, cost, access to imaging, radiation exposure, preferences of treating physicians, availability of expertise, and selecting the best diagnostic imaging modality to assess for the clinical indication.[4] The American

College of Radiology (ACR) Appropriateness Criteria were developed to assist clinicians in making appropriate imaging decisions for a variety of patient clinical conditions. They are the most comprehensive and best evidence-based guidelines for diagnostic imaging selection, radiotherapy protocols, and imaging-guided interventional procedures.[5]

Noncontrast computed tomography (NCCT) can be useful for evaluating disease processes such as ischemic stroke, hemorrhagic stroke, intracranial hemorrhage, or stroke mimickers (e.g., infection, demyelination, tumor, or hydrocephalus). The primary goals of imaging acute stroke include determining stroke type, detecting the presence of intracranial hemorrhage (which would preclude the administration of thrombolytics), detecting ischemia, excluding tumor, and/or identifying other conditions that can mimic stroke. The NCCT is an important first-line imaging test because it is fast; readily available; has high spatial resolution; does not require screening; and is able to detect the presence or absence of intracranial hemorrhage, neoplasm, abscess, or other acute pathology, which guides further management, particularly if the patient is a tPA candidate. The disadvantage of NCCT is the use of ionizing radiation. There are also secondary effects of stroke that must be evaluated, including hemorrhagic transformation, mass effect, herniation, and hydrocephalus, all of which can be readily identified with CT. To detect intracranial hemorrhage, NCCT is the modality of choice, with an overall sensitivity of 91%[6]; however, this is dependent on the time interval between symptom onset and scan time. Sensitivity has been shown in the literature to be 100% for patients imaged within 12 hours, 93% within 24 hours, and 84% after 24 hours.[6,7] With NCCT, hemorrhage progresses from hyperdense to isodense and finally to hypodense over a period of weeks to months due to the breakdown of hemoglobin by macrophages. MRI can also be used to detect hemorrhage but is better used to age hemorrhage. Detection of hemorrhage on MRI is dependent on the age and location of the blood, the strength of the magnet, and the sequence used.[8–15]

Intracranial hemorrhage may be secondary to a variety of causes, such as trauma, hypertension, neoplasm (primary or metastatic), vascular malformation (arteriovenous or cavernous), arterial or venous infarction, amyloid angiopathy in elderly normotensive patients, coagulopathy, or drug ingestion, particularly in younger patients. If intracranial hemorrhage is present, the imaging evaluation in the acute phase may include CTA to assess for an underlying aneurysm in the setting of subarachnoid hemorrhage or an arteriovenous malformation in the setting of an intraparenchymal hemorrhage.[4] Demonstration of the "spot sign" with CTA is indicative of contrast extravasation and active bleeding and has been shown to be an independent predictor of hematoma expansion, portending a poor prognosis. Of those patients scanned within 6 hours of symptoms onset, approximately one-third will show the spot sign.[16–19]

Hypertensive hemorrhage is more commonly a solitary hematoma, rather than a multifocal hemorrhage, and usually occurs in the basal ganglia, thalamus, or cerebellum. This may be differentiated from amyloid angiopathy, the cause of 15%–20% of all spontaneous intracranial hemorrhages in normotensive elderly patients, which is best seen on gradient echo MRI sequences in a subcortical/cortical location. Subarachnoid hemorrhage can also result from trauma, ruptured aneurysm, intracranial arteriovenous malformation, coagulopathy, and other causes.[1,4]

CT often appears normal in patients with "hyperacute" stroke, which is defined as occurring within 6 hours of symptom onset,[19,20] but subtle findings may be detected in as early as 2 to 3 hours. These include hyperattenuating clot within vessels (Figure 4.1A), loss of gray-white differentiation (Figure 4.1 B and C), and sulcal effacement. The hyperdense middle cerebral artery (MCA) sign on NCCT (Figure 4.1A)—which denotes the presence of increased density when compared to the opposite hemisphere along the course of the first and second segments of the MCA—was recognized as one of the earliest signs of ischemic stroke and may appear within 90 minutes after neurological deficits occur.[21–24] The hyperattenuating portion of the vessel measures approximately 80 Hounsfield units and represents intraluminal clot from thrombus.[24,25] This sign is associated with a large MCA territory infarction, severe neurological deficit, and poor clinical outcome.[24,26–28] The specificity of the hyperdense MCA sign is close to 100%, but its sensitivity is low.[27] Hyperdensities along the course of the basilar artery and distal MCA segments, the so-called dot sign, and more recently, the hyperdense posterior cerebral artery (PCA) sign, have been described in the literature to correspond to analogous clots in those vessels and are markers for associated territorial infarctions.[24,29,30] The hyperdense PCA sign has been detected in more than one-third of all patients with PCA ischemia, similar to the incidence of the hyperdense MCA sign, and may not only be helpful for the early diagnosis of PCA infarction, but may also act as a prognostic marker in acute PCA territory ischemic stroke.[24] Previous studies have shown that the length of clot burden, particularly in MCA occlusion, is an independent predictor of successful IV tPA treatment. In fact, Rohan et al and Riedel et al have shown that in acute MCA stroke, IV thrombolysis has nearly zero potential to recanalize occluded vessels if the thrombus exceeds 8 mm.[31,32]

It is important to note that the detection of early signs of ischemia on NCCT varies among experienced observers[33–35] and depends on the size of the infarct, the time between symptom onset and imaging, and the CT level and window settings implemented.[4] The Alberta Stroke Program Early CT Score (ASPECTS)

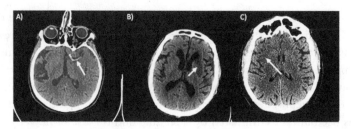

FIGURE 4.1 (A) Hyperdense left middle cerebral artery sign (arrow); (B) hypodensity in the left basal ganglia due to recent infarct (arrow); (C) subtle low attenuation in the right insular ribbon due to recent evolving infarct (arrow)

was developed to serve as a more objective approach for defining the extent of early ischemic changes. ASPECTS is a 10-point scoring system of the MCA vascular territory, with one point deducted for each portion of the territory affected by ischemia.[36–38] The MCA territory regions defined by ASPECTS include the caudate; insular ribbon; internal capsule; lentiform nucleus; anterior MCA cortex at the basal ganglia level (M1); MCA cortex lateral to the insular ribbon (M2); posterior MCA cortex at the basal ganglia level (M3); and M4, M5, and M6, which are the anterior, lateral, and posterior MCA territories immediately superior to M1, M2, and M3, just cranial to the basal ganglia. An ASPECTS score less than or equal to 7 has been shown to predict poor functional outcome with 78% sensitivity and 96% specificity.[39]

There is strong evidence supporting the use of IV tPA as recanalization therapy to improve clinical outcomes during the 0- to 3-hour time window (level 1a)[40–42] and during the 3- to 4.5-hour time window (level 1b).[43–45] This benefit is evident despite an increased risk of symptomatic intracranial hemorrhage after infusion.[4] NCCT prior to administering IV thrombolysis is important not only to exclude intracranial hemorrhage, but also because early signs of ischemia, as discussed earlier, involving more than one-third of the MCA territory in the 0- to 4.5-hour time window, have been associated with large infarcted regions, increased risk of hemorrhagic transformation, and poor outcomes and thus constitute exclusion criteria for IV thrombolysis.[46,47] However, despite this risk, it has been shown that early ischemic changes alone should not be a reason to exclude a patient from treatment within the 3-hour window.[46,48,49]

MRI, especially the diffusion/apparent diffusion coefficient (ADC) sequence, is more sensitive than CT for evaluating an acute recent infarct core and may be considered first line if the neurologic deficit is fixed or worsening and longer than 6 hours in duration.[23] MRI with diffusion may also play an important role in determining infarct core in patients with large-vessel occlusion who have poor collaterals, regardless of the time from ictus.[50] MRI is the best modality to directly image the stroke and evaluate other conditions; however, the downside of MRI is that it may not be able to be performed in patients who are claustrophobic, are morbidly obese, or have cardiac devices or other MRI-incompatible metal implanted within them. One must be cautious when administering IV gadolinium contrast in patients with renal dysfunction due to the risks of contrast allergy or nephrogenic systemic fibrosis (NSF), although the incidence of NSF has been almost eliminated by screening and the use of newer gadolinium agents.[51-53] The ACR documents on MRI safety and contrast media[53,54] provide more detailed safety information as does www.mrisafety.com.

A limited, noncontrast brain MRI can be performed in the acute stroke patient with diffusion-weighted imaging (DWI), an apparent diffusion coefficient (ADC) map, and fluid-attenuated inversion recovery (FLAIR) to evaluate for infarct.[1] Currently, the most common clinical MRI scanners have field strengths of 1.5 Tesla (T) and 3 T.[1] DWI is related to Brownian motion on a molecular level because intracellular water molecules are significantly more limited in motion in comparison to extracellular water molecules. In ischemia, areas of the brain swell after osmosis of water into dying cells. This in turn leads to restricted diffusion or restricted motion, which appears as bright on DWI and dark on the ADC map (Figure 4.2). DWI is positive within minutes to a few hours and remains positive over about 2 weeks. It allows one to distinguish recent strokes as small as 4 mm in diameter from chronic strokes. DWI is more sensitive for detecting ischemic changes compared to NCCT, with a sensitivity of 99% and specificity of 92%.[55-63] In the setting of intracranial hemorrhage, MRI with and without contrast is also useful when evaluating for underlying neoplasm, vascular mass, micro-hemorrhages (which may suggest amyloid angiopathy), multiple cavernomas, or septic emboli, and so on.[4] It is important to note that although MRI is superior to NCCT for confirming stroke in the first 24 hours, there are logistical issues in performing MRI in the emergent setting, and therefore, MRI may be reserved for selected patients for whom the clinical diagnosis is uncertain or for centers that have MRI available 24/7, with streamlined protocols to limit imaging time within the standard-of-care guidelines for thrombolytic therapy.[4]

In the workup of stroke, imaging of the intracranial and extracranial carotid and vertebral vasculature can be performed noninvasively and quickly using MRA and CTA. However, DSA is the gold standard for detecting vascular stenoses or occlusions. CTA is a versatile and very reliable modality to identify areas of vascular stenosis, occlusion, dissection, vasculitis, aneurysm, or vascular malformation. CTA has been reported to have high sensitivity (97%–100%) and specificity (98%–100%) for detecting intracranial stenoses and occlusions

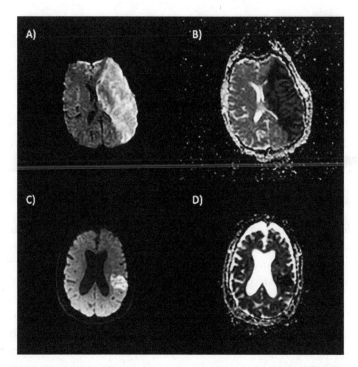

FIGURE 4.2 (A) Large area of hyperintense signal on DWI in the left middle cerebral artery territory compatible with recent infarction; (B) large area of associated hypointense signal on the ADC map in the left middle cerebral artery territory, confirming recent infarction; (C) small area of hyperintense signal on DWI in the left parietal region compatible with recent infarction; (D) small area of associated hypointense signal on the ADC map in the left parietal region, confirming recent infarction

(Figure 4.3) compared to DSA.[64–71] It is also very fast and readily available in comparison to MRA because it can be obtained immediately following NCCT or after initiation of IV thrombolysis, thereby avoiding delay in treatment.[4] However, the downside of CTA is the radiation exposure and artifact from dense calcification and adjacent bone.

In comparison to CTA, noncontrast MRA, including time-of-flight MRA (TOF-MRA), is an excellent tool to evaluate the circle of Willis in acute stroke and relies on flow-related enhancement, with three-dimensional TOF-MRA having outstanding spatial resolution.[1] However, TOF-MRA has difficulty with regions of slow or turbulent flow, which may manifest as partial signal void, leading to an overestimation of stenosis.[4] Contrast-enhanced MRA (CE-MRA) uses the T1-shortening effects of gadolinium agents and is less susceptible to

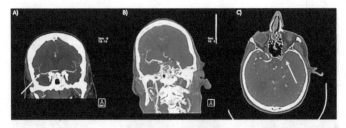

FIGURE 4.3 (A) CT angiogram maximal intensity projection image in the coronal plane demonstrating short segment right M2 branch stenosis (arrow); (B) and (C) long segment stenosis of the entire left middle cerebral artery in the coronal and axial planes, respectively (arrows)

image degradation due to slow and turbulent flow.[1] CTA has been shown to be slightly superior to MRA for the identification of intracranial stenoses or occlusions, especially for distal vascular lesions.[64,65] It is also important to note that these modalities are useful for evaluating the cerebral collateral vasculature, the network of vessels that stabilize blood flow when the major conduits fail. Collateral patterns can differ vastly among patients and are critically necessary to provide flow to ischemic brain. In the literature, patients with robust collateral networks tend to have improved tissue and clinical outcomes in the setting of ischemic stroke (Figure 4.4, A–D).[72] A large stroke and networks of poor collaterals portend a poor functional prognosis as well as poor response to endovascular therapy (Figure 4.4, E–F).[73–77] Souza et al characterized a malignant CTA-based collateral profile as the absence of collaterals in >50% of an MCA M2 superior or inferior division territory. This malignant collateral profile is 97.6% specific for patients with large baseline infarcts (i.e., DWI volume >100 mL) who are at high risk for poor long-term outcome and, therefore, may be unlikely to benefit from revascularization therapy.[78]

Imaging of the cervical arteries is also an important component of the workup for acute ischemic stroke because it may help identify the mechanism of stroke and thus potentially prevent a recurrence.[1,4,79,80] Multiple imaging modalities may be used, such as duplex ultrasound (DUS), CTA, MRA, and DSA.[81–83] Each technique has its own advantages and disadvantages in different clinical scenarios. However, most show general agreement with DSA, which is considered the gold standard technique to assess degree of stenosis/occlusion and thereby determine a patient's eligibility for carotid endarterectomy or other intervention in approximately 90% of cases.[4] Two concordant results from noninvasive DUS, CTA, and/or MRA can be used to determine eligibility for a revascularization procedure, avoiding the risks associated with invasive catheter angiog-

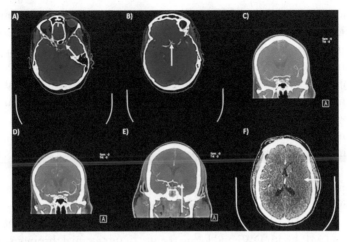

FIGURE 4.4 (A) Axial CTA shows left supraclinoid internal carotid artery (ICA) occlusion (arrow); (B) patent anterior communicating artery (arrow) provides collateral blood flow to the left anterior circulation; (C) and (D) show a favorable collateral circulation profile of the proximal and distal left MCA branches despite left supraclinoid ICA occlusion; (E) and (F) demonstrate a proximal left MCA occlusion (long arrow) with a malignant collateral circulation profile as no distal collateral branches are seen (short arrow)

raphy.[4,84] The "string sign," which is associated with a 99% stenosis, is most accurately detected by DSA, followed closely by CTA, and CE-MRA.[4,85,86]

CTP can be used to identify cerebrovascular reserve and the ischemic penumbra, which is defined as hypoperfused, at-risk, brain tissue that may eventually be recruited into the infarct core if not reperfused quickly enough. CTP time-tracks the IV contrast bolus through the brain and can use this information to make different assessments. To understand these measures, it is helpful to know that cerebral blood flow (CBF) is equal to the cerebral blood volume (CBV) divided by the mean transit time (MTT). With CTP, the penumbra can either show (a) increased MTT with moderately decreased CBF (>60% of normal) and normal or increased CBV (80%–100%) due to autoregulatory mechanisms or (b) increased MTT with markedly reduced CBF (>30%) and moderately reduced CBV (>60%). Infarcted tissue shows severely decreased CBF (<30% of normal) and CBV (<40% of normal) with increased MTT. Clear guidelines on when CTP should be performed and how it should be interpreted are currently lacking. However, there is broad agreement that quantification of perfusion using CTP is not validated, there is high inter-vendor and intra-vendor variability based on the software used, and the efficacy of CTP in improving patient outcomes is unproven.

In addition, the variability in CTP perfusion maps is unquantified with respect to fluctuations in patient heart rate, blood pressure, ejection fraction, rate of contrast infusion, osmolality of contrast, rotation time, and temporal resolution of the scanner.[87] Overall, the role of CTP in the evaluation of acute stroke has been unproven because of sensitivity to motion, low signal-to-noise-ratio, and variation among software packages.[1] However, the utility of CTP is currently being evaluated in various stroke trials.

It is important to note that CTA, CTV, and CTP all use IV iodinated contrast. This may preclude its use in patients who are at risk of contrast-allergy and contrast-induced nephropathy.[1]

In conclusion, it clear that neuroimaging plays a critical role not only in the diagnosis of acute stroke, but also in determining the possibility of intervention through its ability to assess the extent of ischemic or infarcted tissue using NCCT and MRI with DWI and locate the site of intracranial thrombus, as well as evaluate the collateral circulation with CTA or MRA. The value of these tools is immeasurable in the management of the patient with acute stroke when implemented appropriately by the astute clinician in conjunction with the consulting radiologist.

References

1. Salmela MB, Mortazavi S, Jagadeesan BD, et al. Cerebrovascular disease. *ACR Appropriateness Criteria*. 2016. Available at https://acsearch.acr.org/list.
2. Mozaffarian D, Benjamin EJ, Go AS, et al. Heart disease and stroke statistics—2015 update: a report from the American Heart Association. *Circulation*. 2015;131:e29–322.
3. Wippold FJ, Cornelius RS, Aiken AH, et. al. Focal neurologic deficit. *ACR Appropriateness Criteria*. 2012. Available at https://acsearch.acr.org/list
4. Wintermark M, Sanelli PC, Albers GW, et al. Imaging Recommendations for Acute Stroke and Transient Ischemic Attack Patients: A Joint Statement by the American Society of Neuroradiology, the American College of Radiology, and the Society of Neurointerventional Surgery. *AJNR Am J Neuroradiol*. 2013;34:E117-E127.
5. "About the ACR appropriateness criteria." Available at www.acr.org/quality-safety/appropriateness-criteria/about-AC.
6. Sames TA, Storrow AB, Finkelstein JA, et al. Sensitivity of new-generation computed tomography in subarachnoid hemorrhage. *Acad Emerg Med*. 1996;3:16–20.
7. Sidman R, Connolly E, Lemke T. Subarachnoid hemorrhage diagnosis: lumbar puncture is still needed when the computed tomography scan is normal. *Acad Emerg Med*. 1996;3:827–831.
8. Bradley WG Jr., Schmidt PG. Effect of methemoglobin formation on the MR appearance of subarachnoid hemorrhage. *Radiology*. 1985;156:99–103.
9. Edelman RR, Johnson K, Buxton R, et al. MR of hemorrhage: a new approach. *AJNR Am J Neuroradiol*. 1986;7:751–756.
10. Gomori JM, Grossman RI, Goldberg HI, et al. Intracranial hematomas: imaging by high-field MR. *Radiology*. 1985;157:87–93.

11. Hayman LA, Taber KH, Ford JJ, et al. Mechanisms of MR signal alteration by acute intracerebral blood: old concepts and new theories. *AJNR Am J Neuroradiol.* 1991;12:899–907.

12. Kidwell CS, Chalela JA, Saver JL, et al. Comparison of MRI and CT for detection of acute intracerebral hemorrhage. *JAMA.* 2004;292:1823–1830.

13. Linfante I, Llinas RH, Caplan LR, et al. MRI features of intracerebral hemorrhage within 2 hours from symptom onset. *Stroke.* 1999;30:2263–2267.

14. Patel MR, Edelman RR, Warach S. Detection of hyperacute primary intraparenchymal hemorrhage by magnetic resonance imaging. *Stroke.* 1996;27:2321–2324.

15. Schellinger PD, Jansen O, Fiebach JB, et al. A standardized MRI stroke protocol: comparison with CT in hyperacute intracerebral hemorrhage. *Stroke.* 1999;30:765–768.

16. Kim J, Smith A, Hemphill JC, et al. Contrast extravasation on CT predicts mortality in primary intracerebral hemorrhage. *AJNR Am J Neuroradiol.* 2008;29:520–525.

17. Demchuk AM, Dowlatshahi D, Rodriguez-Luna D, et al. Prediction of haematoma growth and outcome in patients with intracerebral haemorrhage using the CT-angiography spot sign (PREDICT): a prospective observational study. *Lancet Neurol.* 2012;11:307–314.

18. Brouwers HB, Falcone GJ, McNamara KA, et al. CTA spot sign predicts hematoma expansion in patients with delayed presentation after intracerebral hemorrhage. *Neurocrit Care.* 2012;17:421–428.

19. Koculym A, Huynh TJ, Jakubovic R, et al. CT perfusion spot sign improves sensitivity for prediction of outcome compared with CTA and postcontrast CT. *AJNR Am J Neuroradiol.* 2013;34:965–970.

20. Bader MK, Palmer S. What's the "hyper" in hyperacute stroke? Strategies to improve outcomes in ischemic stroke patients presenting within 6 hours. *AACN Adv Crit Care.* 2006;17:194–214.

21. Koo CK, Teasdale E, Muir KW. What constitutes a true hyperdense middle cerebral artery sign? *Cerebrovasc Dis.* 2000;10:419–423.

22. Tomsick T, Brott T, Barsan W, et al. Prognostic value of the hyperdense middle cerebral artery sign and stroke scale score before ultraearly thrombolytic therapy. *AJNR Am J Neuroradiol.* 1996;17:79–85.

23. Petitti N. The hyperdense middle cerebral artery sign. *Radiology.* 1998;208:687–688.

24. Krings T, Noelchen D, Mull M, et al. The hyperdense posterior cerebral artery sign: a computed tomography marker of acute ischemia in the posterior cerebral artery territory. *Stroke.* 2006;37:399–403.

25. New PFJ, Aronow S. Attenuation measurements of whole blood and fractions in computed tomography. *Radiology.* 1976;121:635–640.

26. Leys D, Pruvo JP, Godefroy O, et al. Prevalence and significance of hyperdense middle cerebral artery in acute stroke. *Stroke.* 1992;23:317–324.

27. Manelfe C, Larrue V, von Kummer R, et al. Association of hyperdense middle cerebral artery sign with clinical outcome in patients treated with tissue plasminogen activator. *Stroke.* 1999;30:769–772.

28. von Kummer R, Meyding-Lamade U, Forsting M, et al. Sensitivity and prognostic value of early CT in occlusion of the middle cerebral artery trunk. *AJNR Am J Neuroradiol.* 1994;15:9–15.

29. Barber PA, Demchuk AM, Hudon ME, et al. Hyperdense sylvian fissure MCA "dot" sign: a CT marker of acute ischemia. *Stroke.* 2001;32:84–88.

30. Bettle N, Lyden PD. Thrombosis of the posterior cerebral artery (PCA) visualized on computed tomography: the dense PCA sign. *Arch Neurol.* 2004;61:1960–1961.

31. Rohan V, Baxa J, Tupy R. Length of occlusion predicts recanalization and outcome after intravenous thrombolysis in middle cerebral artery stroke. *Stroke.* 2014;45:2010–2017.

32. Riedel CH, Zimmerman P, Jensen-Kondering U, et al. The importance of size: successful recanalization by intravenous thrombolysis in acute anterior stroke depends on clot length. *Stroke.* 2011;42:1775–1777.

33. Schriger DL, Kalafut M, Starkman S, et al. Cranial computed tomography interpretation in acute stroke: physician accuracy in determining eligibility for thrombolytic therapy. *JAMA.* 1998;279:1293–1297.

34. Grotta JC, Chiu D, Lu M, et al. Agreement and variability in the interpretation of early CT changes in stroke patients qualifying for intravenous rtPA therapy. *Stroke.* 1999;30: 1528–1533.

35. Kalafut MA, Schriger DL, Saver JL, et al. Detection of early CT signs of >1/3 middle cerebral artery infarctions: interrater reliability and sensitivity of CT interpretation by physicians involved in acute stroke care. *Stroke.* 2000;31:1667–1671.

36. Barber PA, Demchuk AM, Zhang J, et al. Validity and reliability of a quantitative computed tomography score in predicting outcome of hyperacute stroke before thrombolytic therapy; aspects study group—Alberta Stroke Programme Early CT Score. *Lancet.* 2000;355: 1670–1674.

37. Pexman JH, Barber PA, Hill MD, et al. Use of the Alberta Stroke Program Early CT Score (ASPECTS) for assessing CT scans in patients with acute stroke. *AJNR Am J Neuroradiol.* 2001;22:1534–1542.

38. Demchuk AM, Coutts SB. Alberta Stroke Program Early CT Score in acute stroke triage. *Neuroimaging Clin N Am.* 2005;15:409–419.

39. Wahlgren N, Ahmed N, Eriksson N, et al. Multivariable analysis of outcome predictors and adjustment of main outcome results to baseline data profile in randomized controlled trials: Safe Implementation of Thrombolysis in Stroke-Monitoring Study (SITS-MOST). *Stroke.* 2008;39:3316–3322.

40. Tissue plasminogen activator for acute ischemic stroke: the National Institute of Neurological Disorders and Stroke rt-PA Stroke Study Group. *N Engl J Med.* 1995;333: 1581–1587.

41. Adams HP Jr, Brott TG, Furlan AJ, et al. Guidelines for thrombolytic therapy for acute stroke: a supplement to the guidelines for the management of patients with acute ischemic stroke—a statement for healthcare professionals from a Special Writing Group of the Stroke Council, American Heart Association. *Circulation.* 1996;94:1167–1174.

42. Hacke W, Kaste M, Fieschi C, et al. Intravenous thrombolysis with recombinant tissue plasminogen activator for acute hemispheric stroke: the European Cooperative Acute Stroke Study (ECASS). *JAMA.* 1995;274:1017–1025.

43. Hacke W, Kaste M, Bluhmki E, et al. Thrombolysis with alteplase 3 to 4.5 hours after acute ischemic stroke. *N Engl J Med.* 2008;359:1317–1329.

44. Bluhmki E, Chamorro A, Davalos A, et al. Stroke treatment with alteplase given 3.0–4.5 h after onset of acute ischaemic stroke (ECASS III): additional outcomes and subgroup analysis of a randomised controlled trial. *Lancet Neurol.* 2009;8:1095–1102.

45. Lees KR, Bluhmki E, von Kummer R, et al. Time to treatment with intravenous alteplase and outcome in stroke: an updated pooled analysis of ECASS, ATLANTIS, NINDS, and EPITHET trials. *Lancet.* 2010;375:1695–1703.

46. Miller DJ, Simpson JR, Silver B. Safety of thrombolysis in acute ischemic stroke: a review of complications, risk factors, and newer technologies. *Neurohospitalist.* 2011;1:138–147.

47. Tanne D, Kasner SE, Demchuk AM, et al. Markers of increased risk of intracerebral hemorrhage after intravenous recombinant tissue plasminogen activator therapy for acute ischemic stroke in clinical practice: the Multicenter rt-PA Stroke Survey. *Circulation.* 2002;105:1679–1685.

48. Patel SC, Levine SR, Tilley BC, et al. Lack of clinical significance of early ischemic changes on computed tomography in acute stroke. *JAMA*. 2001;286:2830–2838.
49. Demchuk AM, Hill MD, Barber PA, et al. Importance of early ischemic computed tomography changes using ASPECTS in NINDS rtPA Stroke Study. *Stroke*. 2005;36:2110–2115.
50. Gonzalez RG. Clinical MRI of acute ischemic stroke. *J Magn Reson Imaging* 2012;36: 259–271.
51. Kaewlai R, Abujudeh H. Nephrogenic systemic fibrosis. *AJR Am J Roentgenol*. 2012; 199:W17–23.
52. Yang L, Krefting I, Gorovets A, et al. Nephrogenic systemic fibrosis and class labeling of gadolinium-based contrast agents by the Food and Drug Administration. *Radiology*. 2012;265:248–253.
53. American College of Radiology Manual on Contrast Media. Version 10.2. ACR Committee on Drugs and Contrast Media. 2016. Available at: https://www.acr.org/Quality -Safety/Resources/Contrast-Manual.
54. Kanal E, Barkovich AJ, Bell C, et al. ACR guidance document on MR safe practices: 2013. *J Magn Reson Imaging*. 2013;37:501–530.
55. Chalela JA, Kidwell CS, Nentwich LM, et al. Magnetic resonance imaging and computed tomography in emergency assessment of patients with suspected acute stroke: a prospective comparison. *Lancet*. 2007;369:293–298.
56. Gonzalez RG, Schaefer PW, Buonanno FS, et al. Diffusion-weighted MR imaging: diagnostic accuracy in patients imaged within 6 hours of stroke symptom onset. *Radiology*. 1999;210:155–162.
57. Brazzelli M, Sandercock PA, Chappell FM, et al. Magnetic resonance imaging versus computed tomography for detection of acute vascular lesions in patients presenting with stroke symptoms. *Cochrane Database Syst Rev*. 2009:CD007424.
58. Lövblad KO, Laubach HJ, Baird AE, et al. Clinical experience with diffusion-weighted MR in patients with acute stroke. *AJNR Am J Neuroradiol*. 1998;19:1061–1066.
59. Marks MP, deCrespigny A, Lentz D, et al. Acute and chronic stroke: navigated spin-echo diffusion-weighted MR imaging. *Radiology*. 1996;199:403–408.
60. Kidwell CS, Alger JR, Di Salle F, et al. Diffusion MRI in patients with transient ischemic attacks. *Stroke*. 1999;30:1174–1180.
61. Ay H, Buonanno FS, Rordorf G, et al. Normal diffusion-weighted MRI during stroke-like deficits. *Neurology*. 1999;52:1784–1792.
62. Barber PA, Darby DG, Desmond PM, et al. Identification of major ischemic change: diffusion-weighted imaging versus computed tomography. *Stroke*. 1999;30:2059–2065.
63. Lee LJ, Kidwell CS, Alger J, et al. Impact on stroke subtype diagnosis of early diffusion-weighted magnetic resonance imaging and magnetic resonance angiography. *Stroke*. 2000;31:1081–1089.
64. Hirai T, Korogi Y, Ono K, et al. Prospective evaluation of suspected stenoocclusive disease of the intracranial artery: combined MR angiography and CT angiography compared with digital subtraction angiography. *AJNR Am J Neuroradiol*. 2002;23:93–101.
65. Katz DA, Marks MP, Napel SA, et al. Circle of Willis: evaluation with spiral CT angiography, MR angiography, and conventional angiography. *Radiology*. 1995;195:445–449.
66. Knauth M, vonKummer R, Jansen O, et al. Potential of CT angiography in acute ischemic stroke. *AJNR Am J Neuroradiol*. 1997;18:1001–1010.
67. Shrier DA, Tanaka H, Numaguchi Y, et al. CT angiography in the evaluation of acute stroke. *AJNR Am J Neuroradiol*. 1997;18:1011–1020.
68. Wildermuth S, Knauth M, Brandt T, et al. Role of CT angiography in patient selection for thrombolytic therapy in acute hemispheric stroke. *Stroke*. 1998;29:935–938.

69. Verro P, Tanenbaum LN, Borden NM, et al. CT angiography in acute ischemic stroke: preliminary results. *Stroke*. 2002;33:276–278.

70. Graf J, Skutta B, Kuhn FP, et al. Computed tomographic angiography findings in 103 patients following vascular events in the posterior circulation: potential and clinical relevance. *J Neurol*. 2000;247:760–766.

71. Nguyen-Huynh MN, Wintermark M, English J, et al. How accurate is CT angiography in evaluating intracranial atherosclerotic disease? *Stroke*. 2008;39:1184–1188.

72. Bang OY, Goyal M, Liebeskind DS. Collateral circulation in ischemic stroke assessment tools and therapeutic strategies. *Stroke*. 2015;46:3302–3309.

73. Hill MD, Demchuk AM, Goyal M, et al; IMS3 Investigators. Alberta Stroke Program early computed tomography score to select patients for endovascular treatment: Interventional Management of Stroke (IMS)-III Trial. *Stroke*. 2014;45:444–449.

74. Bang OY, Saver JL, Buck BH, et al; UCLA Collateral Investigators. Impact of collateral flow on tissue fate in acute ischaemic stroke. *J Neurol Neurosurg Psychiatry*. 2008;79:625–629.

75. Bang OY, Saver JL, Kim SJ, et al. Collateral flow predicts response to endovascular therapy for acute ischemic stroke. *Stroke*. 2011;42:693–699.

76. Bang OY, Saver JL, Kim SJ, et al; UCLA-Samsung Stroke Collaborators. Collateral flow averts hemorrhagic transformation after endovascular therapy for acute ischemic stroke. *Stroke*. 2011;42:2235–2239.

77. Kucinski T, Koch C, Eckert B, et al. Collateral circulation is an independent radiological predictor of outcome after thrombolysis in acute ischaemic stroke. *Neuroradiology*. 2003; 45:11–18.

78. Souza LC, Yoo AJ, Chaudhry ZA, et al. Malignant CTA collateral profile is highly specific for large admission DWI infarct core and poor outcome in acute stroke. *AJNR Am J Neuroradiol*. 2012;33:1331–1336.

79. Jauch E, Saver J, Adams HP, et al. Guidelines for the early management of patients with acute ischemic stroke: a guideline for health-care professionals from the American Heart Association/American Stroke Association. *Stroke*. 2013;44:870–947.

80. Adams RJ, Albers G, Alberts MJ, et al. Update to the AHA/ASA recommendations for the prevention of stroke in patients with stroke and transient ischemic attack. *Stroke*. 2008;39:1647–1652.

81. Buskens E, Nederkoorn PJ, Buijs-VanDerWoude T, et al. Imaging of carotid arteries in symptomatic patients: cost-effectiveness of diagnostic strategies. *Radiology*. 2004;233: 101–112.

82. Lovett JK, Dennis MS, Sandercock PA, et al. Very early risk of stroke after a first transient ischemic attack. *Stroke*. 2003;34:e138–e140.

83. Rothwell PM, Giles MF, Flossmann E, et al. A simple score (ABCD) to identify individuals at high early risk of stroke after transient ischaemic attack. *Lancet*. 2005;366:29–36.

84. Johnston DC, Goldstein LB. Clinical carotid endarterectomy decision making: noninvasive vascular imaging versus angiography. *Neurology*. 2001;56:1009–1015.

85. Nederkoorn PJ, Mali WP, Eikelboom BC, et al. Preoperative diagnosis of carotid artery stenosis: accuracy of noninvasive testing. *Stroke* 2002;33:2003–2008.

86. Lev MH, Romero JM, Goodman DN, et al. Total occlusion versus hairline residual lumen of the internal carotid arteries: accuracy of single section helical CT angiography. *AJNR Am J Neuroradiol*. 2003;24:1123–1129.

87. González RG, Copen WA, Schaefer PW, et al. The Massachusetts General Hospital acute stroke imaging algorithm: an experience and evidence based approach. *J Neuro Intervent Surg*. 2013;5(suppl 1):i7–i12.

Cardiac-Based Evaluation of Ischemic Stroke   5

Liliana Cohen and Amardeep Saluja

Ischemic stroke is an increasingly prevalent problem with significant implications on both the mortality and the quality of life in affected patients. In the United States, the number of cases has increased to nearly 700,000 per annum with significant associated disability.[1] The economic consequences of this disease are profound as well, with an estimated $38.6 billion spent annually in the United States on stroke care.[2]

There are five types of ischemic stroke identified by the TOAST (Trial of Org 10172 in Acute Stroke Treatment) criteria as reviewed in Chapter 3.[3] The role of cardiac imaging (echocardiography, cardiac CT, and cardiac MRI) in discerning the etiology of an ischemic stroke and guiding management is significant given the frequency of causative cardiac and vascular pathology. Cardioembolic disease is acknowledged to account for between 20% and 30% of all ischemic strokes.[4] Furthermore, cardioembolic strokes have been found to be associated with a lower 2-year survival than other etiologies[3] and have a higher risk of recurrence.[5]

Potential cardiac sources for ischemic stroke are numerous and include atrial arrhythmia-associated thrombosis (left atrial appendage thrombosis, left atrial thrombosis), prosthetic valve thrombosis, infective endocarditis, marantic endocarditis, cardiac tumors, and paradoxical embolism secondary to the presence of a patent foramen ovale (PFO) or atrial septal defect (ASD).[6] Echocardiography and cardiac computed tomography angiography (CCTA) are pivotal in diagnosing these conditions. In addition, imaging modalities are also sensitive in discerning large artery embolic sources, such as aortic atheroma, which, for the purposes of the TOAST classification, are classified as a cardioaortic etiology.

Echocardiography has been a powerful modality through which to delineate the presence of the previously discussed pathologies after stroke. However, the mode of echocardiography, transthoracic (TTE) versus transesophageal (TEE), has been the topic of significant debate and investigation. TTE is a noninvasive modality of imaging that is relatively less invasive but is limited by acoustic windows. TTE is noted to be sensitive in identifying mitral valve stenosis, mitral annular calcification, and other chamber characteristics, such as left atrial size, which correlates with stroke risk.[5] Studies have also demonstrated that TTE is superior to TEE in the visualization of left ventricular (LV) thrombus.[6,7] However, TTE has been shown to have a decreased sensitivity in the detection of PFOs, ASDs, infective endocarditis, and prosthetic valve thrombosis when compared to TEE.[8,9]

TEE involves the insertion of an echocardiographic probe into the esophagus and allows for modulation of the angle of visualization. This technique allows for improved visualization of posterior cardiac structures, such as the left atrial appendage (LAA), as well as tomographic assessment of prosthetic valves, valvular apparatus, and the descending aorta in multiple views. TEE also allows for measurement of LAA velocities in a majority of patients, which have been correlated with stroke risk.[10] However standardized use of TEE for all patients with ischemic stroke has not been adapted for several reasons, including increased cost, manpower requirements, exposure to light/moderate sedation, and risk of complications.[11,12] Access to TEE is generally limited to weekdays, which potentially prolongs hospitalization and results in a delay in determination of an urgent need for anticoagulation.

There has been conflicting evidence regarding the benefit of TEE over TTE as part of routine evaluation in ischemic stroke patients. Many studies suggest that TEE is more effective in identifying underlying cardiac etiologies for embolism.[8] One study suggested that in patients with cryptogenic stroke, TEE revealed undiagnosed cardiac pathology in 71% of cases in patients who have previously had TTE.[4] However, other studies have found lower incidences of causative cardiac pathology after TEE evaluation.[1,13] There are at least theoretical concerns for anesthesia-related relative hypotension and hypercapnia causing loss of collaterals and stroke progression, but data are limited to justify withholding TEE for these concerns. Rare occurrences of esophageal perforation, bleeding, aspiration, and respiratory failure have been reported.[12]

Despite literature suggesting that cardiac/vascular pathology is frequently identified during TEE, it is unclear whether these results lead to alteration in clinical management enough to justify routine use. Several single-center studies have examined this issue, and there are markedly disparate results. One study found only 4% of patients may have initiation of anticoagulation or PFO closure as a result of TEE findings post-stroke.[4] In contrast, other studies have found higher percentages ranging between 11% and 16.7%.[1,13] These varied results are likely a function of significant heterogeneity and limited sample sizes in the studies conducted. Additionally, there is heterogeneity in the clinical strategy with respect to initiation of anticoagulation and closure of PFO based on TEE results among the studies. Hence, the results must be interpreted with caution, given the small sample size in all included studies as well as variation in clinical strategy employed based on TEE results. Therefore, based on current literature, we are unable to provide a recommendation on the benefit of routine TEE over TTE and recommend consideration in the clinical context for each individual patient.

LEFT ATRIAL THROMBOSIS

The echocardiographic evaluation for cardioembolic stroke in patients with atrial tachyarrythmias merits discussion. Atrial fibrillation is significantly associated with stroke risk and stroke recurrence. This arrhythmia often results in the development of thrombus in the left atrial appendage or the left atrium, which must be detected to mitigate stroke recurrence risk via anticoagulation. From an imaging standpoint, there are several additional parameters that should be evaluated, including left atrial (LA) size, LAA velocities, and LA morphology.

The LA and LAA are evaluated by echocardiography for the presence of thrombus, sludge, or spontaneous echo contrast (smoke). The presence of thrombus or sludge has been significantly associated with an increased risk of ischemic stroke and usually prompts the initiation of anticoagulation.[14] The most frequently noted location of thrombus on TEE is the LAA.[15] Thus, appropriate visualization of the LAA is important to discern potential sources for stroke. The LAA is a posterior structure, which can be multilobed and difficult to evaluate from a transthoracic study. Unfortunately, with TTE, appropriate visualization can only be obtained in approximately 25%–75% of patients.[16] Therefore, TEE is often utilized if there is suspicion for LAA thrombus because it has a reported 100% negative predictive value.[14,15] During TEE, the left atrial appendage is usually found in the midesophageal views and is visualized between 0 degrees and 90 degrees in standard tomographic views.

Multidetector CT (MDCT) has been examined as a method to evaluate the left atrium and left atrial appendage for thrombus.[17] The advantage of MDCT is the ability to acquire a three-dimensional data set with high spatial resolution and isotropic voxels. A recent meta-analysis examined 19 studies conducted in combined atrial fibrillation and post–ischemic stroke patient populations comparing the MDCT including CCTA and TEE. The study noted that overall CCTA had a nearly 100% negative predictive value (NPV) with only a 41% positive predictive value (PPV).[18] However, modulation of imaging protocols to include delayed imaging improved the PPV to 92%. The other limitations of this modality are the requirement for administration of iodinated contrast material and exposure to ionizing radiation. MDCT could thus be utilized in the future with greater frequency in select patient populations in whom TEE is contraindicated due to anatomic/respiratory constraints.[18]

Cardiac MRI (CMR) is also a novel modality that allows for thorough anatomical and functional evaluation of the left atrium and associated structures. The modality's advantages include the acquisition of high-quality imaging comparative to TEE and the ability to define anatomical risk factors for thromboembolism. CMR allows for accurate chamber size quantification and characterization of appendage structure. However, CMR examinations are limited by several patient factors, including the presence of an implantable defibrillator, the inability to hold breath, and a significant arrhythmia. These patient-dependent factors can compromise image quality significantly. Within CMR, three imaging methods have been employed in the evaluation for thromboembolic disease: long-inversion, time-delayed gadolinium enhancement imaging; cine MRI; and three-dimensional, contrast-enhanced magnetic resonance angiography (MRA). It has been shown that long-inversion, time-delayed gadolinium enhancement imaging has the highest sensitivity and specificity (99%) when compared to TEE for detection of thrombus.[19]

Left atrial diameter is also evaluated because it has been significantly associated with the risk of stroke both in patients without known atrial fibrillation (AF) and with known AF.[19] Studies have demonstrated that moderate to severe left atrial enlargement correlates significantly with increased risk for stroke and risk for recurrence of cardioembolic/cryptogenic stroke.[20,21] Prior literature that correlated LA size to risk of thromboembolism was based on M-mode measurements. However, current practice is to measure the LA in two-dimensional imaging as per the most recent American Society of Echocardiography (ASE) guidelines.

In addition, LA appendage velocities are routinely measured. Velocities below 20 cm/sec^2 correlate with an increased risk for ischemic stroke.[10] There is a suggestion that in patients with left atrial thrombosis, there is an increased risk of embolization with increased LA appendage velocities and LA ejection fraction (Figure 5.1).[22]

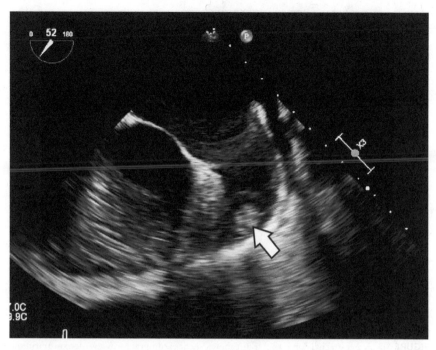

FIGURE 5.1 A midesophageal transesophageal echocardiogram view with a left atrial appendage thrombus

CARDIAC TUMORS

Echocardiography also plays a significant role in defining the presence of cardiac tumors, which may rarely embolize to the cerebral vasculature resulting in ischemic stroke. These occurrences are extremely infrequent given the relatively low incidence of primary cardiac tumors, 0.001% to 0.08% in the population.[23] The majority of cardiac tumors are benign, approximately 80%.[23] The most frequent benign tumor is the myxoma. Cardiac myxomas are frequently found in the left atrium, usually attached to the interatrial septum by a stalk, though they may be found in the right atrium or ventricles. The left-sided myxomas are more frequently associated with systemic and cerebral embolization. However, in the presence of a right-to-left shunt, paradoxical embolization from a right-sided myxoma is possible. Myxoma are more frequently detected by transesophageal echocardiography, with a reported sensitivity of 100%, making this the preferred modality for diagnosis. Surgical resection is often considered in this setting based on other clinical factors.[24] Other cardiac tumors are also detected with greater sensitivity using TEE, including fibroelastoma and malignant tumors with detection of only large tumors on TTE. (Figure 5.2).

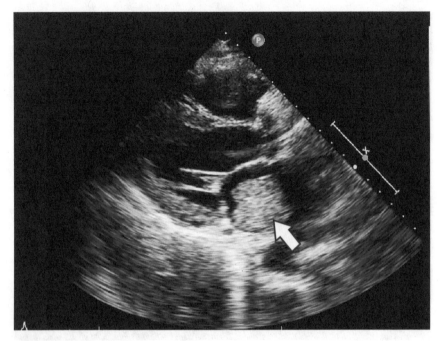

FIGURE 5.2 A parasternal long axis transthoracic echocardiographic view demonstrating a large left atrial myxoma

PATENT FORAMEN OVALE/ATRIAL SEPTAL DEFECT

A patent foramen ovale (PFO) is an abnormal space between the septum primum and secondum leading to the presence of a connection between the right and left atria.[25] It has an approximate 25% prevalence in the general population. However, PFOs have been detected in a higher proportion of younger patients with cryptogenic strokes, up to 61%, though they have not been significantly associated as a risk factor for stroke.[26] One study noted that in patients under the age of 40 with cryptogenic ischemic stroke, 42% were diagnosed with PFO as compared to 7% in the ischemic stroke of undetermined cause group.[25] It has been postulated that the PFO serves a conduit for para-doxical embolism. PFOs can vary in size, and the flow can be bidirectional based on the pressure gradient across the connection. The most widely accepted means of diagnosis is via a bubble echocardiographic study utilizing agitated saline contrast. The diagnostic criteria indicate that at least three bubbles of agitated saline contrast injected into a peripheral vein must appear in the left atrium within three cardiac cycles.[27] Provocative Valsalva maneuvers are also performed during agitated saline injection to improve detection of a PFO in both TTE and TEE.

Despite the postulated relationship between PFOs and ischemic stroke, it is unclear whether medical therapy with antiplatelet therapy versus mechanical closure confers an additional benefit. Three major trials have been conducted on this subject examining optimal medical therapy in contrast to percutaneous closure. The RESPECT trial and PC trial using the Amplatzer occluder device both showed a trend toward benefit with a mechanical closure device. However, a meta-analysis of the data showed no significant reduction in composite endpoint of stroke, transient ischemic attack (TIA), or mortality.[2]

PFOs are also frequently associated with atrial septal aneurysms (ASAs), defined as at least 1.5 cm of the atrial septum, which is highly mobile. Prior studies have previously suggested that PFOs associated with ASAs confer a higher risk for thromboembolism.[2] However, this relationship has been questioned in more recent literature and remains unclear. Chapter 11 will cover the management of PFO, with or without ASA, in detail.

AORTIC ATHEROMA

Cardiac imaging modalities have also been instrumental in the detection of large artery sources for embolic stroke. Specifically, TEE and MDCT have high sensitivity in detection of significant aortic atheroma. Prior studies have demonstrated that the presence of a complex atheroma, or an aortic atheroma with >4-mm thickness, portends a significantly increased risk of recurrent stroke.[28] A recent study has also suggested that standard two-dimensional TEE measurements might underestimate the size of complex atheromas as compared to three-dimensional TEE.[29] MDCT has also been studied for this indication and noted to be less sensitive than TEE but very specific. Chapter 11 will cover secondary prevention of stroke in patients with aortic arch atheroma.

ELECTROCARDIOGRAPHIC MONITORING IN ISCHEMIC STROKE

Basis for Monitoring

Atrial fibrillation (AF) is the most common cause of cardioembolic stroke. Data from the Framingham Heart Study demonstrate this risk to be independent from coexistent coronary heart disease, hypertension, and heart failure.[30]

AF is an arrhythmia characterized by rapid, chaotic atrial depolarization. The lack of synchronized atrial contraction promotes stasis and the development of thrombi, particularly in the LAA, where approximately 90% of thrombus involved in cardioembolic strokes is believed to arise.[31]

The risk of cardioembolic stroke in patients with nonvalvular AF is four to seven times that of patients with normal sinus rhythm, and risk further increases in those with valvular AF (mitral stenosis or a prosthetic heart valve).[32] Interestingly enough, the risk of stroke seems to be equal in patients with persistent and paroxysmal AF.[33]

Previous studies have validated the use of anticoagulation to mitigate stroke risk in patients with AF. This is thought to be due to decreased clot formation in the atria and subsequent embolization.[34,35] Proper electrocardiographic assessment is therefore crucial to the medical workup of patients with ischemic stroke.

While a source of ischemic stroke may be identified in some patients during the index hospitalization, those without an established etiology after an initial evaluation may be classified as having cryptogenic stroke. In this patient subset, a more exhaustive workup is warranted for episodic conditions associated with stroke, such as arrhythmia. Numerous electrocardiographic monitoring modalities, both inpatient and outpatient, are available to screen for AF as a potential etiology of embolism.

Electrocardiogram

The initial cardiac evaluation of patients with a TIA or ischemic stroke should include a 12-lead electrocardiogram (ECG).[36] The ECG can help in the diagnosis of potential concomitant acute cardiac conditions (such as acute coronary syndrome), chronic cardiac pathology associated with cerebrovascular disease, and rhythm disorders associated with thromboembolism.

Abnormalities in presenting ECGs are found in upward of 75% to 90% of patients with TIA or ischemic stroke.[37] As acute myocardial infarction (MI) can either precede or result from ischemic stroke, ST segment changes suggesting myocardial infarction may be present. In addition to the ECG assessment of ischemia, initial laboratory tests should include an assay for troponin because cardiac enzyme elevation is present in approximately 20% of acute stroke patients and is independently associated with death.[38] Abnormalities of the ECG indicating infarction may lead to suspicion of LV thrombus. The overall rate of LV thrombus after acute MI is reported to be 5.1% but is highest in patients with anterior MI (11.5% vs. 2.3% in other coronary territories).[39] The presence of persistent ST elevations may signify LV aneurysm, which can similarly act as a nidus for thrombus formation.

Approximately 25% of patients with first-time stroke have an ECG that shows AF.[40] This seemingly high detection rate is mostly due to patients with known AF. In patients without a known history of AF, the detection rate of AF after an acute stroke or TIA is 2% to 5%.[41]

The clinician needs to be aware of other clues on ECG correlated with increased risk of stroke. For instance, a prolonged corrected QT (QTc) interval is associated with a two-fold increased risk of AF, which increases the risk of stroke.[42] A prolonged QTc may also increase stroke rates independent of an increased risk of AF. Evidence from several large studies, including one study with 27,000 patients, found that prolonged QTc carried a three-fold increased risk of incident stroke independent of traditional stroke risk factors, including AF.[43,44]

Ventricular ectopy and arrhythmias also carry significant prognostic information in stroke patients. The detection of premature ventricular contractions (PVCs) on screening ECGs carries an increased risk of stroke.[45,46] This may be due to PVCs acting as a marker of further arrhythmogenic potential because some evidence correlates PVCs with increased risk of new-onset AF.[47] PVCs could also be a sign of subclinical atherosclerotic disease and, therefore, higher stroke risk.

Continuous Inpatient Telemetry Monitoring

Continuous telemetry monitoring should be performed for at least 24 hours in all patients admitted with stroke. Hospital telemetry is typically a continuous recording of a limited number of ECG leads, which is monitored on site in real time. Continuous telemetry may increase the diagnostic for AF and electrical disorders, which may be intermittent and, therefore, not evident on a single ECG. A recent meta-analysis by Kishore et al showed that after an acute ischemic stroke or TIA, continuous inpatient monitoring was able to detect new-onset AF in 5.5% of unselected patients and 15.0% of patients who met prespecified trial enrollment criteria (selected patients). Furthermore, with every additional 24 hours of monitoring, detection rates increased 2% to 4% up to 72 hours of monitoring. When the data were pooled with all electrocardiographic monitoring modalities, the ability to detect new AF was 6.2% for unselected patients, 13.4% among selected patients, and 15.9% for patients with cryptogenic stroke.[48]

When combining admission ECG with 12 to 24 hours of continuous telemetry, Christensen et al showed that abnormalities in conduction or rhythm were observed in 60% of patients with cerebral infarction and 44% of patients with TIA. In the cerebral infarction subset, multivariable logistic regression analysis demonstrated that AF, atrioventricular block, ST elevation, ST depression, and T-wave inversion were predictive of 3-month mortality independent of stroke severity or age, although ectopic beats >10%, atrial flutter, sinus bradycardia, isoelectric T-waves, and ventricular and sinus tachycardia were not. In the TIA subset, none of the ECG findings were predictive of 3-month mortality.[49]

Holter Monitors

For stroke patients for whom a cause of stroke has not been identified despite a standard vascular workup and inpatient telemetry, additional monitoring may be done on an outpatient basis.

Holter monitors are battery-operated, portable devices that continuously record typically two or three channels of electrocardiographic data for a fixed period of time, usually 24 or 48 hours. Although Holter monitoring may be done in hospitals without the capability for continuous telemetry, it is typically performed on outpatients. Patients have the ability to activate event markers to correlate the recorded rhythm with symptoms. The data are digitally stored and analyzed upon playback at the completion of the monitoring period.

In a systematic review by Liao et al, Holter monitors were collectively able to detect new AF or atrial flutter in 4.6% of 588 patients, with duration of monitoring ranging from 21 to 72 hours.[50] A multicenter study of 1,100 German patients with ischemic stroke by Grond et al showed that by extending Holter monitoring from 24 hours to 72 hours, they were able to nearly double the detection of AF from 29 patients (2.6%) to 49 patients (4.4%), resulting in a number needed to screen of 55 patients for each additional diagnosis of AF.[51] Studies comparing the yield of continuous telemetry with that of Holter monitoring for diagnosing arrhythmia have been mixed.[52,53] These conflicting results may in part be due to the duration of Holter monitor use.

Holter monitoring has also been shown to have utility in identifying populations at risk for AF and, therefore, stroke. Wallmann et al described increased ectopic atrial activity as a marker of future AF. In patients with >70 premature atrial beats in 24 hours, AF was detected in 26% of cases when monitoring was extended to 7 days and in only 6.5% of patients with infrequent ectopic atrial beats.[54]

External Loop Recorders

In some patients with paroxysmal AF, weeks may elapse between episodes. Therefore, it is not uncommon for patients to remain undiagnosed even after several days of continuous monitoring. External loop recorders (ELRs) may be useful in patients with cryptogenic stroke in whom longer rhythm monitoring is warranted. ELRs are external monitoring systems that are typically worn for up to 30 days. Unlike Holter monitors, which continuously record each beat over the monitoring period, ELRs record the ECG over intermittent short intervals. Recording is initiated either automatically by the device upon detection of an arrhythmia or manually by the patient (typically when symptoms such as palpitations are felt). Data are stored on the device, and strips are transmitted (typically by phone) to a central monitoring station for interpretation, freeing the device's memory to be overwritten. ELRs offer the advantage of prolonged detection times in patients with cryptogenic stroke and a high suspicion of paroxysmal arrhythmias. Two earlier studies regarding ELRs include Barthelemy et al, which detected AF in 14.3% of 28 patients with cryptogenic stroke over a mean monitoring duration of 70 hours, and Jabaudon et al, who detected AF in 5.7% of 149 patients monitored on average for 159 hours.[55,56]

More recently, the EMBRACE trial (30-Day Cardiac Event Monitor Belt for Recording Atrial Fibrillation After a Cerebral Ischemic Event) sought to determine if longer monitoring periods improved arrhythmia detection rates. In this trial, 572 patients with cryptogenic ischemic stroke or TIA, but without known AF, were randomly assigned to monitoring with either a 30-day event-triggered monitor or a conventional 24-hour Holter monitor. The primary endpoint of AF lasting 30 seconds or longer was detected in 16.1% in the ELR cohort and 3.2% in the control arm at 30 days ($p < 0.001$). The secondary endpoint of AF lasting 2.5 minutes or longer was detected in 9.9% of the ELR group and 2.5% in the control group ($p < 0.001$). The EMBRACE trial proved that 30-day outpatient noninvasive monitoring was superior to shorter-term ECG monitoring for the detection of AF in those with no known prior AF and cryptogenic stroke or TIA.[57]

Mobile Cardiac Outpatient Telemetry

Mobile cardiac outpatient telemetry (MCOT) provides all the benefits of ELRs while overcoming some of its inherent limitations. These systems are externally worn electrode devices that provide real-time continuous monitoring. The ECG is typically transmitted wirelessly in real time to a continuously monitored central station, where it is analyzed by trained staff.

Advantages of MCOT include faster patient and physician notification of dangerous arrhythmias than either Holter monitors or ELRs, which can only be analyzed when the data are uploaded by the patient. Like Holter monitors, recording all of the rhythm activity for the day allows for a quantification of total arrhythmia burden, which is not possible with ELRs. However, MCOT is typically more expensive than either Holter monitors or ELRs, and the cost can be substantial for prolonged monitoring.

A meta-analysis by Sposato et al showed that out of 417 patients from six studies, MCOT was able to detect AF in 15.3% of patient without known prior AF.[58] One limitation of prolonged monitoring, however, is patient compliance. In one large study by Miller et al in which 30-day MCOT monitoring was suggested, 80% of patients completed 14 days of monitoring, and only 62% completed 21 days. This study also concluded that the optimal duration of use was 21 days because the rate of paroxysmal AF detection significantly increased from 3.9% in the initial 48 hours, to 9.2% at 7 days, 15.1% at 14 days, and finally 19.5% by 21 days.[59]

Implantable Loop Recorders

Implantable loop recorders (ILRs) are subcutaneous monitoring systems with loop memory that record ECG data. These devices typically record a single ECG lead derived from positive and negative terminals located on the device itself. Newer-generation devices have a battery life of several years and can store many minutes of ECG data, including patient-activated events and automatically detected episodes. Unlike implanted devices with leads directly connected to the atrium, ILRs cannot sense atrial activity directly and thus have a lower sensitivity and specificity for AF detection compared to (for example) dual-chamber pacemakers and defibrillators. Proprietary AF detection algorithms that utilize R-R interval variability as well as p-wave sensing discriminatory analysis have been developed, which have improved their accuracy in detecting AF.

The largest trial to date studying ILRs in patients with cryptogenic stroke is the Cryptogenic Stroke and Underlying AF (CRYSTAL AF) trial. In this study by Sanna et al, 441 patients without a history of AF with ischemic stroke or TIA classified as cryptogenic after extensive testing, including at least 24 hours of ECG monitoring, were randomized either to ILR monitoring (Medtronic REVEAL XT) or to the control arm of routine ECG monitoring. The primary endpoint was time to detection of AF lasting >30 seconds within 6 months, and a secondary endpoint was time to detection at 12 months. At 6 months AF was detected in 8.9% of patients in the ILR arm and 1.4% of patients in the control arm ($p < 0.001$). At 12 months AF detection increased to 12.4% in the ILR and 2.0% in the control arm ($p < 0.001$). Of note, the first episode of AF was asymptomatic in 23 of 29 patients in the ILR arm (79%) and 2 of 4 patients in the control arm (50%). During follow-up, ischemic stroke or TIA occurred in 11 patients (5.2%) in the ILR group and 18 patients (8.6%) in the control group at 6 months and subsequently in 15 patients (7.1%) and 19 patients (9.1%) in the ILR versus control group at 12 months, respectively.[60]

Patient Selection for Monitoring

Several clinical risk score calculators have been created to help identify ischemic stroke and TIA patients with increased risk of AF (Table 5.1).[61,62] As previously discussed, many of the meta-analyses and large trials found significantly higher rates of AF in selected versus unselected patients. Preselection of patients for extended cardiac monitoring may improve diagnostic efficiency and may help mitigate the inherent costs that come with extended monitoring modalities.

The choice of monitoring modality will be tailored to individual patient preferences, compliance, financial resources, and demographics. Table 5.2 discusses the advantages and disadvantages of the electrocardiographic monitoring options discussed in this chapter as well as their diagnostic yield for AF based on currently available trial data.

TABLE 5.1 Clinical risk score calculators for predicting AF in ischemic stroke

STAF criteria (Suissa et al)[1]	Points	Fujii et al criteria[2]	Points
Age (years)		Baseline NIHSS score	
>62	2	≥8	1
≤62	0	<8	0
Baseline NIHSS score		Left atrial size	
≥8	1	≥3.8 cm	1
<8	0	<3.8 cm	0
Left atrial dilatation		Mitral valvular disease	
Yes	2	Yes	1
No	0	No	0
Vascular etiology		BNP level	
Yes	0	≥144 pg/mL	1
No	3	<144 pg/mL	0
Total		Total	

1. A total score of ≥5 identifies patients with AF with a sensitivity of 89% (95% CI, 83 to 94) and a specificity of 88% (95% CI, 84 to 91).

2. Frequency of PAF is 0% with a score of 0, 4% with a score of 1, 14% with a score of 2, 26% with a score 3, 50% with a score of 4, and 100% with a score of 5.

TABLE 5.2 Electrocardiographic monitoring modalities

Modality	Advantages	Disadvantages	Diagnostic yield of AF
ECG	• Ease of use • Low cost • Quick interpretation	• Isolated "snapshot" of rhythm with no prolonged monitoring	• 7.7% (admission) • 5.6% (serial)
Continuous inpatient telemetry monitoring	• Standard of care for many hospitalized stroke patients • Detects asymptomatic arrhythmias	• Requires inpatient status • Brief monitoring period • Restricts patient movement	• 4.1%–7.0%
Holter monitor	• Easy to arrange • Continuous recording • Detects asymptomatic arrhythmias	• Brief monitoring period • Need for patient symptom diary	• 4.5% (inpatient) • 10.7% (ambulatory)
External loop recorders	• Prolonged monitoring • Correlates rhythm and symptoms • Detects asymptomatic arrhythmias	• The ability to detect asymptomatic arrhythmias is limited by automatic detection algorithms • Requires long-term patient compliance	• 16.2%
Mobile continuous outpatient telemetry	• Prolonged monitoring • Detects asymptomatic arrhythmias • Real-time continuous monitoring by trained staff	• Requires long-term patient compliance • Expense	• 15.3%
Implantable loop recorders	• Prolonged monitoring, up to 3 years • Does not require active patient compliance • Detects asymptomatic arrhythmias	• Invasive placement and removal • Risk of implant site complications • Expense • The ability to detect asymptomatic arrhythmias is limited by automatic detection algorithms	• 16.9%

References

1. Khariton Y, House JA, Comer L, et al. Impact of transesophageal echocardiography on management in patients with suspected cardioembolic stroke. *Am J Cardiol.* 2014; 114:1912–1916.

2. Khan AR, Bin Abdulhak AA, Sheikh MA, et al. Device closure of patent foramen ovale versus medical therapy in cryptogenic stroke a systematic review and meta-analysis. *JACC: Cardiovasc Interv.* 2013;6:1317–1323.

3. Kolominsky-Rabas PL, Weber M, Gefeller O, et al. Epidemiology of ischemic stroke subtypes according to TOAST criteria incidence, recurrence, and long-term survival in ischemic stroke subtypes: a population-based study. *Stroke.* 2001;32:2735–2740.

4. Galougahi KK, Stewart T, Choong CY, et al. The utility of transoesophageal echocardiography to determine management in suspected embolic stroke. *Int Med J.* 2010; 40:813–818.

5. Ustrell X, Pellisé A. Cardiac workup of ischemic stroke. *Curr Cardiol Rev.* 2010;6: 175–183.

6. Lerakis S, Nicholson WJ. Part I: use of echocardiography in the evaluation of patients with suspected cardioembolic stroke. *Am J Med Sci.* 2005;329:310–316.

7. Loh E, Sutton MS, Wun CC, et al. Ventricular dysfunction and the risk of stroke after myocardial infarction. *N Engl J Med.* 1997;336:251–257.

8. McGrath ER, Paikin JS, Motlagh B, et al. Transesophageal echocardiography inpatients with cryptogenic ischemic stroke: a systematic review. *Am Heart J.* 2014;168:706–712.

9. Morris JG, Fisher M. Cardiac workup of ischemic stroke: can we improve our diagnostic yield? *Stroke.* 2009;40:2893–2898.

10. Goldman ME, Lesly A, Pearce MS, et al. Pathophysiologic correlates of thromboembolism in nonvalvular atrial fibrillation: I. Reduced flow velocity in the left atrial appendage (the Stroke Prevention in Atrial Fibrillation [SPAF-III] study). *J Am Soc Echocardiogr.* 1999;12:1080–1087.

11. Holmes M, Rathbone J, Littlewood C, et al. Routine echocardiography in the management of stroke and transient ischaemic attack: a systematic review and economic evaluation. *Health Technol Assess.* 2014;18(16):1–176.

12. Daniel WG, Kasper W, Visser, CA, et al. Safety of transesophageal echocardiography a multicenter survey of 10,419 examinations. *Circulation.* 1991;83:817–821.

13. Buddhadeb D, Abdul M.A. Hasnie, M.D. et al. Transesophageal echocardiography impacts management and evaluation of patients with stroke, transient ischemic attack, or peripheral embolism. *Echocardiography.* 2006;23:202–207.

14. Rui Providencia M, Trigo J, Paiva L, et al. The role of echocardiography in thromboembolic risk assessment of patients with nonvalvular atrial fibrillation. *J Am Soc Echocardiogr.* 2013;26:801–812.

15. Manning WJ, Waksmonski CA, Hacring JM, et al. Accuracy of transesophageal echocardiography for identifying left atrial thrombi: a prospective intraoperative study. *Ann Int Med.* 1995;123:817–822.

16. Omran HWJ, Rabahieh R, Wirtz P, et al. Imaging of thrombi and assessment of left atrial appendage function: a prospective study comparing transthoracic and transoesophageal echocardiography. *Heart.* 1999;81:192–198.

17. Shapiro MD, Neilan TG, Jassal DS, et al. Multidetector computed tomography for the detection of left atrial appendage thrombus: a comparative study with transesophageal echocardiography. *J Comput Assist Tomogr.* 2007;31:905–909.

18. Romero J, Kelesidis I, Sanz J, et al. Detection of left atrial appendage thrombus by cardiac computed tomography in patients with atrial fibrillation a meta-analysis. *Circ Cardiovasc Imaging.* 2013;6:185–194.

19. Kitkungvan D, Nabi F, Gosh MG, et al. Detection of LA and LAA thrombus by CMR in patients referred for pulmonary vein isolation. *J Am Coll Cardiol Img.* 2016;9: 809–818.

20. Yaghi S, Mora-McLaughlin C, Willey JZ, et al. Left atrial enlargement and stroke recurrence: the Northern Manhattan Stroke Study. *Stroke.* 2015;46:1488–1493.

21. Benjamin EJ, D'Agostino RB, Belanger AJ, et al. Left atrial size and the risk of stroke and death: the Framingham Heart Study. *Circulation.* 1995;92:835–841.

22. Kavlak ESHK, Yigit Z, Okcun B, et al. Clinical and echocardiographic risk factors for embolization in the presence of left atrial thrombus. *Echocardiography.* 2005;24: 515–521.

23. Acampa MFG, Tassi R, D'Andrea R, et al. Thrombolytic treatment of cardiac myxoma-induced ischemic stroke: a review. *Curr Drug Safety.* 2014;9:83–88.

24. Junaid Akhtar MW, Javeria Rauf. Atrial myxoma: a rare cause of cardioembolic stroke. *BMJ Case Rep.* 2012;10:1–3.

25. Di Tullio M, Venketasubramanian N, Sherman D, et al. Comparison of diagnostic techniques for the detection of a patent foramen ovale in stroke patients. *Stroke.* 1993;24: 1020–1024.

26. Pickett CA, Ferguson MA, Hulten EA. Percutaneous closure versus medical therapy alone for cryptogenic stroke patients with a patent foramen ovale: meta-analysis of randomized controlled trials. *Texas Heart Institute J.* 2014;4:357–367.

27. Pinto FJ. When and how to diagnose patent foramen ovale. *Heart.* 2005;91:438–440.

28. Group FSoAP. Atherosclerotic disease of the aortic arch as a risk favor for recurrent ischemic stroke. *N Engl J Med.* 1996;334:1216–1221.

29. Weissler-Snir AGG, Shapira Y, Weisenberg D, et al. Transoesophageal echocardiography of aortic atherosclerosis: the additive value of three-dimensional over two-dimensional imaging. *Eur Heart J—Cardiovascular Imaging.* 2015;16:389–394.

30. Wolf P, Abbott R, Kannel W. Atrial fibrillation as an independent risk factor for stroke: the Framingham Study. *Stroke.* 1991;22:983–988.

31. Manning WJ. Atrial fibrillation, transesophageal echo, electrical cardioversion, and anticoagulation. *Clin Cardiol.* 1995;18:58,114.

32. Walker AM, Bennett D. Epidemiology and outcomes in patients with atrial fibrillation in the United States. *Heart Rhythm.* 2008;5:1365–1372.

33. Nieuwlaat R, Dinh T, Olsson SB, et al. Should we abandon the common practice of withholding anticoagulation in paroxysmal atrial fibrillation? *Eur Heart J.* 2008;29: 915–922.

34. Boston Area Anticoagulation Trial for Atrial Fibrillation Investigators, Singer DE, Hughes RA, Gress DR, et al. The effect of low dose warfarin on the risk of stroke in patients with non-rheumatic atrial fibrillation. *N Engl J Med.* 1990;323:1505–1511.

35. Stroke Prevention in Atrial Fibrillation Study. Final results. *Circulation.* 1991;84:527–539.

36. Jauch EC, Saver JL, Adams HP, et al. Guidelines for the early management of patients with acute ischemic stroke: a Guideline for Healthcare Professionals from the American Heart Association/American Stroke Association. *Stroke.* 2013 Mar;44(3):870–947.

37. Khechinashvii G, Asplund K. Electrocardiographic changes in patients with acute stroke: a systematic review. *Cerebrovasc Dis.* 2002;14:67–76.

38. Kerr G, Ray G, Wu O, et al. Elevated troponin after stroke: a systematic review. *Cerebrovasc Dis.* 2009;28:220–226.

39. Chiarella F, Santoro E, Domenicucci S, et al. Predischarge two-dimensional echocardiographic evaluation of left ventricular thrombosis after acute myocardial infarction in the GISSI-3 study. *Am J Cardiol.* 1998;81:822–827.

40. Marini C, De Santis F, Sacco S, et al. Contribution of atrial fibrillation to incidence and outcome of ischemic stroke: results from a population-based study. *Stroke.* 2005;36: 1115–1119.

41. Bell C, Kapral M. Use of ambulatory electrocardiography for the detection of paroxysmal atrial fibrillation in patients with stroke. Canadian Task Force on Preventive Health Care. *Can J Neurol Sci.* 2000;27:25–31.

42. Mandyam MC, Soliman EZ, Alonso A, et al. The QT interval and risk or incident atrial fibrillation. *Heart Rhythm.* 2013 Oct;10(10):1562–1568.

43. Soliman EZ, Howard G, Cushman M, et al. Prolongation of QTc and risk of stroke: the REGARDS (REasons for Geographic and Racial Differences in Stroke) study. *J Am Coll Cardiol.* 2012 Apr 17;59(16):1460–1467.

44. O'Neal WT, Efird JT, Kamel H, et al. The association of the QT interval with atrial fibrillation and stroke: the Multi-Ethnic Study of Atherosclerosis. *Clin Res Cardiol.* 2015 Mar 10. [Epub ahead of print]

45. Agarwal SK, Chao J, Peace F, et al. Premature ventricular complexes on screening electrocardiogram and risk of ischemic stroke. *Stroke.* 2015 Apr 14. [Epub ahead of print]

46. Ofoma U, He F, Shaffer ML, et al. Premature cardiac contractions and risk of incident ischemic stroke. *J Am Heart Assoc.* 2012 Oct;1(5):e002519. doi: 10.1161/JAHA.112.002519.

47. Watanabe H, Tanabe N, Makiyama Y, et al. ST-segment abnormalities and premature complexes are predictors of new-onset atrial fibrillation: the Niigata Preventive Medicine Study. *Am Heart J.* 2006;152:731–735.

48. Kishore A, Vail A, Majid A, et al. Detection of atrial fibrillation after ischemic stroke or transient ischemic attack a systematic review and meta-analysis. *Stroke.* 2014;45:520–526.

49. Christensen H, Fogh Christensen A, Boysen G. Abnormalities on ECG and telemetry predict stroke outcome at 3 months. *J Neurol Sci.* 2005;234:99–103.

50. Liao J, Khalid Z, Scallan C, et al. Noninvasive cardiac monitoring for detecting paroxysmal atrial fibrillation or flutter after acute ischemic stroke: a systematic review. *Stroke.* 2007;38:2935–2940.

51. Grond M, Jauss M, Hamann G, et al. Improved detection of silent atrial fibrillation using 72-hour Holter ECG in patients with ischemic stroke a prospective multicenter cohort study. *Stroke.* 2013;44:3357–3364.

52. Lazzaro MA, Krishnan K, Prabhakaran S. Detection of atrial fibrillation with concurrent holter monitoring and continuous cardiac telemetry following ischemic stroke and transient ischemic attack. *J Stroke Cerebrovasc Dis.* 2012 Feb;21(2):89–93.

53. Rizos T, Gunter J, Jenetzky E, et al. Continuous stroke unit electrocardiographic monitoring versus 24-hour Holter electrocardiography for detection of paroxysmal atrial fibrillation after stroke. *Stroke.* 2012 Oct;43(10):2689–2694.

54. Wallmann D, Tuller D, Wustmann K, et al. Frequent atrial premature beats predict paroxysmal atrial fibrillation in stroke patients: an opportunity for a new diagnostic strategy. *Stroke.* 2007;38:2292–2294.

55. Barthelemy JC, Feasson-Gerard S, Garnier P, et al. Automatic event recorders reveal paroxysmal atrial fibrillation after unexplained strokes or transient ischemic attacks. *Ann Noninvasive Electrocardiol.* 2003;8:194–199.

56. Jabaudon D, Sztajzel J, Sievert K, et al. Usefulness of ambulatory 7-day ECG monitoring for the detection of atrial fibrillation and flutter after acute stroke and transient ischemic attack. *Stroke.* 2004;35:1647–1651.

57. Gladstone DJ, Spring M, Dorian P, et al. Atrial fibrillation in patients with cryptogenic stroke. *N Engl J Med*. 2014 Jun 26;370(26):2467–2477.

58. Sposato LA, Cipriano LE, Saposnik G, et al. Diagnosis of atrial fibrillation after stroke and transient ischaemic attack: a systematic review and meta-analysis. *Lancet Neurol*. 2015 Apr;14(4):377–387.

59. Miller DJ, Khan MA, Schultz LR, et al. Outpatient cardiac telemetry detects a high rate of atrial fibrillation in cryptogenic stroke. *J. Neurol. Sci*. 2013;324:57–61.

60. Sanna T, Diener HC, Passman R, et al. Cryptogenic stroke and underlying atrial fibrillation. *N Engl J Med*. 2014;370:2478–2486.

61. Suissa L, Bertora D, Lachaud S, et al. Score for the targeting of atrial fibrillation (STAF). A new approach to the detection of atrial fibrillation in the secondary prevention of ischemic stroke. *Stroke*. 2009;40:2866–2868.

62. Fujii S, Shibazaki K, Kimura K, et al. A simple score for prediction paroxysmal atrial fibrillation in acute ischemic stroke. *J Neurol Sci*. 2013 May 15;328(1–2):83–86.

Thrombolytic Therapy for Acute Ischemic Stroke

6

Ava L. Liberman and Michael T. Mullen

INTRODUCTION

Effective therapies exist for the treatment of ischemic stroke. Acute thrombolysis has the potential to re-canalize occluded arteries, restore blood flow to ischemic brain tissue, and reduce disability after stroke. Recombinant tissue plasminogen activator (tPA) can be given intravenously up to 4.5 hours after symptom onset and is effective at reducing morbidity following stroke. It does, however, have some risks—most notably, intracranial and systemic hemorrhage—and therefore may not be appropriate in all patients. This chapter reviews the seminal trials demonstrating the utility of IV tPA, current eligibility and contraindications for this medication, guideline treatment recommendations, risks associated with treatment, and challenges/limitations.

INTRAVENOUS RECOMBINANT TISSUE PLASMINOGEN ACTIVATOR

Fibrinolytic therapy with intravenous recombinant tissue plasminogen activator (IV tPA) is recommended for eligible patients who can be treated within 4.5 hours of symptom onset.[1] Treatment with tPA catalyzes the conversion of plasminogen to plasmin, its activated form. Plasmin dissolves clots by breaking apart fibrin, which reduces thrombus volume and increases the odds of recanalizing occluded arteries.

The first trial to demonstrate the effectiveness of tPA was the National Institute of Neurological Disorders and Stroke (NINDS) Trial, a phase III randomized, placebo-controlled trial of 624 subjects published in 1995.[2] Subjects were enrolled who could be treated within 3 hours of stroke symptom onset. Subjects were excluded from the trial if there was any evidence of hemorrhage on a CT scan of the head. Additional exclusion criteria were established largely by expert opinion and included recent surgery, recent trauma, laboratory values demonstrating coagulopathy, and history of intracranial hemorrhage.[3] To judge whether or not tPA improved clinical outcomes, a number of different scales were used, including the modified Rankin scale (mRS) (see Table 6.1). The mRS is an ordinal scale, where 0 corresponds to no functional limitation and 5 corresponds to severe disability requiring constant nursing care.[4] Treatment with IV tPA resulted in a 16% absolute improvement in the proportion of subjects with minimal or no disability (mRS $\leq$ 1) at 90 days, resulting in a number needed to treat (NNT) of 6. Using a global outcome measure incorporating multiple disability scales, the odds ratio (OR) for a favorable outcome in the tPA treated group was 1.7 [95% confidence interval (CI) 1.2–2.6, $p = 0.008$]. This benefit existed despite an increased risk of symptomatic intracerebral hemorrhage (ICH) in those treated with IV tPA compared to controls (6.4% vs. 0.6%, $p \leq 0.001$). No statistical relationship between IV tPA and mortality was detected.

Since the publication of the NINDS trial, IV tPA has become the standard of care for eligible patients with ischemic stroke. Unfortunately, many stroke patients simply present too late to receive this therapy.[5] Multiple studies have therefore evaluated the use of tPA beyond 3 hours. In 2008, the European Cooperative Acute Stroke Study III (ECASS III) tested the efficacy of IV tPA 3 to 4.5 hours from symptom onset.[6] Exclusion criteria in this trial were similar to those of the NINDS trial, with several notable additions: subjects with age >80, severe stroke as assessed by exam or imaging, and a combined history of both stroke and diabetes were excluded. Treatment with IV tPA significantly improved the proportion of subjects with an excellent outcome (mRS $\leq$ 1) at 90 days compared to placebo (52.4% vs. 45.2%, $p = 0.04$), resulting in an NNT of 14. This benefit existed despite an increased risk of symptomatic ICH in subjects treated with IV tPA (2.4% vs. 0.2%, $p = 0.008$). It is important to note that the hemorrhage rate in ECASS III is not directly comparable to that of the earlier NINDS trial because different definitions of symptomatic ICH (sICH) were used. In the NINDS study, sICH was defined by any neurologic worsening, whereas in ECASS III, sICH required a worsening of 4 or more points on the NIHSS. This definition was thought to be more clinically meaningful than the definition used in the NINDS trial. Using the NINDS definition of sICH on the ECASS III data, sICH occurred in 7.9% of patients treated with IV tPA as compared to 3.5% who were not treated ($p = 0.006$).[6]

TABLE 6.1 Modified Rankin scale (mRS)

Score	Description
0	No symptoms at all
1	No significant disability despite symptoms; able to carry out all usual duties and activities
2	Slight disability; unable to carry out all previous activities but able to look after own affairs without assistance
3	Moderate disability; requiring some help, but able to walk without assistance
4	Moderately severe disability; unable to walk without assistance and unable to attend to own bodily needs without assistance
5	Severe disability; bedridden, incontinent, and requiring constant nursing care and attention
6	Dead

In an attempt to further expand the treatment window for IV tPA to 6 hours, the Third International Stroke Trial (IST-3) was published in 2013.[7] There was no significant difference in functional outcome at 6 months in subjects treated with IV tPA compared to placebo. It is critical to understand that IST-3 excluded subjects who had a clear indication for IV tPA based on the NINDS and ECASS III trials. Many subjects presenting within 4.5 hours of symptom onset therefore were not eligible for the IST-3 trial and, instead, were treated with IV tPA based on the prior, positive trials. This likely biased the results of this trial toward the null.

A meta-analysis using patient level data from nine acute stroke trials, including NINDS, ECASS III, and IST-3, confirmed that IV tPA is beneficial when given within 4.5 hours and reinforced the importance of rapid treatment of eligible patients.[8] In this meta-analysis, treatment with IV tPA within 3 hours was associated with an increased odd of an excellent outcome (32.9% vs. 23.1%, OR 1.75, 95% CI 1.35–2.27, $p < 0.0001$). Treatment between 3 and 4.5 hours was also associated with a significant improvement in outcome, although the benefit was smaller (35.3% vs. 30.1%, OR 1.26, 95% CI 1.05–1.51, $p = 0.0132$). The benefit of IV tPA was similar in patients ≤ 80 and in those > 80 years old. The benefit of IV tPA was also consistent across a range of initial NIHSS scores (0–4, 5–10, 11–15, 16–21, and ≥ 21). IV tPA was beneficial despite a 5.5% absolute increase risk of symptomatic ICH (6.8% vs. 1.3%, OR 5.55, 95% CI 4.01–7.70, $p < 0.0001$). Treatment with IV tPA was not associated with an increased risk of death at 90 days (17.9% vs. 16.5%, hazard ratio [HR] 1.11, 95% CI 0.99–1.25, $p = 0.07$).

Based on the preceding data, IV tPA is recommended by both the American Heart Association/American Stroke Association (AHA/ASA) and the European Stroke Organization (ESO) within 3 hours of stroke symptom onset (Class 1, Level of Evidence A). Thrombolysis with IV tPA is also strongly recommended in the 3- to 4.5-hour window according to both organizations (AHA Class 1, Level of Evidence B; ESO Class 1, Level of Evidence A).[1,9] While patients may be treated up to 4.5 hours, it is critically important to treat with IV tPA as quickly as possible;[1] the typical patient loses up to 1.9 million neurons each minute in which stroke is untreated.[10] IV tPA is dosed at 0.9 mg/kg (maximum dose of 90 mg), with the first 10% administered as an IV push over 1 minute and the remaining 90% administered over 1 hour.[2]

RISKS ASSOCIATED WITH IV tPA

The most important risk associated with IV tPA is symptomatic ICH. As noted above, symptomatic ICH occurred in approximately 6% of treated subjects in the initial IV tPA trials.[2,11] Although relatively rare, symptomatic ICH has a significant impact on morbidity and mortality.[11] Older age, higher stroke severity, higher glucose level, baseline antiplatelet use (particularly dual antiplatelet use[12]), the presence of atrial fibrillation, congestive heart failure, renal impairment, and early ischemic changes on head CT are all associated with an increased risk of symptomatic ICH.[13] A number of predictive models exist to aid in risk stratification for ICH following treatment with IV tPA: the HAT score,[14] SITS-SICH score,[15] iScore,[16] SEDAN score,[17] SPAN-100 index,[18] and GRASPS score.[19] The utility of these scores is limited, and patients with higher scores may still benefit from IV tPA. As a result, no single score is in widespread use, and current AHA/ASA guidelines do not recommend using these scores to select patients for treatment with IV tPA.[1] Treatment with IV tPA also has the potential to cause systemic bleeding. The incidence of systemic hemorrhage is low, occurring in only 1.6% of subjects in the NINDS trial.[2]

In the event of life-threatening bleeding, either systemic or intracranial, protocols exist to reverse coagulopathy after IV tPA. About 50% of tPA is cleared within 3 to 6 minutes after cessation of the infusion, and approximately 80% is cleared within 40 minutes.[20] Despite rapid clearance, the effect of tPA may last up to 24 hours after infusion.[21] If a patient has an acute neurologic deterioration within the first 24 hours of tPA infusion, the infusion should be immediately held (if still infusing) and an emergent, noncontrast head CT obtained. If ICH is detected, cryoprecipitate (10 units over 10-30 minutes) and tranexamic acid (1000 mg over 10 minutes) or epsilon-aminocaproic acid (4-5 grams over 1 hour) should be infused.[22] Our protocol is to transfuse 2 units of thawed plasma, which is immediately available at our institution, followed by 10 units of cryoprecipitate and 8 units of pooled platelets. Fibrinogen levels are then checked, with administration of more cryoprecipitate if levels remain low. There may also be a role for surgical hematoma evacuation depending on the size and location of the hemorrhage and the patient's overall clinical condition.[1,23]

Orolingual angioedema is another important, but rare, complication of IV tPA administration, with an incidence of 0.2% to 5.1%.[24] This anaphalyactoid reaction causes swelling of the tongue, lips, and/or oropharynx, which is likely due to plasmin activation of bradykinin. The swelling is often unilateral and contralateral to the ischemic hemisphere. It is typically mild and transient.[25,26] However, orolingual angioedema can, at times, be severe and cause airway obstruction. All patients treated with IV tPA should have inspection of the tongue, lips, and oropharynx after treatment. If orolingual angioedema develops, tPA should be discontinued and methylprednisolone 125 mg, diphenhydramine 50 mg, and ranitidine 50 mg or famotidine 20 mg IV should be administered.[1] Intramuscular epinephrine 0.01 mg/kg, up to a maximum of 0.5 mg, can also be administered.[1,27] Intubation should be considered if the patient develops stridor due to airway obstruction but should be performed by an experienced clinician due to the risk of trauma and bleeding during the iatrogenic coagulopathy of IV tPA. Direct visual inspection of the oropharynx and/or CT of the tongue may be useful to differentiate angioedema from hematoma formation.

PATIENT SELECTION FOR IV tPA

The AHA/ASA-recommended guidelines for tPA eligibility are listed (see Table 6.2). A comprehensive review of the evidence and scientific rationale for these guidelines was published by the AHA/ASA in 2016.[28] This document was partially a response to changes made by the U.S. Food and Drug Administration (FDA) to the prescribing information for alteplase. The FDA changed the prescribing information in order to be compliant with the Physician Labeling Rule, not due to new information about the risks/benefits of IV tPA. Because the Physician Labeling Rule requirements include very specific definitions for contraindications and precautions, the FDA prescribing information for alteplase has removed, or made less specific, many of the exclusion criteria. Differences between the FDA prescribing information and the AHA/ASA guidelines are a potential source of confusion to clinicians and may pose a barrier to treatment with IV tPA treatment. We strongly support the AHA/ASA guidelines because they provide clear and specific guidance, and we encourage providers

TABLE 6.2 Indications and contraindications for IV tPA

Indications 3 Hours From Symptom Onset

Diagnosis of ischemic stroke causing disabling symptoms

Onset of symptoms <3 hours before beginning treatment

Age ≥18 years

Contraindications

Imaging reveals acute intracranial hemorrhage

Significant head trauma or prior stroke in previous 3 months

Symptoms suggest subarachnoid hemorrhage

History of previous intracranial hemorrhage

Intra-axial intracranial neoplasm

Intracranial or intraspinal surgery in previous 3 months

Infective endocarditis

Aortic arch dissection

Elevated blood pressure (systolic >185 mm Hg or diastolic >110 mm Hg) despite aggressive BP-lowering therapy

Active internal bleeding

GI malignancy or GI bleeding event in previous 21 days

Acute bleeding diathesis, including but not limited to platelet count <100 000/mm^3, heparin received within 48 hours, resulting in abnormally elevated aPTT >40 s

Current use of anticoagulant with INR > 1.7 or PT > 15 seconds

Use of direct thrombin inhibitors or direct factor Xa inhibitors within 48 hours (unless appropriate lab parameters are normal) or treatment dose of low molecular weight heparin within 24 hours (prophylactic dose is permitted)

Blood glucose concentration <50 mg/dL (2.7 mmol/L)

CT demonstrates extensive regions of clear hypoattenuation

Additional Contraindications in 3–4.5 Hours From Symptom Onset for Class I Indication

Age >80 years

Severe stroke (NIHSS > 25)

Taking an oral anticoagulant regardless of INR

Imaging evidence of ischemic injury involving more than one-third of the MCA territory

History of both diabetes and prior ischemic stroke

to use these criteria when making treatment decisions in clinical practice. Probably the most important contribution of the 2018 ischemic stroke guidelines is abandonment of the terms inclusion and exclusion criteria and the confusing "relative exclusion" term in deference to indications, contraindications, and "additional recommendations."

Some of the additional recommendations in the 2018 Guidelines require additional discussion and clarification. In the 3- to 4.5-hour time period, for Class I indication, guidelines list additional contraindications: age >80 years, severe stroke defined by NIHSS > 25, taking an oral anticoagulant regardless of international normalized ratio (INR), and history of both diabetes and prior ischemic stroke. These additional criteria mimic the exclusion criteria in the ECASS III trial.[6] However, large observational studies[29-31] have failed to demonstrate an increased risk of sICH or worse clinical outcome in patients who were treated despite these additional exclusion criteria. A recent survey of practicing vascular neurologists found that only 51% adhere to the additional ECASS III exclusion criteria when treating patients in the 3- to 4.5-hour time window.[32] The latest AHA/ASA guidelines recommend treatment in the 3- to 4.5-hour window for patients >80 years old (Class IIa; Level of Evidence B) and those taking warfarin with an INR < 1.7 (Class IIb; Level of Evidence B). They further note that in the extended window, treating patients with a history of prior stroke and diabetes may be effective and is a reasonable option (Class IIb; Level of Evidence B) but that the benefit of thrombolysis in patients with an NIHSS of >25 is uncertain (Class IIb; Level of Evidence C).[28]

Additional consideration is required for major surgery or severe trauma within the previous 14 days.[1] In these patients, fibrin clot formation either at the surgical site or at a site of prior trauma could be disrupted by tPA. Unfortunately, major surgery and major trauma have not been defined, and it is likely that the risk of systemic bleeding varies considerably with the extent of injury and the vascularity of the injured organ. Patients who have had minor procedures at readily compressible sites (e.g., cardiac catheterization, digit amputation, and skin biopsies) can likely receive IV tPA soon, or even immediately, after surgery. For example, IV tPA treatment within 36 hours of cardiac catheterization has been associated with a significant improvement in functional outcome without a significant increase in bleeding events or mortality and is considered reasonable by the 2018 Guidelines.[33] For patients who have had minor surgeries, where the risk of bleeding is low and the potential for disability after stroke is high, we recommend treatment with IV tPA if they are otherwise eligible.

Patients who have had surgeries in which surgical site bleeding is expected to be severe or difficult to control (e.g., organ transplantation or high-risk vascular surgery) or where a small amount of bleeding could be catastrophic (e.g., cardiac surgery and otolaryngology procedures) should not be treated with IV tPA within 14 days.[34] Risk of serious bleeding following major surgery may in fact extend beyond 14 days. For instance, hemopericardium has been reported in a patient who received IV tPA 16 days after coronary artery bypass grafting.[35] Neurosurgery is another instance in which the risk of bleeding is likely to be extremely high. Neurosurgery could be considered a form of head trauma, and it is reasonable to exclude patients from IV tPA if they have had neurosurgery in the past 3 months. Eligible patients with major surgery within 14 days, and potentially beyond that time if there is a very high risk for serious bleeding, should not receive IV tPA and should instead be considered for endovascular thrombectomy (see Chapter 7).[1]

Recent MI was previously a relative exclusion to IV tPA. The 2018 Guidelines consider tPA reasonable in the setting of acute MI, recent non-ST segment elevation MI (non-STEMI), or STEMI of inferior wall and may be reasonable for STEMI of left anterior wall.[1] There are a few case reports of IV tPA causing hemopericardium via cardiac rupture or cardiac tamponade in patients who have recently experienced an MI.[35–37] The incidence of cardiac rupture following MI in IV tPA treated patients is not known. Indirect histopathologic evidence indicates that the risk of cardiac rupture is highest within the first 5 days after MI, and then the risk falls over 7 weeks as fibrosis and scarring progress.[38] Treatment decisions should be individualized based on time from MI and the severity of the stroke. Other cardiac conditions worth mentioning include infective endocarditis and cardiac thrombus. Acute stroke symptoms that occur in the setting of infective endocarditis should not be treated with IV tPA because doing so has been associated with significant risk of sICH.[39] In contrast, patients with cardiac thrombi likely can be safely treated with IV tPA.[40]

Patients who are therapeutically anticoagulated were excluded from IV tPA trials given concern for an increased risk of sICH. Large observational studies have shown that patients with INR ≤ 1.7 are not at increased risk of ICH compared to other IV tPA treated patients.[41,42] Current guidelines note that IV tPA can be given to patients who have been taking warfarin if the INR directly prior to treatment is ≤1.7.[1]

Direct oral anticoagulants (DOACs), including both direct thrombin inhibitors and direct factor Xa inhibitors, are not as well studied as warfarin in acute ischemic stroke. The reliability of thrombin time (TT), ecarin clotting time (ECT), and partial thromboplastin time (PTT) to evaluate direct thrombin inhibitor effect[43] and prothrombin time (PT)/international normalized ratio (INR), PTT, and anti-Xa activity assays to evaluate the effect of direct factor Xa inhibitors are not well understood.[1] Most of these tests are also not available in the acute setting. While there are case reports of successful treatment with IV tPA in patients on DOACs,[44,45] there is a significant potential for increased risk.[46] Current guidelines do not recommend IV tPA in those taking DOACs unless either appropriate, sensitive tests for anticoagulant effect are normal or the patient has not received a dose for ≥48 hours. Endovascular therapy could be considered in these patients.[1] Additional recommendations are provided in the 2018 Guidelines for how to approach patients with pre-existing disability, arterial dissection, unruptured intracranial aneurysms and vascular malformations, cerebral microbleeds, pregnancy, menstruation, ophthalmological conditions, and sickle cell disease.[1]

The initial trials of IV tPA explicitly excluded patients with "rapidly improving" or "minor symptoms." Minor deficits, generally defined as National Institutes of Health Stroke Scale (NIHSS) score of ≤5, and rapid improvement in symptoms are commonly cited reasons for exclusion from IV tPA treatment.[47] However, there is evidence that a significant proportion of untreated minor stroke patients do not return to their neurological baseline.[48] Based on these data and the proven benefit of IV rtPA in treatment, the most recent AHA/ASA guidelines note that "there should be no exclusion for patients with mild but nonetheless disabling stroke symptoms in the opinion of the treating physician" (Class I; Level of Evidence A). Similarly, IV rtPA treatment is reasonable for patients with improving symptoms if they remain "potentially disabled in the judgment of the examiner" at the time of the treatment decision (Class IIa; Level of Evidence A).[28] Disabling symptoms that should prompt consideration of treatment, despite a low NIHSS score, could include, but are not limited to, visual field deficits, isolated weakness (particularly hand weakness, which is not scored in the NIHSS), neglect, aphasia, or gait impairment.

Stroke Mimics and IV tPA

Differentiating ischemic stroke from stroke mimics, which are conditions that simulate acute ischemic stroke but are due to a non-vascular cause, can be challenging in the acute setting. In the largest study to date of 8,187 consecutive patients referred for evaluation of a suspected stroke in the Emergency Department, 30% were stroke mimics.[49] Common stroke mimic diagnoses include migraine; seizures/post-ictal states; conversion disorder; toxic-metabolic abnormalities, including hyperglycemia; and systemic infection and demyelinating disease.[28,50–53] It may not be possible to differentiate stroke and stroke mimics on the basis of history and examination. For example, in a study of 326 suspected acute stroke patients, five out of nine patients who had seizures at stroke onset also had an ischemic stroke.[54] Unfortunately, diagnostic tests that can help to differentiate stroke mimics from true ischemic stroke, such as magnetic resonance imaging, often take an unacceptable amount of time, and so clinicians must make the best judgment possible given the data that are available to them.

Evidence suggests that the risk of intracerebral hemorrhage after IV tPA is significantly lower in stroke mimics. In a pooled study of 392 stroke mimics treated with IV tPA, the rate of sICH was 0.5%.[51] Because the benefit of IV tPA is time dependent, the AHA/ASA notes that using IV tPA in possible stroke mimics is "probably recommended over delaying treatment to pursue additional diagnostic studies" (Class IIa; Level of Evidence B).[28] Further, AHA/ASA also states that IV rtPA is "reasonable in patients with a seizure at the time of onset of acute stroke if evidence suggests that residual impairments are secondary to stroke and not a post-ictal phenomenon (Class IIa; Level of Evidence C)."[28] When there is diagnostic uncertainty and there are disabling symptoms that may be due to ischemic stroke, it is often preferred to proceed with rapid treatment with IV tPA rather than spending time on more definitive diagnostic testing.

Communication of IV tPA Risks and Benefits

Delays in thrombolytic treatment may be due in part to challenges communicating the risks and benefits of acute IV tPA treatment.[55] It is recommended that the risks and benefits of IV tPA be discussed using a neutral tone to encourage shared decision making.[56] Additionally, the discussion should be conducted in phases.[57] First, the diagnosis of probable ischemic stroke must be established. Then, there should be a discussion of the risks and benefits of treatment. It is helpful to explicitly note that although there is an increased risk of sICH with IV tPA, treatment is still associated with a significant reduction in morbidity. Established visual aids may be useful to speed the decision-making process,[58] and their use is recommended by the AHA/ASA (Class IIa; Level of Evidence B).[28] With practice, obtaining consent for tPA can be easily streamlined. One study noted that an acceptable consent process took an average of 2.8 minutes.[59] The presumption of consent for emergency acute stroke treatment is also well established,[60] and for incompetent patients without available healthcare proxy, the AHA/ASA recommends proceeding with intravenous treatment in an otherwise eligible acute ischemic stroke patient (Class I; Level of Evidence C).[28]

Challenges and Limitations of IV tPA

Despite the proven benefit for intravenous tPA for reducing morbidity after stroke, only a minority of patients receive this therapy. Population-based studies have suggested that nationally <10% of patients with ischemic stroke are treated.[61,62] Multiple factors contribute to this low utilization. Patient delays from symptom onset to presentation are a major limitation, but there are also numerous hospital- and provider-level factors that contribute to underutilization, including missed diagnosis of stroke, inadequate stroke expertise at some hospitals, and in-hospital delays in evaluation and management of acute stroke.

Missed diagnosis of acute ischemic stroke, or even delayed diagnosis of stroke, can preclude patients from treatment with IV tPA. A population-based retro-spective cohort study found that 14% of hospitalized ischemic stroke patients were missed in the emergency department.[63] Other single-center studies reported emergency department false-negative rates of 2% to 26%.[64–67] Patients with atypical symptoms (generalized weakness, altered mental status, headache, gait impairment, and dizziness) are more likely to be missed than those with focal weakness and speech impairment.[68] Though bedside diagnostic testing exists to rapidly distinguish central versus peripheral vertigo,[69–71] additional rapid ischemic stroke detection strategies for atypical stroke symptoms would be beneficial.[72] Until such tools are developed, it is critical for providers to maintain a high suspicion for stroke in all cases where there is a sudden onset of neurologic deficits.

Bringing greater stroke-specific expertise to the patient can improve diag-nostic accuracy and tPA utilization. Telestroke, in which a stroke neurologist evaluates a patient remotely using audio–video teleconferencing, provides access to stroke care at hospitals that do not have vascular neurologists on site. Telestroke has been shown to improve diagnostic accuracy and increase the utilization of IV tPA.[73,74] It is also an important part of regionalized stroke care systems and has the potential to improve patient triage and reduce unnecessary transfers across hospitals. Mobile stroke units (MSUs) take the concept of bringing stroke care to the patient one step farther. An MSU is an ambulance that contains a mobile CT scanner, point-of-care laboratory testing, and either a physician with expertise in stroke or a telemedicine connection to such an expert. MSUs have significant potential to increase IV tPA treatment rates and to reduce treatment time.[75] Clinical trials are currently being conducted to prove their effectiveness.

Finally, it is important to note that although IV tPA is an effective treatment and should be administered to all eligible patients who present within 4.5 hours of symptom onset, tPA alone is not sufficient treatment for patients with large-vessel occlusions. A meta-analysis of recanalization rates found that with IV tPA, there is recanalization of the occluded artery 46.2% of the time. Recana-lization rates may vary by vessel, and with internal carotid artery occlusion recanalization occurred in only 13.9% of cases treated with IV tPA alone.[76] Endovascular techniques have much higher rates of recanalization, can be used after IV tPA, and have been shown to improve both recanalization rates and functional outcomes.[77] These techniques will be further discussed in Chapter 7. It is critical to rapidly identify patients who have a large-vessel occlusion and consider endovascular thrombectomy in a process that is concurrent with determination of eligibility for IV tPA.

CONCLUSION

Acute thrombolysis has been shown to reduce disability after stroke. Treatment with IV tPA for eligible patients is safe and effective within 4.5 hours of symptom onset. All ischemic stroke patients who present within 4.5 hours of symptom onset and who are eligible for IV tPA should be treated as quickly as possible.

References

1. Powers WJ, Rabinstein AA, Ackerson T, et al. 2018 guidelines for the early management of patients with acute ischemic stroke: a guideline for healthcare professionals from the American Heart Association/American Stroke Association, http://stroke.ahajournals.org /content/early/2018/01/23/STR.0000000000000158. *Stroke* 2018; 49(3):509–551.
2. Tissue plasminogen activator for acute ischemic stroke. The National Institute of Neurological Disorders and Stroke rt-PA Stroke Study Group. *N Engl J Med*. 1995;333:1581–1587.
3. Re-examining Acute Eligibility for Thrombolysis Task Force, Levine SR, Khatri P, et al. Review, historical context, and clarifications of the NINDS rt-PA stroke trials exclusion criteria: Part 1: rapidly improving stroke symptoms. *Stroke*. 2013;44:2500–2505.
4. van Swieten JC, Koudstaal PJ, Visser MC, et al. Interobserver agreement for the assessment of handicap in stroke patients. *Stroke*. 1988;19:604–607.
5. Schwamm LH, Ali SF, Reeves MJ, et al. Temporal trends in patient characteristics and treatment with intravenous thrombolysis among acute ischemic stroke patients at Get With The Guidelines-Stroke hospitals. *Circ Cardiovasc Qual Outcomes*. 2013;6: 543–549.
6. Hacke W, Kaste M, Bluhmki E, et al. Thrombolysis with alteplase 3 to 4.5 hours after acute ischemic stroke. *N Engl J Med*. 2008;359:1317–1329.
7. The IST-3 collaborative group. Effect of thrombolysis with alteplase within 6 h of acute ischaemic stroke on long-term outcomes (the third International Stroke Trial [IST-3]): 18-month follow-up of a randomised controlled trial. *Lancet Neurol*. 2013;12:768–776.
8. Emberson J, Lees KR, Lyden P, et al. Effect of treatment delay, age, and stroke severity on the effects of intravenous thrombolysis with alteplase for acute ischaemic stroke: a meta-analysis of individual patient data from randomised trials. *Lancet*. 2014; 384(9958): 1929–1935.
9. European Stroke Organisation Executive C, Committee ESOW. Guidelines for management of ischaemic stroke and transient ischaemic attack 2008. *Cerebrovas Dis*. 2008; 25:457–507.
10. Saver JL. Time is brain—quantified. *Stroke* 2006;37:263–266.
11. Hacke W, Donnan G, Fieschi C, et al. Association of outcome with early stroke treatment: pooled analysis of ATLANTIS, ECASS, and NINDS rt-PA stroke trials. *Lancet*. 2004; 363:768–774.

12. Cucchiara B, Kasner SE, Tanne D, et al. Factors associated with intracerebral hemorrhage after thrombolytic therapy for ischemic stroke: pooled analysis of placebo data from the Stroke-Acute Ischemic NXY Treatment (SAINT) I and SAINT II Trials. *Stroke.* 2009;40:3067–3072.

13. Whiteley WN, Slot KB, Fernandes P, Sandercock P, Wardlaw J. Risk factors for intracranial hemorrhage in acute ischemic stroke patients treated with recombinant tissue plasminogen activator: a systematic review and meta-analysis of 55 studies. *Stroke.* 2012;43:2904–2909.

14. Lou M, Safdar A, Mehdiratta M, et al. The HAT Score: a simple grading scale for predicting hemorrhage after thrombolysis. *Neurology.* 2008;71:1417–1423.

15. Mazya M, Egido JA, Ford GA, et al. Predicting the risk of symptomatic intracerebral hemorrhage in ischemic stroke treated with intravenous alteplase: safe Implementation of Treatments in Stroke (SITS) symptomatic intracerebral hemorrhage risk score. *Stroke.* 2012;43:1524–1531.

16. Saposnik G, Fang J, Kapral MK, et al. The iScore predicts effectiveness of thrombolytic therapy for acute ischemic stroke. *Stroke.* 2012;43:1315–1322.

17. Strbian D, Engelter S, Michel P, et al. Symptomatic intracranial hemorrhage after stroke thrombolysis: the SEDAN score. *Ann Neurol.* 2012;71:634–641.

18. Saposnik G, Guzik AK, Reeves M, et al. Stroke Prognostication using Age and NIH Stroke Scale: SPAN-100. *Neurology.* 2013;80:21–28.

19. Menon BK, Saver JL, Prabhakaran S, et al. Risk score for intracranial hemorrhage in patients with acute ischemic stroke treated with intravenous tissue-type plasminogen activator. *Stroke.* 2012;43:2293–2299.

20. Acheampong P, Ford GA. Pharmacokinetics of alteplase in the treatment of ischaemic stroke. *Expert Opin Drug Metab Toxicol.* 2012;8:271–281.

21. Yaghi S, Eisenberger A, Willey JZ. Symptomatic intracerebral hemorrhage in acute ischemic stroke after thrombolysis with intravenous recombinant tissue plasminogen activator: a review of natural history and treatment. *JAMA Neurol.* 2014;71:1181–1185.

22. Morgenstern LB, Hemphill JC, 3rd, Anderson C, et al. Guidelines for the management of spontaneous intracerebral hemorrhage: a guideline for healthcare professionals from the American Heart Association/American Stroke Association. *Stroke.* 2010;41:2108–2129.

23. Frontera JA, Lewin JJ 3rd, Rabinstein AA, et al. Guideline for reversal of antithrombotics in intracranial hemorrhage: a statement for healthcare professionals from the Neurocritical Care Society and Society of Critical Care Medicine. *Neurocrit Care.* 2016;24:6–46. doi: 10.1007/s12028-015-0222-x.

24. Correia AS, Matias G, Calado S, Lourenco A, Viana-Baptista M. Orolingual angiodema associated with alteplase treatment of acute stroke: a reappraisal. *J Stroke Cerebrovasc Dis.* 2015;24:31–40.

25. Hill MD, Lye T, Moss H, et al. Hemi-orolingual angioedema and ACE inhibition after alteplase treatment of stroke. *Neurology.* 2003;60:1525–1527.

26. Hill MD, Barber PA, Takahashi J, Demchuk AM, Feasby TE, Buchan AM. Anaphylactoid reactions and angioedema during alteplase treatment of acute ischemic stroke. *CMAJ.* 2000;162:1281–1284.

27. Fugate JE, Kalimullah EA, Wijdicks EF. Angioedema after tPA: what neurointensivists should know. *Neurocrit Care.* 2012;16:440–443.

28. Demaerschalk BM, Kleindorfer DO, Adeoye OM, et al. Scientific Rationale for the Inclusion and Exclusion Criteria for Intravenous Alteplase in Acute Ischemic Stroke: A Statement for Healthcare Professionals From the American Heart Association/American Stroke Association. *Stroke.* 2016;47:581–641.

29. Cronin CA, Sheth KN, Zhao X, et al. Adherence to third European cooperative acute stroke study 3- to 4.5-hour exclusions and association with outcome: data from get with the guidelines-stroke. *Stroke*. 2014;45:2745–2749.

30. Wahlgren N, Ahmed N, Davalos A, et al. Thrombolysis with alteplase 3–4.5 h after acute ischaemic stroke (SITS-ISTR): an observational study. *Lancet*. 2008;372:1303–1309.

31. Mishra NK, Ahmed N, Andersen G, et al. Thrombolysis in very elderly people: controlled comparison of SITS International Stroke Thrombolysis Registry and Virtual International Stroke Trials Archive. *BMJ*. 2010;341:c6046.

32. De Los Rios F, Kleindorfer DO, Guzik A, et al. Intravenous fibrinolysis eligibility: a survey of stroke clinicians' practice patterns and review of the literature. *J Stroke Cerebrovasc Dis*. 2014;23:2130–2138.

33. Khatri P, Taylor RA, Palumbo V, et al. The safety and efficacy of thrombolysis for strokes after cardiac catheterization. *J Am Coll Cardiol*. 2008;51:906–911.

34. Mullen MT, McGarvey ML, Kasner SE. Safety and efficacy of thrombolytic therapy in postoperative cerebral infarctions. *NeurolClin*. 2006;24:783–793.

35. Kasner SE, Villar-Cordova CE, Tong D, et al. Hemopericardium and cardiac tamponade after thrombolysis for acute ischemic stroke. *Neurology*. 1998;50:1857–1859.

36. Kremen SA, Wu MN, Ovbiagele B. Hemopericardium following intravenous thrombolysis for acute ischemic stroke. *Cerebrovas Dis*. 2005;20:478–479.

37. Dhand A, Nakagawa K, Nagpal S, et al. Cardiac rupture after intravenous t-PA administration in acute ischemic stroke. *Neurocrit Care*. 2010;13:261–262.

38. De Silva DA, Manzano JJ, Chang HM, Wong MC. Reconsidering recent myocardial infarction as a contraindication for IV stroke thrombolysis. *Neurology*. 2011;76: 1838–1840.

39. Ong E, Mechtouff L, Bernard E, et al. Thrombolysis for stroke caused by infective endocarditis: an illustrative case and review of the literature. *J Neurol*. 2013;260:1339–1342.

40. Derex L, Nighoghossian N, Perinetti M, Honnorat J, Trouillas P. Thrombolytic therapy in acute ischemic stroke patients with cardiac thrombus. *Neurology*. 2001;57:2122–2125.

41. Mazya MV, Lees KR, Markus R, et al. Safety of intravenous thrombolysis for ischemic stroke in patients treated with warfarin. *Ann Neurol*. 2013;74:266–274.

42. Xian Y, Liang L, Smith EE, et al. Risks of intracranial hemorrhage among patients with acute ischemic stroke receiving warfarin and treated with intravenous tissue plasminogen activator. *JAMA*. 2012;307:2600–2608.

43. Blommel ML, Blommel AL. Dabigatran etexilate: a novel oral direct thrombin inhibitor. *Am J Health Syst Pharm*. 2011;68:1506–1519.

44. De Smedt A, De Raedt S, Nieboer K, De Keyser J, Brouns R. Intravenous thrombolysis with recombinant tissue plasminogen activator in a stroke patient treated with dabigatran. *Cerebrovasc Dis*. 2010;30:533–534.

45. De Smedt A, Cambron M, Nieboer K, et al. Intravenous thrombolysis with recombinant tissue plasminogen activator in a stroke patient treated with apixaban. *Int J Stroke*. 2014;9:E31.

46. Casado Naranjo I, Portilla-Cuenca JC, Jimenez Caballero PE, Calle Escobar ML, Romero Sevilla RM. Fatal intracerebral hemorrhage associated with administration of recombinant tissue plasminogen activator in a stroke patient on treatment with dabigatran. *Cerebrovasc Dis*. 2011;32:614–615.

47. Reeves MJ, Grau-Sepulveda MV, Fonarow GC, et al. Are quality improvements in the get with the guidelines: stroke program related to better care or better data documentation? *Circ Cardiovasc Qual Outcome*. 2011;4:503–511.

48. Sangha RS, Caprio FZ, Askew R, et al. Quality of life in patients with TIA and minor ischemic stroke. *Neurology*. 2015;85:1957–1963.

49. Merino JG, Luby M, Benson RT, et al. Predictors of acute stroke mimics in 8187 patients referred to a stroke service. *J Stroke Cerebrovasc Dis*. 2013;22:e397–403.

50. Zinkstok SM, Engelter ST, Gensicke H, et al. Safety of thrombolysis in stroke mimics: results from a multicenter cohort study. *Stroke*. 2013;44:1080–1084.

51. Tsivgoulis G, Zand R, Katsanos AH, et al. Safety of intravenous thrombolysis in stroke mimics: prospective 5-year study and comprehensive meta-analysis. *Stroke*. 2015;46: 1281–1287.

52. Libman RB, Wirkowski E, Alvir J, Rao TH. Conditions that mimic stroke in the emergency department. Implications for acute stroke trials. *Arch Neurol*. 1995;52:1119–1122.

53. Gargalas S, Weeks R, Khan-Bourne N, et al. Incidence and outcome of functional stroke mimics admitted to a hyperacute stroke unit. *J Neurol Neurosurg Psychiatry*. 2017;88:2–6.

54. Sylaja PN, Dzialowski I, Krol A, et al. Role of CT angiography in thrombolysis decision-making for patients with presumed seizure at stroke onset. *Stroke*. 2006;37:915–917.

55. Prabhakaran S, Khorzad R, Brown A, Nannicelli AP, Khare R, Holl JL. Academic-Community Hospital Comparison of Vulnerabilities in Door-to-Needle Process for Acute Ischemic Stroke. *Circ Cardiovasc Qual Outcome*. 2015;8:S148–54.

56. Gong J, Zhang Y, Feng J, et al. How best to obtain consent to thrombolysis: Individualized decision-making. *Neurology*. 2016;86:1045–1052.

57. Lie ML, Murtagh MJ, Watson DB, et al. Risk communication in the hyperacute setting of stroke thrombolysis: an interview study of clinicians. *Emerg Med J*. 2015;32:357–363.

58. Gadhia J, Starkman S, Ovbiagele B, Ali L, Liebeskind D, Saver JL. Assessment and improvement of figures to visually convey benefit and risk of stroke thrombolysis. *Stroke*. 2010;41:300–306.

59. Thomas L, Viswanathan A, Cochrane TI, et al. Variability in the Perception of Informed Consent for IV-tPA during Telestroke Consultation. *Front Neurol*. 2012;3:128.

60. Chiong W, Kim AS, Huang IA, Farahany NA, Josephson SA. Testing the presumption of consent to emergency treatment for acute ischemic stroke. *JAMA*. 2014;311: 1689–1691.

61. Reeves MJ, Arora S, Broderick JP, et al. Acute stroke care in the US: results from 4 pilot prototypes of the Paul Coverdell National Acute Stroke Registry. *Stroke*. 2005;36: 1232–1240.

62. Mullen MT, Kasner SE, Kallan MJ, Kleindorfer DO, Albright KC, Carr BG. Joint commission primary stroke centers utilize more rt-PA in the nationwide inpatient sample. *J Am Heart Assoc*. 2013;2:e000071.

63. Madsen TE, Khoury J, Cadena R, et al. Potentially Missed Diagnosis of Ischemic Stroke in the Emergency Department in the Greater Cincinnati/Northern Kentucky Stroke Study. *Acad Emerg Med*. 2016;23:1128–1135.

64. Richoz B, Hugli O, Dami F, Carron PN, Faouzi M, Michel P. Acute stroke chameleons in a university hospital: risk factors, circumstances, and outcomes. *Neurology*. 2015;85: 505–11.

65. Arch AE, Weisman DC, Coca S, Nystrom KV, Wira CR, 3rd, Schindler JL. Missed Ischemic Stroke Diagnosis in the Emergency Department by Emergency Medicine and Neurology Services. *Stroke*. 2016;47:668–673.

66. Lever NM, Nystrom KV, Schindler JL, Halliday J, Wira C, 3rd, Funk M. Missed opportunities for recognition of ischemic stroke in the emergency department. *J Emerg Nurs*. 2013;39:434–439.

67. Dupre CM, Libman R, Dupre SI, et al. Stroke chameleons. *J Stroke Cerebrovasc Dis.* 2014;23:374–378.

68. Tarnutzer AA, Lee SH, Robinson KA, et al. ED misdiagnosis of cerebrovascular events in the era of modern neuroimaging: a meta-analysis. *Neurology.* 2017;88:1468–1477.

69. Tarnutzer AA, Berkowitz AL, Robinson KA, Hsieh YH, Newman-Toker DE. Does my dizzy patient have a stroke? A systematic review of bedside diagnosis in acute vestibular syndrome. *CMAJ.* 2011;183:E571–92.

70. Newman-Toker DE, Kerber KA, Hsieh YH, et al. HINTS outperforms ABCD2 to screen for stroke in acute continuous vertigo and dizziness. *Acad Emerg Med.* 2013; 20:986–996.

71. Kattah JC, Talkad AV, Wang DZ, Hsieh YH, Newman-Toker DE. HINTS to diagnose stroke in the acute vestibular syndrome: three-step bedside oculomotor examination more sensitive than early MRI diffusion-weighted imaging. *Stroke.* 2009;40:3504–3510.

72. Liberman AL, Prabhakaran S. Stroke Chameleons and Stroke Mimics in the Emergency Department. *Curr Neurol Neurosci Rep.* 2017;17:15.

73. Meyer BC, Raman R, Hemmen T, et al. Efficacy of site-independent telemedicine in the STRokE DOC trial: a randomised, blinded, prospective study. *Lancet Neurol.* 2008;7:787–795.

74. Switzer JA, Hall C, Gross H, et al. A web-based telestroke system facilitates rapid treatment of acute ischemic stroke patients in rural emergency departments. *J Emerg Med.* 2009;36:12–18.

75. Fassbender K, Grotta JC, Walter S, Grunwald IQ, Ragoschke-Schumm A, Saver JL. Mobile stroke units for prehospital thrombolysis, triage, and beyond: benefits and challenges. *Lancet Neurol.* 2017;16:227–237.

76. Rha JH, Saver JL. The impact of recanalization on ischemic stroke outcome: a meta-analysis. *Stroke.* 2007;38:967–973.

77. Saver JL, Goyal M, van der Lugt A, et al. Time to Treatment With Endovascular Thrombectomy and Outcomes From Ischemic Stroke: A Meta-analysis. *JAMA.* 2016;316: 1279–1288.

Endovascular Management of Acute Ischemic Stroke

Vikas Patel and Igor Rybinnik

The standard of care for management of acute, large-vessel, anterior circulation ischemic stroke has been revolutionized over the past several years with technological advancements in endovascular therapies. For decades, intravenous tissue plasminogen activator (IV tPA) has been the only U.S. Food and Drug Administration (FDA)–approved effective medical therapy for acute ischemic stroke.[1,2] Unfortunately the efficacy of IV tPA is time-sensitive, diminishing rapidly with increasing symptom onset to treatment time, and lesion-sensitive, with low recanalization rates in patients with more severe strokes due to proximal clots, such as those in the terminal internal carotid.[3] Endovascular treatments were explored because more than half of patients treated with IV tPA still had poor outcomes.[4]

EARLY INTRA-ARTERIAL TPA TREATMENT

Intra-arterial stroke treatment was investigated early with administration of an intra-arterial thrombolytic in the PROACT II (Prolyse in Acute Cerebral Thromboembolism II) trial.[5] This North American double-blinded study randomized a total of 180 patients with acute ischemic stroke in the middle cerebral artery (MCA) territory causing disabling deficits (National Institutes of Health Stroke Scale [NIHSS] score of 4 or greater) within 6 hours of symptom onset to receive heparin alone or in combination with 9 mg of intra-arterial recombinant pro-urokinase (proUK). Large-vessel occlusion was verified using digital subtraction cerebral angiography. The primary endpoint of favorable neurologic functional recovery (defined as a modified Rankin scale [mRS] of

0–2 at 90 days) was nearly double in the IA proUK treatment arm—a difference that was statistically significant. Subgroup analysis showed that larger strokes with NIHSS scores greater than 10 drove the positive response. Mortality rates were similar between the two arms, although symptomatic intracranial hemorrhage (sICH) was more common in the group receiving IA proUK (10% of patients) compared to the control arm (2% of patients). Unfortunately, this early study highlighted several concerns with endovascular reperfusion therapies, including significantly delayed treatment and increased symptomatic intracranial hemorrhage. Although proUK was never approved by FDA due to limited supporting evidence, based on the extrapolation of these positive results, intra-arterial tPA became a common intravascular intervention in the United States.[6]

FIRST WAVE OF ENDOVASCULAR THERAPY TRIALS

Intra-arterial treatment of acute ischemic stroke was further investigated in several randomized controlled trials, with the first three—SYNTHESIS, IMS III, and MR RESCUE—published in 2013 with disappointing results and failing to show any benefit of endovascular therapy over standard treatment.[7–9] The major reasons cited for negative results included (a) device choice, with predominant use of first-generation devices with lower recanalization rates, and (b) inappropriate patient selection, with interventions potentially carried out without confirmation of proximal large-vessel occlusive lesions and in patients with mild to moderate strokes or those with large completed ischemic core infarcts, both of which were less likely to benefit from endovascular therapy. Time to reperfusion was also a major factor, with extensive delays in treatment introduced by the catheter-based procedures themselves as well as multimodal imaging.

SYNTHESIS Expansion was a prospective, randomized, open-label, blinded-endpoint (PROBE) trial that enrolled 362 patients with acute ischemic stroke predominantly in the anterior circulation eligible for intravenous r-tPA within 4.5 hours of onset and for whom endovascular treatment was possible within 6 hours.[8] The trial was designed to assess for the superiority of endovascular reperfusion therapy as compared to the standard of care, intravenous r-tPA. Confirmation of large-vessel occlusion was not required, and the patients were randomized 1:1 to standard-dose intravenous r-tPA 0.9 mg/kg or endovascular therapy, including intra-arterial r-tPA, mechanical thrombectomy, or a combination of the two. Median symptom onset to treatment time was nearly 4 hours, 1 hour longer than in the intravenous r-tPA group, and more effective second-generation clot retriever devices were used infrequently. Primary endpoint of death or disability (defined as a modified Rankin scale score of 0–1) at 3 months was not significantly different between the two groups. Interestingly, endovascular therapy appeared to be as safe as intravenous r-tPA, with no significant difference in the rates of sICH at 7 days. Subgroup analyses of time to treatment (0–3 and 3–4.5 hours), stroke severity (NIHSS <11 or ≥11) and age (≤67 years) similarly showed no significant difference. The authors concluded that on the basis of this trial, endovascular therapy was not superior to standard treatment with intravenous thrombolysis for patients with acute ischemic stroke.[8]

The Interventional Management of Stroke Trial III (IMS III) was a PROBE, two-arm, superiority trial that enrolled patients with a major ischemic stroke defined by an NIHSS score ≥10 who received intravenous r-tPA within 3 hours and were likely to or known to have occlusion of a major cerebral artery, with overwhelming predominance of anterior circulation infarctions.[7] The aim of this trial was to investigate the efficacy of bridging endovascular therapy with IV tPA in the treatment of acute ischemic stroke to mitigate treatment delays. Large completed infarctions involving more than one-third of the MCA territory on non-enhanced CT were excluded.[10] Although confirmation of large-vessel occlusion was not required, screening with CT angiography (CTA) for patients with moderate strokes (NIHSS score >8) was allowed midway through the trial. Patients were randomly assigned in a 1:2 ratio to receive standard dose intravenous r-tPA (0.9 mg/kg) alone or a reduced dose (0.6 mg/kg) of intravenous r-tPA in combination with catheter-based therapy selected at the discretion of the treating physician. The angiographic procedure had to begin within 5 hours and be completed within 7 hours after the onset of stroke. With less than 2% of interventions employing second-generation stent retriever devices, resulting in poor recanalization rates of less than 50% and a median time of recanalization greater than 5 hours, there was no statistically significant difference in primary outcomes of death or disability (defined as an mRS score of 2 or below) at 90 days. However, time to treatment within 2 hours of symptom onset and superior recanalization resulted in a trend toward improving outcomes in the endovascular group. Safety was comparable between the two groups, with similar rates of sICH at 30 hours post-intervention. The trial was aborted prematurely due to futility after enrollment of 656 out of projected 900 patients. In conclusion, the trial showed that despite similar safety outcomes, supplementing IV tPA with endovascular therapy for the treatment of acute ischemic stroke did not significantly benefit mortality or functional independence.

MR and Recanalization of Stroke Clots Using Embolectomy (MR RESCUE) was a PROBE, two-arm, superiority trial that enrolled 118 patients with large-artery occlusion and anterior circulation ischemic stroke within 8 hours who were ineligible for or failed intravenous thrombolysis, with persistent vessel occlusion after IV r-tPA.[9] The primary aim of this trial was to use multimodal imaging to improve patient selection for endovascular interventions in hopes of improving outcomes. Patients were stratified into two groups by the presence or absence of a favorable penumbral pattern, defined as substantial salvageable tissue and a small infarct core on pretreatment CT or MRI of the brain, randomized 1:1 to standard-care or catheter-based therapy with a variety of first-generation devices with optional addition of intra-arterial r-tPA. Emblematic of an early endovascular trial, favorable recanalization rates—reperfusion of more than half of the occluded vascular territory—was very poor at 25% in the endovascular group, and median time to intervention was over 6 hours. Mean scores on the mRS at 3 months did not differ between embolectomy and standard care, even in patients with favorable penumbral patterns.[9] In summary, a favorable penumbral pattern on neuroimaging unfortunately did not identify patients who would preferentially benefit from endovascular therapy for acute ischemic stroke.

MODERN ENDOVASCULAR TRIALS AND THE CHANGING STANDARD OF CARE

In 2015 and 2016, seven landmark modern endovascular trials—MR CLEAN, EXTEND-IA, ESCAPE, SWIFT PRIME, REVASCAT, THRACE, and THERAPY—aimed to rectify the criticisms of early trial designs and finally demonstrated the efficacy of catheter-based therapies for patients with large-artery occlusions (Table 7.1).[11–17] Patient selection was improved by mostly enrolling moderate to severe strokes with a vascular imaging requirement to confirm large-vessel occlusion, with optional additional standardized imaging paradigms. Pragmatic selection avoided multimodal imaging in favor of a widely available CTA to confirm large-vessel occlusion in combination with a predefined time window for intervention and standardized assessment of core infarct on CT by Alberta Stroke Program Early CT Score (ASPECTS), where the entire MCA vascular territory is subdivided into 10 segments and 1 point is deducted from the maximal score of 10 for every region with early infarct signs. One trial stratified patients for intervention based on collateral imaging with multiphase CTA, with the contrast bolus in the initial phase timed with the peak arterial flow per routine CTA protocols and two additional phases acquired in the venous phases to capture collaterals with delayed flow. Some trials employed penumbral imaging, but unlike the earlier MR RESCUE trial, an automated and swift RApid processing of Perfusion and Diffusion (RAPID) was used to expedite patient stratification. In addition to the standardization of patient selection, initial CT to reperfusion time was limited to less than 2 hours to expedite recanalization. Beyond patient selection, modern trials addressed the poor recanalization rates seen in the early trials by almost exclusively employing superior second-generation retrievable stent devices. Neurological outcomes were generally measured at 90 days by the modified Rankin scale, with favorable outcome considered at or below 2, which corresponds to slight disability but functional independence.[13–17]

The Multicenter Randomized Clinical Trial of Endovascular Treatment for Acute Ischemic Stroke in the Netherlands (MR CLEAN) was a PROBE, two-arm, superiority trial that enrolled 500 patients with acute ischemic stroke in the anterior circulation and imaging-confirmed occlusion of the distal internal carotid artery (ICA), MCA (M1 or M2 segments), or anterior cerebral artery (A1 or A2 segments).[17] This trial was unique in its selection and intervention criteria as well as enrollment. Patient selection was pragmatic, omitting multimodal imaging in favor of a non-enhanced CT (ASPECTS score) for estimation of core infarct, CTA for confirmation of large-vessel occlusion, and presence of at least minor deficits (NIHSS ≥2) for enrollment, but otherwise adhering to the preexisting treatment criteria for IV tPA. Reperfusion criteria were standardized to permit endovascular intervention within 6 hours of stroke onset, and lack of prespecified observation time to ascertain improvement post–IV tPA was intended to speed treatment. Furthermore, it was the only study that ran to completion of planned enrollment, whereas the positive results from MR CLEAN led to premature termination of all other ongoing endovascular trials. Selection bias was minimized because endovascular therapy in the Netherlands was not reimbursed by insurers when performed outside of a trial setting. Without a prespecified upper age restriction, the mean age of study participants was 65 years, with a 96-year-old being the oldest patient enrolled. The vast majority of the patients were eligible for and received IV tPA, with average symptom onset to treatment time of 85 minutes, but randomization occurred at 3 hours (median time of 204 min), and groin puncture in the interventional group followed 1 hour post-randomization at 4 hours after symptom onset (median 260 minutes). Patients receiving endovascular therapy had a median ASPECT score of 9 (range 7–10), mostly distal ICA or MCA stem occlusions, and a median NIHSS of 17 (interquartile range, 14–21). Therefore, with high ASPECT scores and persistent large-vessel occlusions documented at randomization 2 hours after IV tPA, the MR CLEAN interventional group essentially represented IV tPA failures with relatively small pre-intervention core infarcts.

Although the endovascular treatment was relatively delayed and moderately effective despite the use of modern stent retrievers in 80% of the interventions (only two-thirds of patients had favorable reperfusion), intervention improved

TABLE 7.1 Seven landmark modern endovascular trials

	MR CLEAN	ESCAPE	EXTEND-IA
Number of patients	500	315	70
Control arm	Best medical management, IV tPA	Best medical management, IV tPA	IV tPA only
Interventional arm	Intra-arterial therapy (82% with stentriever)	Intra-arterial therapy (87% with stentriever)	Thrombectomy with stentriever
Key inclusion criteria	NIHSS ≥ 2, Age ≥ 18	NIHSS > 5, ASPECTS > 5, moderate-good collaterals	Ischemic core <70 mL, mismatch
Imaging criteria (in addition to confirmation of LVO)	Noncontrast CT (ASPECTS)	Noncontrast CT (ASPECTS), collateral imaging with mCTA	RAPID perfusion imaging
Target vessels	ICA, M1, M2, A1, A2	ICA, M1 or "M1 equivalent" with ≥2 M2 segments	ICA, M1, M2
Median age in years (IQR)	66 (55–76)	71 (60–81)	70 ± 12
Median NIHSS (IQR)	17 (14–21)	16 (13–20)	13 (9–19)
Median ASPECTS	9 (7–10)	9 (8–10)	Not reported
Received IV tPA	89%	73%	100%
Time window for intervention from symptom onset	<6 hours	<12 hours	<6 hours
Median time from stroke onset to groin puncture (IQR), min	260 (210–313)	Not reported	210 (166–251)
Median time to reperfusion (IQR), min	Not reported	241 (176–359)	248 min (204–277)
TICI grade 2b/3 recanalization	59%	72%	86%
Symptomatic ICH (vs. control)	7.7% vs. 6.4% ($p < 0.05$)	3.6% vs. 2.7 (OR 1.4, 95% CI 0.4–4.7)	0% vs. 6% ($p = 0.49$)
90-day mortality (vs. control)	19% vs. 18% ($p > 0.05$)	10% vs. 19% (OR 0.5, 95% CI 0.3–1.0)	9% vs. 20% ($p = 0.18$)
Functional independence at 90 days, (mRS ≥2), vs. control	33% vs. 19% (OR 2.05, 95% CI 1.36–3.09)	53% vs. 29% (OR 1.8, 95% CI 1.4–2.4)	71% vs. 40% ($p = 0.009$)

SWIFT PRIME	REVASCAT	THRACE	THERAPY
196	206	385	108
IV tPA only	Best medical management, IV tPA	IV tPA only	IV tPA only
Thrombectomy with stentriever	Thrombectomy with stentriever	Mechanical thrombectomy	Thrombectomy with aspiration system
Age 18–80, NIHSS 8–29, ASPECTS ≥6	Age 18–80, NIHSS ≥6, ASPECTS ≥7, prespecified waiting period post–IV tPA	Age 18–80, NIHSS 10–25	Age 18–85, NIHSS ≥8, Clot length ≥8mm
Noncontrast CT (ASPECTS) or RAPID perfusion imaging	Noncontrast CT (ASPECTS) or MRI	Noncontrast CT (ASPECTS)	Noncontrast thin-section CT (ASPECTS, clot length)
ICA, M1	ICA, M1	ICA, M1, BA	ICA, M1, M2
65 ± 11	66 ± 11	66 (54–74)	Not reported
17 (13–19)	17 (14–20)	18 (15–21)	Not reported
9 (8–10)	7 (6–9)	Median not reported. 8–10 (48% of patients), 5–7 (41%), 0–4 (11%)	7.5 (6–9)
100%	68%	100%	100%
<6 hours	<8 hours	<5 hours	<4.5 hours
224 (165–275)	269 (201–340)	250 (210–290)	227 (184–263)
252 (190–300)	355 (269–430)	303 (261–345)	Not reported
88%	66%	69%	70%
0% vs. 3% ($p = 0.12$)	1.9% vs. 1.9% (RR 1.0, 95% CI 0.1–7.0)	2% vs. 2% ($p = 0.71$)	9.3% vs. 9.7% ($p = 1.0$)
9% vs. 12% ($p = 0.5$)	19% vs. 16% (RR 1.2, 95% CI 0.6–2.2)	12% vs. 13% ($p = 0.7$)	12% vs. 24% ($p = 0.18$)
60% vs. 35% ($p < 0.001$)	44% vs. 28% (OR 2.0, 95% CI 1.1–3.5)	53% vs. 42% ($p = 0.03$)	38% vs. 30% ($p = 0.52$)

the odds of functional independence as defined by mRS 0–2 at 90 days by 1.7 times (95% confidence interval [CI] of 1.21–2.30) without worsening sICH rates or improving mortality. Although reperfusion typically occurred at 5.5 hours, the clinical benefit markedly declined if reperfusion was delayed beyond just after 6 hours.[18]

The Endovascular Treatment for Small Core and Anterior Circulation Proximal Occlusion with Emphasis on Minimizing CT to Recanalization Times (ESCAPE) was a PROBE, two-arm superiority trial of 315 patients worldwide with disabling acute ischemic stroke (NIHSS score >5) and occluded proximal intracranial artery in the anterior circulation (ICA, M1 MCA, or "MCA equivalent" with ≥2 occluded M2 branches). The trial was terminated early after the presentation of MR CLEAN results. ESCAPE was one of the most inclusive trials, increasing the interventional window to up to 12 hours after stroke onset. Although it relied on the ASPECT score of 6–10 to select patients with small core infarcts, similar to MR CLEAN, multiphase CTA was used instead of a traditional CTA to identify patients with preserved collateral flow in more than half of the MCA territory. Multiphase CTA, as described earlier in this chapter, improved sensitivity for detection of collaterals and probably resulted in inclusion of patients that would otherwise be excluded from intervention in MR CLEAN.[19] ESCAPE focused on speed of intervention, requiring the fastest time from imaging to groin puncture of less than 60 minutes and encouraging rapid recanalization with retrievable stents within 90 minutes from the initial CT. Despite broad inclusion criteria, this strategy led to effective recanalization in more than 70% of patients in the interventional group, with median time of stroke onset to reperfusion of 4 hours (interquartile range [IQR] of 176–359 minutes), 1.5 hours earlier than in MR CLEAN. Functional independence (mRS 0–2) was achieved in 53% of interventional patients, nearly double that of the standard therapy group, resulting in a number needed to treat of 4. The sICH rates were similar between the two groups, and mortality nearly halved with intervention.[20]

The Extending the Time for Thrombolysis in Emergency Neurological Deficits–Intra-Arterial (EXTEND-IA) was the smallest of all the recent endovascular trials, randomizing a total of 70 patients, predominantly in Australian and New Zealand centers, before being prematurely terminated short of the projected 100-patient mark in light of MR CLEAN results.[16] Patients with acute ischemic stroke were randomized in a 1:1 fashion to standard of care alone (intravenous thrombolysis within 4.5 hours from symptom onset) or in combination with endovascular therapy exclusively with stent retriever within 6 hours of stroke onset. Verification of large-vessel occlusion was required with enrollment of predominantly terminal ICA and MCA stem occlusions in patients with moderate to severe strokes (median NIHSS 13, IQR 9–19), as typical of a modern endovascular trial. However, EXTEND-IA was the only trial to rely on automated RAPID penumbral imaging for patient selection rather than non-contrast CT.[13–16] The rationale was to select patients with large-vessel occlusion but also presence of salvageable tissue beyond the core infarction, which would have the best chance of response to reperfusion. As a result, approximately a quarter of the patients were excluded on the basis of perfusion imaging that would otherwise have been appropriate based on ASPECTS. Similar to ESCAPE, there was an emphasis on speed of reperfusion, with median initial imaging to groin puncture of 93 minutes (IQR 71–138 minutes) and median time from stroke onset to reperfusion of 4 hours (IQR 204–277 minutes). Excellent recanalization results approaching 90% were achieved in at least half of the MCA territory, corresponding to a highly significant 30% increase in functional independence (mRS 0–2) in the endovascular group, with number needed to treat of 3.2.

Solitaire FR with the Intention for Thrombectomy as Primary Endovascular Treatment of Acute Ischemic Stroke (SWIFT PRIME) was a PROBE global trial randomizing 196 patients in the United States and Europe[13] and was aborted short of the planned 200-patient interim analysis after MR CLEAN results were published. Design of the SWIFT PRIME trial was very similar to EXTEND-IA. Patients with moderate to severe strokes (NIHSS scores 8–29) and confirmed anterior circulation large-vessel occlusion were randomized to the standard of care or endovascular treatment with retrievable stents on the basis of either ASPECT scoring on noncontrast CT or perfusion imaging with RAPID. Treatment was initiated within 6 hours from stroke onset and within 90 minutes of qualifying imaging. Unique to SWIFT PRIME was the fact that nearly all patients received intravenous thrombolysis prior to intervention, and recanalization rates, as well as median times from stroke onset to reperfusion, were comparable to those in the EXTEND-IA trial, although initiation of endovascular therapy after initial imaging occurred at a median time of 1 hour rather than 90 minutes. Functional independence (mRS 0–2) at 90 days was nearly double in the interventional group, and that difference was statistically significant with a number needed to treat of 4.

REVASCAT (Endovascular Revascularization with Solitaire Device versus Best Medical Therapy in Anterior Circulation Stroke within 8 Hours) was yet another modern endovascular trial with a design very similar to SWIFT PRIME but conducted in a small homogeneous group of investigators and centers in Spain.[14] There were 206 patients with acute ischemic stroke and an NIHSS score of ≥6 with documented intracranial ICA or MCA stem occlusion; they were randomized to medical management or additional catheter-based reperfusion with retrievable stent, with early enrollment termination due to emerging results of the aforementioned trials. Imaging inclusion criteria included ASPECTS of ≥7 on noncontrast CT or ≥6 on hyperacute MRI. There were several notable elements of REVASCAT trial design: extended time window for intervention of 8 hours (although not as long as the 12-hour window of the ESCAPE trial), an upper age limit of 80 years (with amendment toward the end of enrollment, allowing randomization of 85-year-olds with very favorable ASPECT scores >8), an experienced interventional team, and a prespecified 30-minute waiting period after intravenous thrombolysis to monitor for significant neurological improvement contrary to the enrollment practices of all previously discussed trials. However, despite this artificial delay, median time from initial imaging to the start of intervention was 74 minutes, which was comparable to other modern endovascular trials. Despite the relatively lower recanalization rates of 66%, a favorable outcome of functional independence (mRS of 0–2) at 90 days was reached in 44% in the interventional group and 28% in the control group (adjusted odds ratio [OR] 2.1; 95% CI, 1.1–4.0).[14]

The sixth trial of endovascular therapy for acute ischemic stroke, the Trial and Cost Effectiveness Evaluation of Intra-arterial Thrombectomy in Acute Ischemic Stroke (THRACE) conducted in France, terminated early and published in 2016.[12] There were 414 patients presenting with moderate acute ischemic stroke (NIHSS score 10–25) and confirmed occlusion of intracranial ICA, MCA stem, or superior third of the basilar artery; they were enrolled within 5 hours of symptom onset. Similarly to MR CLEAN, this trial used pragmatic imaging criteria for patient selection. All thrombectomies were done with modern stent retriever or aspiration devices, and the rate of favorable recanalization was nearly 70%, which was within the range of rates reported in the aforementioned trials. Unique to the THRACE trial was the initial limitation of intravenous thrombolysis time window to 3 hours (instead of 4.5 hours as in the previously discussed trial), with a prespecified clinical assessment period after infusion, and a clinical improvement of NIHSS score ≥4 points precluded endovascular therapy. Later in the trial, the intravenous thrombolysis window was increased to 4 hours, and clinical assessment was done during the infusion rather than at its completion in an effort to reduce time to reperfusion to potentially avoid fast responders to intravenous alteplase. THRACE results echoed the findings of previously discussed modern endovascular trials that mechanical thrombectomy is beneficial in improving functional independence in a wide range of patients with large-vessel occlusion of the anterior circulation, although there were no significant differences in 3-month mortality among groups. The other unique feature of THRACE is a prespecified economic analysis of cost effectiveness of endovascular therapy as compared to intravenous reperfusion, which is forthcoming at the time of this writing.[12]

Finally, the last study in the wave of modern reperfusion trials was Trial to Assess the Penumbra System in the Treatment of Acute Stroke (THERAPY).[11] Although the majority of trials discussed earlier primarily or exclusively used stent retriever thrombectomy, THERAPY was an international industry-sponsored PROBE trial, which used pragmatic enrollment criteria, without a requirement of advanced multimodal imaging, to evaluate reperfusion by an aspiration system specifically for the poorest-prognosis patients with a severe clot burden of ≥8 mm. The trial was halted prematurely after 108 patients, following the results from MR CLEAN because providing intravenous tPA alone would plausibly have been unethical, yielding an underpowered sample. Although THERAPY did not achieve its primary endpoint of highlighting improvement in functional independence (mRS 0–2) at 90 days in patients receiving intervention, there was a trend toward benefit.[11]

PATIENT SELECTION

Taken as a whole, the modern catheter-based reperfusion trials established superiority of rapid, early endovascular thrombectomy with second-generation stent retrievers alone or in combination with intravenous thrombolysis over standard care in patients with acute ischemic strokes caused by large-vessel occlusions in the anterior circulation, with a number needed to treat of 3 to 4 to achieve functional independence. In its 2015 focused update to the 2013 guidelines for the management of acute ischemic stroke, the American Stroke Association/American Heart Association (ASA/AHA) concluded that endovascular reperfusion therapy, in combination with intravenous thrombolysis whenever possible, is the new standard of care in appropriate patients.[10] However, what constitutes an ideal endovascular patient is somewhat nebulous given variability in trial design, and we will attempt to analyze selection criteria with respect to age, stroke severity, time windows for reperfusion, imaging selection, location of occlusion, and device choice. It is critical to recognize that more than two-thirds of the patients received intravenous thrombolytic prior to catheter-based therapies per standard of care and that intravenous reperfusion can be administered much more rapidly and should never be delayed in eligible patients while considering endovascular thrombectomy.

Regarding age, most modern trials other than REVASCAT and SWIFT PRIME did not have an upper age limit, although the median age in the interventional groups was 68 (interquartile range of 57–77), and the oldest patient enrolled in MR CLEAN was 96 years of age. Older patients typically developed more severe strokes and worse outcomes, although treatment effect of intervention versus standard of care remained constant over the entire age range in a meta-analysis.[21] On the opposite side of the age spectrum, there are no randomized trials of endovascular therapy enrolling patients <18 years of age, and favorable outcomes are limited to case series subjected to selection bias.[22] Therefore, when it comes to age, it is reasonable to be all inclusive for patients ≥18 years old.

Stroke severity is perhaps the most controversial. All trials selected patients with functional independence prior to the index stroke, and the majority required, at most, a minimal baseline disability (mRS 0–1). The median NIHSS score at enrollment was 17, with an interquartile range of 14 to 20, predominantly reflecting moderate to severe strokes. However, the inclusion NIHSS score varied widely from the lowest in MR CLEAN of 2 to the highest in SWIFT PRIME of 29. EXTEND-IA included patients with any NIHSS score, although it was, by far, the smallest of all the modern endovascular trials. In the 2016 meta-analysis, strokes with NIHSS >10 clearly benefited from intervention, and although statistical significance was lost with NIHSS scores ≤10, there was a trend toward benefit in that milder stroke group.[21] The 2015 ASA/AHA guidelines selected NIHSS score criteria of ≥6, reflecting the prevalence of data; the guidelines also aimed to improve identification of patients with large-vessel occlusion, especially at primary stroke centers, to facilitate appropriate transfers for intervention. However, one-fifth of the patients eligible for intervention may still be mistriaged on the basis of clinical score alone, and thus urgent vessel imaging is very important in identification of large-vessel occlusions, regardless of NIHSS score.[23] At our institution, we apply the pragmatic MR CLEAN criteria and offer endovascular therapy to otherwise appropriate patients with any disabling deficit of NIHSS score ≥2, such as isolated significant aphasia, although stroke severity should be carefully considered in the context of all other selection criteria.

The time window for anterior circulation reperfusion was most commonly set at 6 hours. Although REVASCAT and ESCAPE widened that window to 8 and 7 hours, respectively, the median time to reperfusion across all trials was just over 4.5 hours in the HERMES meta-analysis (interquartile range of 210–362 minutes), and benefits became nonsignificant at just over 7 hours from known time of stroke onset when modern endovascular trial data were analyzed with a specific focus on time to treatment and outcomes.[21,24] Therefore, ASA/AHA stipulated that treatment (groin puncture) should be initiated within 6 hours of symptom onset. However, in carefully selected patients with otherwise favorable criteria and a firm last known normal time, applying the 12-hour window of the ESCAPE trial may be possible. This extended time window may be specifically applicable to patients with unknown time of onset, such as wake-up strokes, which were excluded from the trials.

Assessment of core infarction and collaterals is paramount because it suggests the extent and potential viability of at-risk brain tissue in an individual patient beyond the somewhat arbitrary population-based time windows. Although selection criteria vary with respect to use of perfusion imaging, all modern endovascular trials required at least a noncontrast head CT for a crude assessment of core infarction and vascular imaging for confirmation of large-vessel occlusion. The median ASPECT score was 9 (range 6–10), and most trials enrolled patients with ASPECTS ≥6, representing a population with non-infarcted MCA territory of at least 60%. Beyond the pragmatic criteria, ESCAPE used collateral imaging (multiphase CTA) to select patients with preserved collateral flow in at least half of the MCA territory. EXTEND-IA relied on automated RAPID penumbral imaging, and the same imaging technique was accepted but not required for the bulk of patients in SWIFT PRIME. Although multimodal imaging is a promising technique in individualizing catheter-based interventions, it should be limited to experienced centers, where the time cost of obtaining and interpreting such imaging is minimal. At our institution, we follow the pragmatic approach of MR CLEAN whenever possible and recommend selecting patients with large-vessel occlusion on the basis of ASPECTS ≥6 on a noncontrast head CT. However, we also routinely estimate collateral flow with standard rather than multimodal CTA, adhering to ESCAPE criteria.

Confirmation of large-vessel occlusion was a requirement in all the modern endovascular trials. Here, 90% of enrolled patients had either distal ICA or MCA stem occlusions, and although second-order MCA branches and other vessels (including posterior circulation in some trials) were allowed, they constituted only 10% of the total trial population.[21] In the 2015 guidelines, AHA/ASA concluded that endovascular thrombectomy may be reasonable for carefully selected patients with occlusions of distal MCA, anterior cerebral arteries, or posterior circulation vessels, although the benefits were uncertain for that group.[10]

Device choice is perhaps the most straightforward interventional criterion. More than two-thirds of the patients in the modern endovascular trials received intervention with stent retriever devices, which had double the rate of recanalization compared to the use of first-generation devices. As a result, stent retrievers are recommended as the first-line intervention. The use of an aspiration system for patients with a severe clot burden of ≥8 mm may be reasonable based on THERAPY trial results, although the benefit was implied rather than proven in an underpowered sample population. Finally, although the PROACT II trial established a small but significant benefit of intra-arterial fibrinolysis within a 6-hour window, the trial methodology no longer reflects current practice, including the use of pro-urokinase, which is no longer available.[10]

ENDOVASCULAR INTERVENTION IN THE EXTENDED WINDOW

Recently, two additional modern endovascular trials—DEFUSE 3, and DWI or CTP Assessment with Clinical Mismatch in the Triage of Wake-Up and Late Presenting Strokes Undergoing Neurointervention with Trevo (DAWN)— demonstrated extraordinary efficacy of catheter-based stroke intervention, extending the endovascular reperfusion window to 24 hours from last seen at baseline in select patients, which was reflected in the 2018 update of ASA/AHA guidelines for the management of acute ischemic stroke.[25]

Both trials employed the PROBE design, treated anterior circulation occlusions (M1 and terminal ICA) within 6 to 24 hours from symptom onset in the case of DAWN, and 6 to 16 hours in DEFUSE 3 with modern thrombectomy devices (retrievable stents and aspiration systems), and were halted early due to overwhelming evidence of success in the prespecified interim analyses. The hallmark feature of these trials is the standardized use of perfusion imaging (predominantly RAPID) to identify patients with salvageable brain tissue (Target Mismatch Profile). DAWN trial pre-specified a less than one-third of MCA territory infarction at presentation with clinical-imaging mismatch, and stratified eligible patients into three groups: Two younger age groups ≤80 years old with moderate (NIHSS ≥ 10) and severe (NIHSS ≥ 20) deficits corresponding to core infarctions of ≤30 mL and 31–51 mL, respectively, as well as an older age group (age ≥80) with significant neurological deficit (NIHSS ≥ 10) and a smaller core infarction of ≤20 mL. DEFUSE 3 pre-specified NIHSS ≥ 6, ≤70 mL core infarction (ASPECTS ≥ 6 on initial NCCT), and core/perfusion mismatch ratio of ≥1.8 (mismatch volume of ≥15 mL).

It is important to note that over half of the patients enrolled in these trials were so-called wake-up strokes, with deficits noted on awakening. Although the time last known at baseline puts these patients within the extended window, there is mounting evidence in the literature that these strokes likely occur shortly before presentation, and may in fact be within the "standard" endovascular window. Nevertheless, the outcome in DAWN and DEFUSE 3 is an unprecedented number needed to treat of 2 to 3—among the lowest of all medical treatments—to achieve functional independence at 90 days. Therefore, we recommend that every patient with acute ischemic stroke presenting within the extended window (6–24 hours from last known at baseline) with significant neurological deficits (NIHSS ≥10), ASPECTS ≥6 on initial head CT, and confirmed M1 or ICA occlusion, should be evaluated with perfusion imaging and treated with endovascular therapy when the target mismatch profile is identified in accordance with DAWN and DEFUSE 3 selection criteria.[26,27]

SAFETY OF MODERN ENDOVASCULAR THERAPIES

With respect to safety, risks of symptomatic intracerebral hemorrhage post-intervention in the modern endovascular trials were 4% to 5%, comparable to those in patients receiving the standard of care.[21] Considering that a vast majority of patients in these trials have also received intravenous thrombolysis, catheter-based therapy after thrombolysis is likely safe and considered routine. Large observational studies suggest that hemorrhage risks do not substantially increase in patients receiving thrombolysis while on vitamin K antagonists (with international normalized ratio [INR] ≤1.7) or direct oral anticoagulants.[28,29] Use of IV abciximab appears to increase risk of symptomatic intracranial hemorrhage in the setting of concurrent endovascular mechanical thrombectomy and carotid stenting for acute ischemic stroke.[30] Numerous studies have shown an unfavorable risk–benefit ratio of using full-dose anticoagulation in the setting of acute ischemic stroke, and intravenous anticoagulation should generally be avoided.

Endovascular Intervention in Posterior Circulation Strokes

Despite the wealth of recent data in favor of endovascular reperfusion therapy for large-vessel occlusion in the anterior circulation, evidentiary support for posterior circulation interventions is deficient. Posterior circulation strokes constitute approximately one-fifth of all ischemic stokes.[31–33] Although less frequent, these cerebral infarctions, especially when caused by basilar artery occlusion (BAO) may be even more devastating than anterior circulation infarctions with significant morbidity and mortality.[34] Unfortunately, as expected, patient populations of the modern endovascular trials predominantly reflected anterior circulation, large-vessel occlusions, with inadequate numbers of patients enrolled with vertebrobasilar occlusions to allow for clinically significant assessment of efficacy.

Most treatment strategies directed at managing acute BAO rely on the results from registries, case series, and data extrapolated from stroke interventional trials focused on other cerebrovascular regions. A prospective observational cohort noted high rates of severe disability or mortality nearing 70% in patients with BAO without a statistically significant improvement in outcomes after reperfusion therapy, although trending toward benefit in patients with severe deficits.[34] Although mortality with BAO still remains high at 30%, single-center cohort and meta-analysis suggest that mechanical thrombectomy with a stent retriever for basilar artery occlusion is safe, with symptomatic hemorrhage rates comparable to those of the endovascular arms of the trials discussed earlier in this chapter, and resulted in functional independence in nearly half of the treated patients.[35] In the absence of randomized clinical trial data for the endovascular treatment of posterior circulation stroke, we conclude that catheter-based therapy is a reasonable and safe option for the treatment of BAO, especially considering the high mortality of this disease, and may contribute to improved outcomes.

Medical Management Post-Intervention

Post-procedure management following intravascular mechanical thrombectomy involves the same basic principles of care as those following intravenous thrombolysis for acute ischemic stroke. Key features in post-procedure care include serial and frequent neurologic examinations in an intensive care unit setting, follow-up neuroimaging, continuous ECG monitoring, hemodynamic monitoring and blood pressure control, glycemic control, and temperature control.[36–38] A detailed, baseline neurological exam is paramount, and changes in neurological status (especially decreased arousal and NIHSS score increase of 4 or more points) warrant emergent repeat neuroimaging. Otherwise, routine post-procedural imaging can be repeated within 24 hours with noncontrast head CT or MRI. Post-thrombectomy blood pressure control goals have been largely adapted from intravenous thrombolysis guidelines, with target blood pressure of less than 180/105 following endovascular reperfusion, with further adjustments to be made as necessary given the clinical context.[36] Rapid thrombectomy with sudden restoration of blood flow through more proximal cerebral vessels may increase the risk of reperfusion injury, and additional blood pressure lowering may be warranted in that clinical situation.[39] Cardiac monitoring for at least 24 hours is critical to screen for atrial fibrillation and other cardiac arrhythmias that are frequently associated with acute stroke.[37] Continued evaluation of the groin access site to look for any signs of infection, edema, or hematoma is also important.[36] Finally, glycemic and temperature control remains an intrinsic part of acute stroke care, and it is reasonable to target normoglycemia with a glucose goal of <180 mg/dL and avoid hypoglycemia, as well as address hyperthermia by identifying the source and aggressively treating to a normothermic goal of <38°C.[40]

Prehospital Patient Selection, Triage, and Stroke Systems of Care

Despite the central role of endovascular reperfusion therapy in the new standard of acute ischemic stroke treatment, two major challenges to timely delivery of this therapy persist—namely, identification of appropriate patients and access to care. Accurate identification and triage of stroke patients in the prehospital setting are paramount because direct transfer of patients with suspected large-vessel occlusion to comprehensive stroke centers, or primary stroke centers with continuous endovascular capability, ultimately results in improvement in outcomes.[41] Prehospital and emergency department triage providers in the United States employ multiple structured stroke assessment tools, which are largely oversimplifications of the NIHSS, for the identification and triage of acute stroke patients; chief among them are the Face Arm Speech Test (FAST), Recognition of Stroke in the Emergency Room (ROSIER), Los Angeles Prehospital Stroke Screen (LAPSS), and the Cincinnati Prehospital Stroke Scale (CPSS). Although these scales are reasonably reliable, valid, and reproducible, they show poor performance in identifying patients with posterior circulation strokes and were established prior to the publication of modern endovascular therapy trials.[42-44] Recently, the Cincinnati Prehospital Stroke Severity Scale (CPSSS or C-STAT), Los Angeles Motor Scale (LAMS), and Rapid Arterial Occlusion Evaluation (RACE) have improved assessment of stroke severity and identification of large-vessel occlusion to greater than two-thirds of the patients.[45-47] Another new and promising stroke assessment, VAN (Vision, Aphasia, Neglect), incorporated cortical signs expected to be present with an anterior circulation large-vessel occlusion, and outperformed the NIHSS ≥6 criteria relied upon by most modern endovascular trials, boasting greater than 90% sensitivity and specificity, excellent interobserver reliability, and a high negative predictive value, albeit derived from a small patient sample. This dichotomized scale (deficits are either recorded as present or absent) has an added benefit of being easier to administer.[48] The ASA/AHA has not yet endorsed a singular tool for prehospital identification of large-vessel occlusion.

However, a sizable number of large-vessel occlusions are missed by clinical scales alone.[49,50] Furthermore, imaging-based exclusion of intracranial hemorrhage and confirmation of large-vessel occlusion remain crucial requirements for initiation of reperfusion therapy, which clinical scales cannot displace. Over the past decade, the advent and clinical implementation of mobile stroke units (MSUs)—which are mobile emergency rooms delivering essential brain imaging and point-of-care laboratory testing capabilities, as well as intravenous reperfusion therapy, directly to the emergency site—is a promising novel strategy to speed intravenous thrombolysis and more accurately and appropriately triage patients with large-vessel occlusion to comprehensive stroke centers where catheter-based therapies can be delivered.[50] Prehospital stroke thrombolysis utilizing the MSU concept is not only feasible but also improves treatment rates and substantially reduces treatment delays.[51–53]

For acute stroke patients arriving to primary stroke centers and other healthcare facilities with the capability of intravenous but not catheter-based reperfusion, telemedicine is yet another useful screening tool for identification of patients with potential large-vessel occlusion, and initiation of rapid transport to comprehensive stroke centers for catheter-based salvage therapy. Outcomes are similar among patients reperfused intravenously directly at a stroke center or reperfused with remote supervision and subsequently transported to a regional stroke center.[54] Early experience with telestroke triage for endovascular therapy internationally yielded mixed but largely positive results with respect to outcomes, and times to initiation of intervention were significantly reduced.[55–57] Ultimately, availability of telestroke was paramount in influencing state-based stroke legislation to promote development and advancement of stroke systems of care.[58]

While it is estimated that more than 80% of the U.S. population has geographical access to intravenous reperfusion–capable hospitals within 60 minutes by ground transport, only half of the population has access to endovascular-capable hospitals within that time frame. Access improves significantly when using costly air transport, although timely access to endovascular therapies remains a challenge requiring further optimization of stroke systems in the United States.[59] However, despite the challenges, safe and effective modern endovascular reperfusion therapies have revolutionized the standard of care and forecast a promising future for the treatment of acute ischemic stroke.

References

1. National Institute of Neurological Disorders and Stroke rt-PA Stroke Study Group. Tissue plasminogen activator for acute ischemic stroke. *N Engl J Med*. 1995;333(24): 1581–1587.
2. Hacke W, et al. Thrombolysis with alteplase 3 to 4.5 hours after acute ischemic stroke. *N Engl J Med*. 2008;359(13):1317–1329.
3. Saqqur M, et al. Site of arterial occlusion identified by transcranial Doppler predicts the response to intravenous thrombolysis for stroke. *Stroke*. 2007;38(3):948–954.
4. Albers GW, et al. Intravenous tissue-type plasminogen activator for treatment of acute stroke: the Standard Treatment with Alteplase to Reverse Stroke (STARS) study. *JAMA*. 2000;283(9):1145–1150.

5. Furlan A, et al. Intra-arterial prourokinase for acute ischemic stroke. The PROACT II study: a randomized controlled trial. Prolyse in Acute Cerebral Thromboembolism. *JAMA*. 1999;282(21):2003–2011.

6. Powers WJ. Cerebrovascular diseases: controversies and challenges. *Neurol Clin*. 2015; 33(2):xiii.

7. Broderick JP, et al. Endovascular therapy after intravenous t-PA versus t-PA alone for stroke. *N Engl J Med*. 2013;368(10):893–903.

8. Ciccone A, et al. Endovascular treatment for acute ischemic stroke. *N Engl J Med*. 2013;368(10):904–913.

9. Kidwell CS, et al. A trial of imaging selection and endovascular treatment for ischemic stroke. *N Engl J Med*. 2013;368(10):914–923.

10. Powers WJ, et al. 2015 American Heart Association/American Stroke Association Focused Update of the 2013 Guidelines for the Early Management of Patients with Acute Ischemic Stroke Regarding Endovascular Treatment: A Guideline for Healthcare Professionals from the American Heart Association/American Stroke Association. *Stroke*. 2015;46(10):3020–3035.

11. Mocco J, et al. Aspiration thrombectomy after intravenous alteplase versus intravenous alteplase alone. *Stroke*. 2016;47(9):2331–2338.

12. Bracard S, et al. Mechanical thrombectomy after intravenous alteplase versus alteplase alone after stroke (THRACE): a randomised controlled trial. *Lancet Neurol*. 2016;15(11): 1138–1147.

13. Saver JL, et al. Stent-retriever thrombectomy after intravenous t-PA vs. t-PA alone in stroke. *N Engl J Med*. 2015;372(24):2285–2295.

14. Jovin TG, et al. Thrombectomy within 8 hours after symptom onset in ischemic stroke. *N Engl J Med*. 2015;372(24):2296–2306.

15. Goyal M, et al. Randomized assessment of rapid endovascular treatment of ischemic stroke. *N Engl J Med*. 2015;372(11):1019–1030.

16. Campbell BC, et al. Endovascular therapy for ischemic stroke with perfusion-imaging selection. *N Engl J Med*. 2015;372(11):1009–1018.

17. Berkhemer OA, et al. A randomized trial of intraarterial treatment for acute ischemic stroke. *N Engl J Med*. 2015;372(1):11–20.

18. Fransen PS, et al. Time to reperfusion and treatment effect for acute ischemic stroke: a randomized clinical trial. *JAMA Neurol*. 2016;73(2):190–196.

19. Menon BK, et al. Multiphase CT angiography: a new tool for the imaging triage of patients with acute ischemic stroke. *Radiology*. 2015;275(2):510–520.

20. Hill MD, Goyal M, Demchuk AM. ESCAPE: Endovascular treatment for Small Core and Anterior circulation Proximal occlusion with Emphasis on minimizing CT to recanalization times. URL: http://professional.heart.org/idc/groups/ahamah-public/@wcm/@sop/@scon/documents/downloadable/ucm_471808.pdf. 2015. University of Calgary Cumming School of Medicine.

21. Goyal M, et al. Endovascular thrombectomy after large-vessel ischaemic stroke: a meta-analysis of individual patient data from five randomised trials. *Lancet*. 2016;387(10029): 1723–1731.

22. Satti S, et al. Mechanical thrombectomy for pediatric acute ischemic stroke: review of the literature. *J Neurointerv Surg*. 2016.

23. Heldner MR, et al. Clinical prediction of large vessel occlusion in anterior circulation stroke: mission impossible? *J Neurol*. 2016;263(8):1633–1640.

24. Saver JL, et al. Time to treatment with endovascular thrombectomy and outcomes from ischemic stroke: a meta-analysis. *JAMA*. 2016;316(12):1279–1288.

25. Powers WJ, Rabinstein AA, Ackerson T, et al. 2018 Guidelines for the early management of patient with acute ischemic stroke: a guideline for healthcare professionals from the American Heart Association/American Stroke Association, http://stroke.ahajournals.org /content/early/2018/01/23/STR.0000000000000158. *Stroke.* 49(3):509–551.

26. Nogueira RG, Jadhav AP, Haussen DC, et al. for the DAWN Trial Investigators. Thrombectomy 6 to 24 hours after stroke with a mismatch between deficit and infarct. *N Engl J Med.* 2018; 378:11–21.

27. Albers GW, Marks MP, Kemp S, et al. for the DEFUSE 3 Investigators. Thrombectomy for stroke at 6 to 16 hours with selection by perfusion imaging. *N Engl J Med.* 2018; 378:708–718.

28. Xian Y, et al., Risks of intracranial hemorrhage among patients with acute ischemic stroke receiving warfarin and treated with intravenous tissue plasminogen activator. *JAMA.* 2012;307(24):2600–2608.

29. Seiffge DJ, et al. Recanalization therapies in acute ischemic stroke patients: impact of prior treatment with novel oral anticoagulants on bleeding complications and outcome. *Circulation.* 2015;132(13):1261–1269.

30. Heck DV, Brown MD. Carotid stenting and intracranial thrombectomy for treatment of acute stroke due to tandem occlusions with aggressive antiplatelet therapy may be associated with a high incidence of intracranial hemorrhage. *J Neurointerv Surg.* 2015;7(3):170–175.

31. Gulli G, et al. Stroke risk after posterior circulation stroke/transient ischemic attack and its relationship to site of vertebrobasilar stenosis: pooled data analysis from prospective studies. *Stroke.* 2013;44(3):598–604.

32. Labropoulos N, Nandivada P, Bekelis K. Stroke of the posterior cerebral circulation. *Int Angiol.* 2011;30(2):105–114.

33. Nouh,A, Remke J, Ruland S. Ischemic posterior circulation stroke: a review of anatomy, clinical presentations, diagnosis, and current management. *Front Neurol.* 2014;5:30.

34. Schonewille WJ, et al. Treatment and outcomes of acute basilar artery occlusion in the Basilar Artery International Cooperation Study (BASICS): a prospective registry study. *Lancet Neurol.* 2009;8(8):724–730.

35. Gory B, Eldesouky I, Sivan-Hoffmann R, et al. Outcomes of stent retriever thrombectomy in basilar artery occlusion: an observational study and systematic review. *J Neurol Neurosurg Psychiatry.* 2016 May;87(5):520–525.

36. Lazzaro MA, et al. Developing practice recommendations for endovascular revascularization for acute ischemic stroke. *Neurology.* 2012;79(13 Suppl 1):S243-S255.

37. Froehler MT, Geocadin RG. Postprocedure intensive care management of stroke patients appropriate postprocedure management improves outcomes in stroke patients. *Endovascular Today.* 2007 May 19;6(9):81–84.

38. Willinsky RA, et al. Neurologic complications of cerebral angiography: prospective analysis of 2,899 procedures and review of the literature. *Radiology.* 2003;227(2):522–528.

39. Moulakakis KG, et al. Hyperperfusion syndrome after carotid revascularization. *J Vasc Surg.* 2009;49(4):1060–1068.

40. Mohlenbruch M, et al. Mechanical thrombectomy with stent retrievers in acute basilar artery occlusion. *AJNR Am J Neuroradiol.* 2014;35(5):959–564.

41. Mohamad NF, Hastrup S, Rasmussen M, et al. Bypassing primary stroke centre reduces delay and improves outcomes for patients with large vessel occlusion. *Eur Stroke J.* 2016; 1:85–92.

42. Nor AM, McAllister C, Louw SJ, et al. Agreement between ambulance paramedic- and physician-recorded neurological signs with Face Arm Speech Test (FAST) in acute stroke patients. *Stroke.* 2004;35(6):1355.

43. Kothari RU, Pancioli A, Liu T, et al. Cincinnati Prehospital Stroke Scale: reproducibility and validity. *Ann Emerg Med*. 1999;33(4):373.
44. Kidwell CS, Starkman S, Eckstein M, et al. Identifying stroke in the field. Prospective validation of the Los Angeles prehospital stroke screen (LAPSS). *Stroke*. 2000;31(1):71.
45. Katz BS, McMullan JT, Sucharew H, et al. Design and validation of a prehospital scale to predict stroke severity: Cincinnati Prehospital Stroke Severity Scale. *Stroke*. 2015 Jun;46(6):1508–1512.
46. Llanes JN, Kidwell CS, Starkman S, et al. The Los Angeles Motor Scale (LAMS): a new measure to characterize stroke severity in the field. *Prehosp Emerg Care*. 2004 Jan-Mar;8(1): 46–50.
47. Pérez de la Ossa N, Carrera D, Gorchs M, et al. Design and validation of a prehospital stroke scale to predict large arterial occlusion: the rapid arterial occlusion evaluation scale. *Stroke*. 2014 Jan;45(1):87–91.
48. Heldner MR, Hsieh K, Broeg-Morvay A, et al. Clinical prediction of large vessel occlusion in anterior circulation stroke: mission impossible? *J Neurol*. 2016;263:1633–1640.
49. Teleb MS, Ver Hage A, Carter J, et al. Stroke vision, aphasia, neglect (VAN) assessment—a novel emergent large vessel occlusion screening tool: pilot study and comparison with current clinical severity indices. *J NeuroIntervent Surg*. 2017;9:122–126.
50. Turc G, Maier B, Naggara O, et al. Clinical scales do not reliably identify acute ischemic stroke patients with large-artery occlusion. *Stroke*. 2016;47:1466–1472.
51. Walter S, Kostopoulos P, Haass A, et al. Bringing the hospital to the patient: first treatment of stroke patients at the emergency site. *PLoS ONE*. 2010;5:e13758.
52. Ebinger M, Winter B, Wendt M, et al. Effect of the use of ambulance-based thrombolysis on time to thrombolysis in acute ischemic stroke: a randomized clinical trial. *JAMA*. 2014;311:1622–1631.
53. Bowry R, Parker S, Rajan SS, et al. Benefits of stroke treatment using a mobile stroke unit compared with standard management: the BEST-MSU study run-in phase. *Stroke*. 2015;46:3370–3374.
54. Pervez MA, Silva G, Masrur S, et al. Remote supervision of IV-tPA for acute ischemic stroke by telemedicine or telephone before transfer to a regional stroke center is feasible and safe. *Stroke*. 2010;41:e18–e24.
55. Pfefferkorn T, Holtmannspötter M, Schmidt C, et al. Drip, ship, and retrieve: cooperative recanalization therapy in acute basilar artery occlusion. *Stroke*. 2010;41:722–726.
56. Pedragosa A, Alvarez-Sabín J, Rubiera M, et al. Impact of telemedicine on acute management of stroke patients undergoing endovascular procedures. *Cerebrovasc Dis*. 2012;34:436–442.
57. Kepplinger J, Dzialowski I, Barlinn K, et al. Emergency transfer of acute stroke patients within the East Saxony telemedicine stroke network: a descriptive analysis. *Int J Stroke*. 2014;9:160–165.
58. Silva GS, Schwamm LH. Use of telemedicine and other strategies to increase the number of patients that may be treated with intravenous thrombolysis. *Curr Neurol Neurosci Rep*. 2012;12:10–16.
59. Adeoye O, Albright KC, Carr BG, et al. Geographic access to acute stroke care in the United States. *Stroke*. 2014;45:3019–3024.

Critical Care Management of Ischemic Stroke

Christina Mijalski Sells and Linda C. Wendell

Ischemic stroke can be a devastating disease, and therapies such as tissue plasminogen activator (tPA) and endovascular therapy can significantly decrease permanent disability. However, acute ischemic stroke patients can be at risk for both medical and neurological complications and poor out-comes. The following discussion will explore specific medical and neurological considerations for optimal management of patients with acute ischemic stroke.

MEDICAL MANAGEMENT

Blood Pressure Management

Hypertension has an important role in the setting of ischemic stroke and should be monitored closely. There are allowances made permitting elevated blood pressure (BP) in the setting of acute ischemic stroke with the goal of optimizing cerebral perfusion of penumbra; however, strong evidence is lacking.[1] Further, patients who received thrombolytic therapy have specific BP goals.

When patients are candidates for IV thrombolysis, one of the contraindications to the administration of tPA is a BP >185/110 mm Hg. Hypertension should be treated in order to administer tPA safely. Intravenous labetalol and nicardipine infusion can both be considered to control blood pressure. After the administration of IV tPA, the BP goal is less than 180/105 mm Hg for at least the first 24 hours.[1] A retrospective analysis showed an increase in symptomatic intracerebral hemorrhage after tPA with a pretreatment blood pressure greater than 185/110 mm Hg.[2]

While there have been some studies that demonstrate a benefit in the early lowering of BP after acute strokes, larger randomized trials have found data to support that early and aggressive lowering of blood pressure after acute stroke can lead to worse outcomes.[3-6] A post hoc analysis of National Institute of Neurological Disorders and Stroke (NINDS) data found worse outcomes at 3 months among patients who had a systolic BP reduction greater than 30 mm Hg from baseline and increased risk of death in patients who had more than a 60 mm Hg decline in systolic BP.[4] A nonsignificant trend toward increased risk of poor outcomes has also been shown with acute lowering of BP in stroke patients.[5] In the setting of patients presenting with an acute ischemic stroke who are not eligible for thrombolytic or endovascular treatment, hypertension up to 220/120 mm Hg may be permitted with the goal of perfusing the surrounding penumbra.[4] The current recommendations suggest that allowing hypertension without correction within the first 24 hours after an ischemic stroke may be beneficial unless it will be harmful in the setting of specific medical comorbidities such as acute myocardial infarction.[1]

Patients with a perfusion-dependent exam may require BP augmentation using vasopressors, typically phenylephrine. Several small studies have shown raising the BP by 20% above the patient's baseline can be done safely with improvement in the patient's neurologic symptoms.[7-9] Patients who may benefit the most are those with severe stenosis or occlusion of the middle cerebral artery (MCA) or distal internal carotid artery.[9] Patients with recurrent neurologic deficits due to hypoperfusion should be considered for surgical or endovascular revascularization.[10,11]

Glycemic Control

Blood glucose is an important consideration in the management of stroke because severe hypoglycemia can compromise brain tissue.[1] Blood glucose less than 57 mg/dL can cause autonomic symptoms and, when less than 47 mg/dL, can manifest as severe neurologic dysfunction. In the setting of an acute stroke, suspected blood glucose less than 60 mg/dL should be treated to rule out a possible stroke mimic or exacerbation of stroke symptoms. Hypoglycemia may further compromise brain tissue in the setting of acute stroke by limiting the energy supply to already ischemic tissue. Alternatively, hyperglycemia may exacerbate stroke by predisposing to acidosis and the formation of reactive oxygen species and an amplified inflammatory reaction to ischemia.[12] Hyperglycemia has also been associated with increased odds of hemorrhagic transformation—specifically, parenchymal hematoma, which has an increased risk of disability and death.[13] A recent Cochrane Review on glycemic control in acute ischemic stroke supported that aggressive control of hyperglycemia within hours of ischemic stroke does not confer any benefit to patients. Among patients in whom a narrow level of blood glucose was maintained, there were more symptomatic and asymptomatic hypoglycemic events.[14] Targeting specific glucose levels after stroke is not needed, but hypoglycemia and hyperglycemia should be avoided.[1,13]

Hemoglobin Goals

Anemia has been described as having a similar effect on brain tissue as hypoglycemia or hypoxia. This condition deprives transport of energy and nutrients that may predispose penumbra to further injury in the setting of an acute stroke. A retrospective analysis found that anemia is more common in stroke patients compared to controls; it is associated with greater frequency and severity of comorbidities and independently predicts increased morbidity and mortality from 7 days to 12 months after the occurrence of a stroke.[15] Lower hemoglobin concentration is also associated with severity of stroke.[16] While there are no formal guidelines for hemoglobin goals in neurologically injured patients, it is reasonable to extrapolate data from a critical care study of medically ill patients in the Transfusion Reactions in Critical Care (TRICC) trial. In this trial, critically ill patients were randomly assigned to groups where they would receive a transfusion if the hemoglobin fell below 7 g/dL versus 10 g/dL. While there was a similar mortality between the two groups at 30 days, in-hospital mortality was significantly less among patients transfused only if hemoglobin fell below 7 g/dL ($p = 0.05$).[17]

Albumin Therapy

Albumin was first studied in the setting of acute ischemic stroke as a potential neuroprotectant, with the goal of decreasing permanent damage to ischemic neurons by modulating oxidative stress. High-dose albumin treatment was studied in patients with acute ischemic stroke. Patients who received albumin were more likely to develop pulmonary edema or congestive heart failure within 48 hours compared to those who only received normal saline, 13% versus 1% (ratio rate [RR] 10.8, confidence interval [CI] 4.37–26.72). Patients who received albumin also had a higher rate of symptomatic intracranial hemorrhage, 4% versus 2% (RR 2.42, CI 1.02–5.78). This trial was terminated early due to medical futility as well as these harmful effects.[18] At this time, albumin is considered ineffective for the treatment of stroke and is potentially harmful, which is also reflected in the 2013 Guidelines for the Early Management of Patients with Acute Ischemic Stroke.[1,19]

Temperature Goals

Temperature has many effects on the brain and its metabolism. There are several studies that have linked hyperthermia to poor outcomes in stroke patients. Increased permeability of the blood–brain barrier (BBB) with hyperthermia predisposes to cerebral edema. Similar to effects of blood glucose, hyperthermia can increase the brain's metabolism, thereby decreasing available oxygen and increasing reactive oxygen species, which may perpetuate injury.[20] Because hyperthermia is an independent risk factor for poor outcome and is associated with increased mortality, normothermia is recommended in the setting of acute stroke.[21,22] Normothermia can be maintained with either acetylsalicylic acid or acetaminophen in patients to a temperature less than 38°C.[23] For those who fail antipyretic medications, a surface cooling blanket or endovascular cooling can be considered to maintain normothermia.[24]

Early Tracheostomy

The American Heart Association recommends that patients with recent stroke or cardiac arrest maintain an oxygen saturation greater than 94%.[1,25] Patients with severe stroke are at increased risk of airway compromise due to neurologic deficits, including impaired consciousness and weakness of bulbar and respiratory muscles. Many of these patients will need ventilator support, and there has been some debate regarding the appropriate time for tracheostomy. Primary neurologically injured patients have unique deficits that may predispose to higher rates of failure of extubation, including compromised alertness and awareness. Prior studies have demonstrated extubation failure rates of 5% to 20%; however, this may be greater in patients who have suffered neurological injury.[26] Further, traditional weaning parameters in neurocritical care patients are not reliable predictors of extubation.[27] Therefore, if patients are not able to extubate safely, a proactive approach should be taken due to risk of prolonged intubation.

Early tracheostomy in stroke patients may decrease morbidity. Stroke patients needing prolonged ventilatory support are more likely to experience pulmonary complications before tracheostomy. Patients who undergo early tracheostomy have shorter hospital stays and decreased risk of developing ventilator-associated pneumonia.[28,29] A prospective randomized controlled trial also showed a decrease in mortality and use of sedation in patients undergoing early tracheostomy. Generalization of findings from this trial is limited, however, due to a small sample size.[30] If a patient will require prolonged ventilator support, tracheostomy within the first 10 days should be considered and may avoid infections and prolonged hospital stays.

MANAGEMENT OF NEUROLOGIC COMPLICATIONS

Hemorrhage Following Ischemic Stroke

Ischemic stroke results from a disruption in the local blood-brain barrier, which can also predispose to hemorrhage within the damaged tissue.[31] Hemorrhage after stroke can be subdivided into *hemorrhagic infarction* (HI) and *parenchymal hemorrhage* (PH), each having different hypothesized mechanisms and clinical implications. In the European Cooperative Acute Stroke Study (ECASS) trials, HI was defined as hemorrhage within the margins of an infarct and further classified by small petechiae along the margins (HI1) or confluent petechiae without mass effect (HI2). Alternatively, PH was defined as a hematoma with some mass effect, less than or equal to 30% of the infarct with minimal mass effect (PH1) or more than 30% of the infarction with significant mass effect (PH2).[32,33] Risk of hemorrhage after ischemic stroke is influenced by location and extent of ischemic tissue, age, premorbid medications, blood pressure, body temperature, blood glucose, treatment with tPA, and endovascular intervention.[34]

Newer studies are showing that there may also be some genetic component associated with hemorrhagic transformation after ischemic stroke. The expression of certain proteins may exhibit a neuroprotective effect and decrease the likelihood of this complication.[35] Researchers are also studying possible biomarkers to stratify risk further. There may be an association between levels of neuron-specific enolase (NSE) and hemorrhagic transformation as well as incidence of atrial fibrillation.[36] Future studies are needed, but this association may have important implications for monitoring patients.

Patients who receive tPA are required to have a noncontrast head CT prior to treatment in order to ensure the absence of hemorrhage. In addition, tPA protocol requires that patients also receive a 24-hour post-tPA surveillance scan to evaluate for any hemorrhagic transformation (HT) before proceeding with antiplatelet or anticoagulant therapy. In addition to the predictors of hemorrhage mentioned earlier in the section, initial CT scan within 5 hours of symptom onset with a focal hypodensity has been shown to be predictive of HT. In a case series, hypodensity was associated with eventual HT in 77% of patients (95% CI, 68%–86%) and the absence of a hypodensity correlated with absence of HT in 94% of patients (95% CI, 89%–99%).[37] This finding is an important consideration in early management of acute stroke, and some centers have taken this into further consideration as a determinant for eligibility for endovascular treatment using Alberta Stroke Program Early CT Score (ASPECTS) imaging tool.[34]

Medical Management of Cerebral Edema

There are generally two classifications of cerebral edema: vasogenic and cytotoxic. *Vasogenic edema* refers to fluid that accumulates around cells as a result of disruption of the blood–brain barrier. *Cytotoxic edema* describes fluid that accumulates within cells secondary to injury, most often associated with ischemic stroke.[38] During ischemic stroke, there is a failure of transportation systems on the cellular level, resulting in fluid accumulation within cells. Later in the ischemic process, reactive oxygen species are released and can affect the cerebral capillaries, leading to compromise of the blood vessel walls and, therefore, the BBB. This process may also lead to a secondary vasogenic edema.[39]

Neurologic deterioration after ischemic stroke may occur in up to 20% to 40% of patients after ischemic stroke. Data from the ECASS found that 38% of patients with acute ischemic stroke experienced early worsening in the first 24 hours, and 20% of patients experienced later worsening between 24 hours and 7 days. When decline in neurologic function occurs secondary to brain edema, it most often occurs between days 2 and 5 after the initial ischemic event and can be a significant predictor of morbidity and mortality.[40,41] Specifically, the time to maximum cytotoxic edema after stroke is usually between 24 and 72 hours after ictus.[39] The most common manifestations of cerebral edema after stroke include increased drowsiness, decreased pupillary responses, and a change in breathing pattern. Drowsiness is most likely to occur 1 to 4 days after ischemic stroke and often preceded the onset of the aforementioned physical exam findings by only hours.[42]

Several studies have examined predictors of poor outcome in the setting of cerebral edema after ischemic stroke. Consistent findings include large stroke volume of greater than half of the MCA territory, observable clot in the MCA on CT, severe motor deficits, older age, nausea, vomiting, elevated systolic BP (greater than 180 mm Hg), and poor respiratory status.[41,43] Patients with large MCA territory infarcts are at greatest risk for cerebral edema after stroke, and mortality secondary to herniation may approach 80%.[44]

General recommendations for the treatment of cerebral edema are similar to management of elevated intracranial pressure (ICP) from other causes. Specific therapies include maintaining adequate analgesia and sedation in order to minimize the metabolic demand of the brain, decreasing stress, and sympathetic responses to pain and mechanical ventilation.[45] The occurrence of fever and seizures may have a significant impact on metabolic demand and should be urgently treated. Increased ICP can also be mitigated by optimizing cerebral venous draining in keeping the head above the heart, usually 30 degrees, and maintaining blood pressure for a cerebral perfusion pressure (CPP) goal greater than 60 mm Hg.[46]

It is important to institute close monitoring of patients at risk for cerebral edema with frequent neurological checks so that these signs and symptoms can be recognized in a timely fashion. It is advisable to monitor high-risk patients in a stroke unit or intensive care setting in order to initiate the appropriate interventions.

Osmotherapy is the mainstay for the treatment of cerebral edema. Mannitol and hypertonic saline are recommended for the treatment of elevated ICP due to cerebral edema (Table 8.1). There is no class I evidence comparing the two;

TABLE 8.1 Use of hypertonic saline and mannitol for the management of cerebral edema

	Mannitol	Hypertonic saline
Dosing	0.25 g/kg/dose to 1 g/kg/dose IV bolus over 1 min to 30 min	Different concentrations available as boluses or infusion
	May be given repeatedly every 4 h to 8 h	3% dosing: Initial infusion at 1 mL/kg/h to 2 mL/kg/h, 250 mL bolus over 30 min may be administered
		Bolus can be repeated after 30 min
		23% dosing for refractory elevated intracranial pressure (ICP): 30 mL to 60 mL IV given over 2 min to 20 min
		Bolus can be repeated after 15 min
Recommended maximum dosing	2 g/kg/dose	3%: 1 mEq/kg/h = 1.9 mL/kg/h
		23.4%: May be repeated in 6 h if target sodium level not met
Route	Peripheral IV or central IV	Central IV
Onset of action	Diuretic effect 1 h to 3 h Reduction of ICP 15 min	Rapid
Duration of action	Diuretic effect 4 h to 6 h Reduction of ICP 3 h to 8 h	2 h to 6 h
Targets	ICP, radiographic midline shift, clinical examination	ICP, radiographic midline shift, clinical examination
Monitoring	1. Follow osmolar gap (goal <20 before next dose)	Prespecified sodium ranges (e.g., 150 mEq/L to 160 mEq/L)
	2. Achieve hypernatremia (without systemic hypovolemia)	Avoid exceeding 160 mEq/L
	3. Blood urea nitrogen/creatinine	
Advantages	1. Rapid effect in reducing ICP even before the onset of osmotic diuresis	1. 30 mL bolus of 23.4% has an immediate effect on ICP reduction
	2. No need for central venous access	2. High-throughput screening permeability coefficient 1 vs. 0.9 for mannitol (intact blood–brain barrier [BBB])
		3. Volume expander
		4. Positive inotropy
		5. Mixed immunomodulatory results
Disadvantages	1. Could lead to reduction of intravascular volume and compromise of mean arterial pressure and cerebral perfusion pressure	1. Hypervolemia and pulmonary edema

(continued)

TABLE 8.1 Use of hypertonic saline and mannitol for the management of cerebral edema (*continued*)

	Mannitol	Hypertonic saline
	2. Impaired clearance can lead to nephrotoxicity	2. Hyperchloremic metabolic acidosis (consider 50:50 solutions with sodium acetate)
	3. Accumulation into injured brain via disrupted BBB and rebound edema	3. Accumulation into injured brain via disrupted BBB and rebound edema
		4. Hyperoncotic hemolysis
		5. Requires central venous access (peripheral administration may lead to vein sclerosis)
		6. Bolus administration (especially 23.4%) can lead to transient hypotension
		7. Mixed immunomodulatory results
Maximum serum osmolality	330 mOsm/kg	60 mOsm/kg
Effectiveness	May cause tolerance with repeated administration	Effective after repeated administration and when tolerance of mannitol has occurred
		Beneficial as a rescue therapy to induce hyperosmolality rapidly
Change in mean arterial pressure	Moderate increase initially	Greater, more prolonged
Diuretic effect	Osmotic diuretic, may necessitate volume replacement to avoid hypovolemia and hypotension	Diuresis through the stimulation of atrial natriuretic peptide release
Other suggested interactions	Antioxidant effects	Restoration of resting membrane potential and cell volume, inhibition of inflammation
Cautions	Transient volume overload, pulmonary edema, osmotic nephrosis, congestive heart failure, hypertension, sodium depletion, electrolyte abnormalities, acidosis, increased cerebral blood flow, and risk of postoperative bleeding	1. Hypotension (infusion related)
		2. Thrombophlebitis tissue necrosis if extravasated
		3. Rebound ICP elevated, central pontine myelinolysis, coagulopathy (bleeding), electrolyte abnormalities (hypokalemia, hyperchloremia, hypernatremia), metabolic acidosis, congestive heart failure, and pulmonary edema

Source: Adapted from Reference 49.

however, each has advantages and disadvantages depending on the specific patient. Hypertonic saline has an immediate effect on ICP reduction and can also exercise positive inotropic effects. Administration of 23.4% hypertonic saline is associated with a decrease in ICP by more than 50% and a reversal of transtentorial herniation.[47,48] Hypertonic saline has less tachyphylaxis compared to mannitol, but it has additional risks such as hypotension if administered rapidly, thrombophlebitis in tissue extravasation, and the requirement of central venous access. Alternatively, mannitol also has a rapid effect without the need for central access, but it can be nephrotoxic in the setting of kidney injury. Impaired clearance may build tolerability with repeated administration and cause hypotension via volume depletion and diuretic effects.[49] Recommendations for monitoring mannitol include a goal of less than 330 mOsm/L and an osmolar gap of less than 20 before administering a second dose. Hypertonic saline may be used for goal serum sodium ranging from 140 to 160 mEq/L; however, the serum sodium should not exceed 160 mEq/L.

A meta-analysis evaluating mannitol versus hypertonic saline for the treatment of cerebral edema and elevated ICP demonstrated that hypertonic saline was more effective in decreasing ICP by an average of 2 mm Hg. This study was able to show efficacy but did not evaluate data on patient outcomes.[50] Prospective data on patients treated with mannitol for cerebral edema found that severe hypernatremia (greater than 160 mEq/L) was associated with an increased mortality.[51] There was also an increased incidence of mechanical ventilation and renal failure.

Glucocorticoids are not recommended for the treatment of cytotoxic cerebral edema and elevated ICP after ischemic stroke. A Cochrane Review demonstrated that treatment with glucocorticoids does not improve patient outcome. Hyperglycemia, infection, and gastrointestinal bleeds were among the reported complications.[52]

Surgical Management of Cerebral Edema

The Monro-Kellie hypothesis states that the intracranial space is incompressible and contains a fixed volume. The primary contents of the cranium include brain parenchyma, cerebral spinal fluid, and blood that may shift to accommodate additional volume. In the setting of severe cerebral edema that cannot be physiologically compensated by these measures, decompressive craniectomy to alter the fixed space may be lifesaving.

A planned pooled analysis from three trials evaluating decompressive hemicraniectomy (DHC) in malignant MCA infarcts found that DHC within 48 hours had a 50% risk reduction in mortality, and patients were more likely to have a modified Rankin score (mRS) of 0 to 4 compared to the control group (51% absolute risk reduction). Further, patients in the surgical group were more likely to have an mRS of 0 to 3 compared to those conservatively managed (43% vs. 21%, respectively).[53] In patients over 60 years of age, DHC also has a survival benefit (decrease in mortality from 70% to 33%), but most patients who survive have an mRS of 4 or 5 (severe disability requiring assistance with bodily needs). The decision for DHC should be made on an individual basis dependent on acceptable quality of life to the patient.

CONCLUSIONS

Treatment of ischemic stroke is complex; however, the data are growing to help guide optimal therapy. It is important that acute treatment of stroke include considerations of general medical critical care and neurocritical care to provide patients with the best possible outcomes.

References

1. Jauch EC, Saver JL, Adams HP Jr, et al. Guidelines for the early management of patients with acute ischemic stroke: a guideline for healthcare professionals from the American Heart Association/American Stroke Association. *Stroke.* 2013;44:870–947.
2. Georgios Tsivgoulis, Frey JL, Flaster M, et al. Pre–tissue plasminogen activator blood pressure levels and risk of symptomatic intracerebral hemorrhage. *Stroke* 2009: 3631–3634.
3. Potter JF, Robinson TG, Ford GA, et al. Controlling hypertension and hypotension immediately post-stroke (CHHIPS): a randomised, placebo-controlled, double-blind pilot trial. *Lancet Neurol.* 2009:48–56.
4. Silver B, Lu M, Morris DC, et al. Blood pressure declines and less favorable outcomes in the NINDS tPA stroke study. *J Neurol Sci.* 2008:61–67.
5. Sandset EC, Bath PM, Boysen G, et al. The angiotensin-receptor blocker candesartan for treatment of acute stroke (SCAST): a randomised, placebo-controlled, double-blind trial. *Lancet.* 2011:741–750.
6. Robinson TG, Potter JF, Ford GA, et al. Effects of antihypertensive treatment after acute stroke in the Continue Or Stop post-Stroke Antihypertensives Collaborative Study (COSSACS): a prospective, randomised, open, blinded-endpoint trial. *Lancet Neurol.* 2010: 767–775.
7. Rordorf G, Koroshetz WJ, Ezzeddine MA, et al. A pilot study of drug-induced hypertension for treatment of acute stroke. *Neurology.* 2001;56:1210–1213.
8. Koenig MA, Geocadin RG, de Grouchy M, et al. Safety of induced hypertension therapy in patients with acute ischemic stroke. *Neurocrit Care.* 2006;4:3–7.
9. Hillis AE, Ulatowski JA, Barker PB, et al. A pilot randomized trial of induced blood pressure elevation: effects on function and focal perfusion in acute and subacute stroke. *Cerebrovasc Dis.* 2003;16:236–246.
10. Klopfenstein JD, Ponce FA, Kim LJ, et al. Middle cerebral artery stenosis: endovascular and surgical options. *Skull Base.* 2005;15:175–189.
11. Romero JR, Pikula A, Nguyen TN, et al. Cerebral collateral circulation in carotid artery disease. *Curr Cardiol Rev.* 2009;5:279–288.

12. Robbins NM. Opposing Effects of glucose on stroke and reperfusion injury acidosis, oxidative stress, and energy metabolism. *Stroke*. 2014:1881–1886.

13. Paciaroni M, Agnelli G, Caso V, et al. Acute hyperglycemia and early hemorrhagic transformation in ischemic stroke. *Cerebrovasc Dis*. 2009;28:119–123.

14. Bellolio MF, Gilmore RM, Ganti L. Insulin for glycaemic control in acute ischaemic stroke (Review). *Cochrane Database Syst Rev*. 2014. Jan. 23;(1):CD005346.

15. Milionis H, Papavasileiou V, Eskandari A, et al. Anemia on admission predicts short- and long-term outcomes in patients with acute ischemic stroke. *Int J Stroke*. 2015;10:224–230.

16. Bill O, Zufferey P, Faouzi M, et al. Severe stroke: patient profile and predictors of favorable outcome. *J Thromb Haemost*. 2013;11:92–99.

17. Hébert PC, Wells G, Blajchman MA, et al. A multicenter, randomized, controlled clinical trial of transfusion requirements in critical care. *N Engl J Med*. 1999;340:409–417.

18. Ginsberg MD, Palesch YY, Hill MD, et al. High-dose albumin treatment for acute ischaemic stroke (ALIAS) part 2: a randomised, double-blind, phase 3, placebo-controlled trial. *Lancet Neurol*. 2013;12:1049–1058.

19. Bath PMW. Albumin for hyperacute stroke: another failed neuroprotectant. *Lancet Neurol*. 2013;12:1036–1037.

20. Wang H, Wang B, Normoyle KP, et al. Brain temperature and its fundamental properties: a review for clinical neuroscientists. *Front Neurosci*. 2014;8:307.

21. Azzimondi G, Bassein L, Nonino F, et al. Fever in acute stroke worsens prognosis. A prospective study. *Stroke*. 1995;26:2040–2043.

22. Hajat C, Hajat S, Sharma P. Effects of poststroke pyrexia on stroke outcome: a meta-analysis of studies in patients. *Stroke*. 2000;31:410–414.

23. Sulter G, Elting JW, Maurits N, et al. Acetylsalicylic acid and acetaminophen to combat elevated body temperature in acute ischemic stroke. *Cerebrovasc Dis*. 2004;17:118–122.

24. Wrotek SE, Kozak WE, Hess DC, Fagan SC. Treatment of fever after stroke: conflicting evidence. *Pharmacotherapy*. 2011;31:1085–1091.

25. Peberdy MA, Callaway CW, Neumar RW, et al. Part 9: post-cardiac arrest care: 2010 American Heart Association Guidelines for Cardiopulmonary Resuscitation and Emergency Cardiovascular Care. *Circulation*. 2010;122:S768–786.

26. King CS, Moores LK, Epstein SK. Should patients be able to follow commands prior to extubation? *Respir Care*. 2010;55:56–62.

27. Ko R, Ramos L, Chalela JA. Conventional weaning parameters do not predict extubation failure in neurocritical care patients. *Neurocrit Care*. 2009;10:269–273.

28. Rabinstein AA, Wijdicks EFM. Outcome of survivors of acute stroke who require prolonged ventilatory assistance and tracheostomy. *Cerebrovasc Dis*. 2004;18:325–331.

29. Villwock JA, Villwock MR, Deshaies EM. Tracheostomy timing affects stroke recovery. *J Stroke Cerebrovasc Dis*. 2014;23:1069–1072.

30. Bösel J, Schiller P, Hook Y, et al. Stroke-related Early Tracheostomy versus Prolonged Orotracheal Intubation in Neurocritical Care Trial (SETPOINT): a randomized pilot trial. *Stroke*. 2013;44:21–28.

31. Wang X, Lo EH. Triggers and mediators of hemorrhagic transformation in cerebral ischemia. *Mol Neurobiol*. 2003;28:229–244.

32. Hacke W, Fieschi C, Toni D, et al. Intravenous thrombolysis with recombinant tissue plasminogen activator for acute hemispheric stroke. The European Cooperative Acute Stroke Study (ECASS). *JAMA*. 1995;274:1017–1025.

33. Hacke W, Kaste M, Fieschi C, et al. Randomised double-blind placebo-controlled trial of thrombolytic therapy with intravenous alteplase in acute ischaemic stroke (ECASS II). Second European-Australasian Acute Stroke Study Investigators. *Lancet*. 1998;352:1245–1251.

34. Álvarez-Sabín J, Maisterra O, Santamarina E, et al. Factors influencing haemorrhagic transformation in ischaemic stroke. *Lancet Neurol.* 2013;12:689–705.

35. Mallolas J, Rodríguez R, Gubern C, et al. A polymorphism in the promoter region of the survivin gene is related to hemorrhagic transformation in patients with acute ischemic stroke. *Neuromol Med.* 2014;16:856–861.

36. Kim BJ, Kim YJ, Ahn SH, et al. The second elevation of neuron-specific enolase peak after ischemic stroke is associated with hemorrhagic transformation. *J Stroke Cerebrovasc Dis.* 2014;23:2437–2443.

37. Toni D, Fiorelli M, Bastianello S, et al. Predictability in the first 5 hours from stroke onset and influence on clinical outcome. *Neurology.* 1996;46:341–345.

38. Marmarou A. A review of progress in understanding the pathophysiology and treatment of brain edema. *Neurosurg Focus.* 2007;22:1–10.

39. Rosenberg GA. Ischemic brain edema. *Prog Cardiovasc Dis.* 1999;42:209–216.

40. Dávalos A, Toni D, Iweins F, et al. Potential predictors and associated factors in the European Cooperative Acute Stroke Study (ECASS) I. *Stroke.* 1999;30:2631–2636.

41. Ayata C, Ropper AH. Ischaemic brain oedema. *J Clin Neurosci.* 2002;9:113–124.

42. Ropper AH, Shafran B. Brain edema after stroke. Clinical syndrome and intracranial pressure. *Arch Neurol.* 1984;41:26–29.

43. Wijdicks EF, Diringer MN. Middle cerebral artery territory infarction and early brain swelling: progression and effect of age on outcome. *Mayo Clin Proc.* 1998;73:829–836.

44. Hacke W, Schwab S, Horn M, et al. "Malignant" middle cerebral artery territory infarction: clinical course and prognostic signs. *JAMA Neurol.* 1996;53:309–315.

45. Lassen NA, Christensen MS. Physiology of cerebral blood flow. *Br J Anaesth.* 1976;48: 719–734.

46. Rosner MJ, Rosner SD, Johnson AH. Cerebral perfusion pressure: management protocol and clinical results. *J Neurosurg.* 1995;83:949–962.

47. Lazaridis C, Neyens R, Bodle J, et al. High-osmolarity saline in neurocritical care: systematic review and meta-analysis. *Crit Care Med.* 2013;41:353–360.

48. Koenig MA, Bryan M, Lewin JL III, et al. Reversal of transtentorial herniation with hypertonic saline. *Neurology.* 2008;70:1023–1029.

49. Fink ME. Osmotherapy for intracranial hypertension: mannitol versus hypertonic saline. *Continuum* (Minneap Minn). 2012;18(3):640–654.

50. Kamel H, Navi BB, Nakagawa K, et al. Hypertonic saline versus mannitol for the treatment of elevated intracranial pressure: a meta-analysis of randomized clinical trials. *Crit Care Med.* 2011;39:554–559.

51. Aiyagari V, Deibert E, Diringer MN. Hypernatremia in the neurologic intensive care unit: how high is too high? *J Crit Care.* 2006;21(2):163–172.

52. Sandercock PA, Soane T. Corticosteroids for acute ischaemic stroke. *Cochrane Database Syst Rev.* 2011 Sep 7;(9):CD000064.

53. Vahedi K, Hofmeijer J, Juettler E, et al. Early decompressive surgery in malignant infarction of the middle cerebral artery: a pooled analysis of three randomised controlled trials. *Lancet Neurol.* 2007;6:215–222.

Stroke Rehabilitation   9

Monica Verduzco-Gutierrez and Nneka Ifejika

Stroke is the leading preventable cause of disability.[1] Approximately 800,000 new or recurrent strokes occur annually in the United States. Given the increasing incidence of stroke, as well as the increasing number of stroke survivors as a result of greater availability of acute stroke interventions, stroke rehabilitation is an imperative part of the stroke continuum of care.

Forty percent of stroke survivors experience moderate to severe impairments requiring specialized care.[2] Furthermore, another 10% require placement in a skilled nursing facility or long-term care. Even patients with transient ischemic attacks (TIAs) and minor ischemic stroke had a high rate of disability, up to 23% at 5 years after stroke in one population-based study.[3] In this study, at 5 years post-event, 70% of patients with stroke and 48% of patients with TIA were either disabled or deceased. The 5-year risk of institutionalization was 11% after TIA and 19% after stroke. That being said, there is considerable room for improvement to reduce post-stroke disability and institutionalization.

Rehabilitation medicine is a diverse field that encompasses the first days of inpatient care to years of chronic care in many settings.[4] Stroke is considered a chronic and long-duration disease by the World Health Organization.[5] Stroke rehabilitation is a multidisciplinary concept that minimizes the deleterious effects of immobility and facilitates restoration of function. Included in the rehabilitation team are the physician, rehabilitation nurses, physical and occupational therapists, speech–language pathologists, social workers, and case management nurses. International guidelines recommend that stroke rehabilitation be provided to restore independence and maximize community integration.[6]

Therefore, stroke rehabilitation should improve recovery years after a stroke and decrease long-term disability.

Rehabilitation is a problem-solving, educational process aimed at reducing disability and handicap experienced by someone as a result of disease or injury. Due to advancements in the field, stroke rehabilitation has undergone a major shift in therapeutic strategies. Historically, stroke rehabilitation focused on using the intact limb to compensate for the impaired limb. Now, the rehabilitation team utilizes a variety of techniques to promote neurologic recovery based on adaptive neuroplasticity. Neuroplasticity is the ability for the central nervous system to reorganize and remodel after central nervous system injury. This advancement has allowed the development of new technologies and strategies focused on enhancing neurologic recovery and functional ability.

Integration of stroke rehabilitation as a part of standard practice has occurred on the national level. In one large study, 90% of patients with stroke ($n = 616,982$) were assessed for, or received, rehabilitation.[7] The hospitals in the study were comprehensive stroke centers involved in Get with the Guidelines, a program that requires the reporting of rehabilitation assessments.[8] The Centers for Medicare and Medicaid Services financially incentivizes physicians to promote specific quality information, including rehabilitation services received after a stroke.[9] It has been proposed to integrate neurorehabilitation services earlier in the comprehensive stroke center program, referring patients for rehabilitation during the first days of admission and not at the time of discharge.[10] This would allow for the continuity of care from the multidisciplinary rehabilitation team, paying careful attention to neurorehabilitation. With a systematically integrated assessment of progress for early comprehensive discharge planning, this model of post-stroke care can theoretically improve patient outcomes, decrease financial burdens, and improve the hospital-to-home transition.

LEVELS OF NEUROREHABILITATION CARE

A neurorehabilitation program needs to be customized to the stroke patient, based on the severity of disease, degree of deviation from baseline, and the nature of impairments. For individuals with moderate to severe stroke, an appropriate level of rehabilitation services would be a comprehensive multidisciplinary program in an inpatient rehabilitation facility (IRF).

IRFs are either free-standing or hospital-based units that provide a minimum of 3 hours of rehabilitation services per day.[11] Stroke patients in an IRF can get therapeutic services from an interdisciplinary team that includes a rehabilitation physician, physical therapist, occupational therapist, speech and language pathologist, neuropsychologist, nutritionist/dietary specialist, pharmacist, therapeutic recreation specialist, respiratory therapist, case management specialist, neurologic music therapist, social worker, and chaplain.

As a result of daily medical rehabilitation care, the complication rates of stroke patients receiving IRF care are substantially lower than those receiving care at a skilled nursing facility. Furthermore, patients who go to an IRF for continued care have higher functional independence measure scores compared to those who go to skilled nursing facilities.[12] Therefore, if a stroke patient has significant limitations in mobility, self-care, communication, or cognition, and is capable of participating in and benefiting from 3 or more hours of therapy per day, the patient should undergo an inpatient rehabilitation stay for maximal improvement of outcomes.

Time to inpatient rehabilitation hospital admission has also been shown to affect the functional outcome of stroke patients. A retrospective cohort study showed shorter periods from stroke onset to inpatient rehabilitation hospital admission were significantly associated with greater functional gains for those patients.[13] Moderately impaired patients achieved a greater functional gain when admitted to an inpatient rehabilitation hospital within 21 days of stroke. Severely impaired patients had significantly different functional gain if admitted to an inpatient rehabilitation hospital within 30 days versus 60 days.

After discharge from an IRF, stroke patients can continue rehabilitation services through home care (i.e., home health services) or outpatient programs with physical therapy, occupational therapy, and/or speech and language pathology. Patients with less severe deficits should be assessed by rehabilitation services in the acute care hospital and may be discharged directly from hospital to home to participate in an outpatient rehabilitation or home health program.[14] If the patient cannot participate in the aggressive 3-hour or more per day inpatient rehabilitation program because of poor motivation, severe cognitive deficits, encephalopathy, or poor prognosis, he or she can receive inpatient rehabilitation at a subacute program (skilled nursing facility).

There is some practice variation regarding referral to an inpatient rehabilitation facility versus a skilled nursing facility.[12,15] These studies are suggestive of better outcomes for patients receiving care at inpatient rehabilitation; thus, stroke patients who meet admission criteria and have insurance/payor benefits for this type of care should be preferentially referred to inpatient rehabilitation facilities when possible. Barriers to IRF include not receiving acute care in a multidisciplinary, specialized acute stroke unit, which has been shown to have reduced stroke mortality and improved patient outcomes. Furthermore, healthcare payors continue to constrain access to IRF. Because there is little research comparing outcomes in post–acute care settings, it is difficult to inform policymakers who facilitate patient access to proven standards of rehabilitative care.

STROKE RECOVERY

Initial studies that observed motor recovery after stroke showed a vast majority of patients had a motor impairment. In 1951, Thomas Twitchell studied 121 patients and had some of the initial observations of motor recovery.[16] Early in the recovery course, he observed a phase of diminished proprioceptive reflexes that progressed to abnormally increased reflexes. Prior to recovery of voluntary control, there were nonfunctional flexor or extensor synergistic muscle contraction patterns. He also noted that limb recovery occurred proximally to distally; the leg recovered earlier and more completely than the arm, and most recovery occurred in the first 3 months. Brunnstrom further studied motor recovery after stroke and defined six specific stages: Stage 1 is the initial flaccidity post-stroke; stage 2 is when recovery begins with developing spasticity and synergies; stage 3 is characterized by more pronounced spasticity and strong obligatory synergies with voluntary control through the synergies; stage 4 is characterized by a decrease in the influence of spasticity and synergies; stage 5 has less spasticity and more volitional control with complex movement combinations; stage 6 is resolution of spasticity with near-normal to normal movement and coordination.[17] The flagship Copenhagen Stroke Study followed patterns of recovery in more than 1,100 patients.[18] In this study, motor impairments and autonomy post-stroke were evaluated from admission to the neurology unit to discharge from the rehabilitation center. The study validated the existence of motor recovery in all stroke patients. Even with the most severe motor impairments after stroke, 40% of these patients end up with mild or moderate motor impairments after the recovery process. Further relevance of this study was its analysis of the time course of recovery. Functional recovery was completed within 12.5 weeks from stroke onset in 95% of the patients. Furthermore, the time course of functional recovery was strongly related to initial stroke severity. Jorgensen et al concluded that a reliable prognosis can be made within 12 weeks from stroke onset, and neurological and functional recovery should not be expected after the first 5 months.

Thoughts that functional recovery is "complete" within 3 to 5 months are highly disputed among neurorehabilitation physicians. There are a number of publications and meta-analyses on the impact of rehabilitation or physiotherapy on the post-stroke recovery process. Conclusions of these reviews have been consistent: Rehabilitation positively affects the post-stroke motor recovery process.

There are at least 467 controlled studies on this topic involving 25,373 patients.[19] This meta-analysis concluded that there is strong evidence for physical therapy interventions favoring intensive, high-repetitive, task-oriented and task-specific training in all phases post-stroke. The effects were mostly restricted to the actually trained functions and activities.

NEUROPLASTICITY

Neuroplasticity is our central nervous system's ability to reorganize and remodel after injury. It was originally thought that neuroplasticity could only occur before adulthood. More recent advances have shown that the adult human brain is capable of adaptive plasticity after injury. Now, stroke rehabilitation techniques can be applied, even during the chronic stage, to maximize restoration.

The post-stroke injured brain has the potential for extensive reorganization. Mechanisms of neuroplasticity include dendritic sprouting, new synapse formation/alterations in effectiveness, long-term potentiation, and depression of redundant neuronal networks. Functional neuroimaging has validated these mechanisms of motor recovery.[20] Imaging techniques measure local blood flow via radiotracer in PET scan or paramagnetic properties in oxyhemoglobin in functional MRI (fMRI)—local blood flow is thought to correlate to neuronal activation. Furthermore, advances in noninvasive brain stimulation techniques (transcranial magnetic stimulation [TMS]) give us an understanding of some of the processes that might underlie the recovery of function post-stroke.

Diaschisis is the functional deactivation or depression of blood flow of an undamaged area of the central nervous system that is distant to the lesioned area.[21] Part of post-stroke impairment is correlated with deafferentation of brain areas that are not impaired but receive projections from the injured area. Imaging studies post-stroke have shown patients with lesions in motor areas have diaschisis in cerebellar structures.[22] Crossed cerebellar diaschisis could explain the ataxic nature of some types of motor impairments after middle cerebral artery (MCA) stroke. Resolution of cerebellar diaschisis is proposed to be one of the mechanisms by which there is motor recovery after stroke.

Another mechanism of neuroplasticity is peri-infarct reorganization, also known as vicarious reorganization. This form of plasticity deals with alterations in cortical motor output maps after a lesion in the motor cortex.[23] In this type of plasticity, a healthy region of the brain could take over the function of the lesioned brain area. There are both human and animal studies, but some have failed to show correlations with magnitude of recovery.

Increased activation in both the ipsilesional and contralesional hemisphere is another mechanism of plasticity after stroke. Levels of increased activation have been found in a distributed ipsilesional network, including primary motor cortex, premotor cortex, supplementary motor area, and bilateral Brodmann area.[24] The neuroimaging studies suggest that activation in the ipsilateral motor areas plays an important role in the recovery process for motor performance of a paretic hand. There is also reorganization after stroke in the contralesional hemisphere. Activity in the unaffected hemisphere and its effect on neuroplasticity is not as clear. Regardless of the role of each hemisphere, recovery requires the operation of more extensive ensembles of neurons organized in neural networks linking both hemispheres.

THERAPEUTIC APPROACHES

Prior neurorehabilitation techniques historically were about using the intact upper limb to compensate for the hemiparetic impaired limb. These compensatory strategies were not based on the science of promotion of neurologic recovery. The acceptance that the adult human brain could undergo neuroplasticity has changed the face of rehabilitation. There are now many new therapy techniques that focus on recovery of the impaired upper limb.

Prior rehabilitation techniques were based more on tradition than on medical research, but they are worth mentioning in an overview of stroke rehabilitation. Commonly referred to as sensorimotor techniques, these approaches include strengthening, range-of-motion exercises, balance training, and postural control,[25] well-known traditional rehabilitation techniques that have been taught as fundamentals of neurorehabilitation. Proprioceptive neuromuscular facilitation (PNF) uses quick stretches and diagonal movement patterns to maximize proprioceptive input.[26] The neurodevelopmental technique (NDT) was originally conceived for children with spastic cerebral palsy and aims to inhibit abnormal postures and movement and to facilitate isolated muscle control with handling techniques.[27] Brunnstrom's therapeutic technique encourages early movement and is based on his described patterns of motor recovery in stroke patients.[28] The technique uses primitive synergistic patterns through central facilitation. The sensorimotor, or Rood, technique incorporates cutaneous sensorimotor stimulation to encourage movement.[29] Lastly, Carr and Shepherd developed a motor relearning program based on a problem-solving and task-oriented approach during functional tasks.[30]

These traditional sensorimotor techniques may be adapted to aid in neuroplasticity, but more studies are needed. Many therapists trained in these techniques revise them to the current knowledge of forced use of the paretic limb, massed practice, shaping, skill acquisition, and task-specific movement.[25] The emerging strategies must be functional, meaningful, and challenging to the patient.

A recent Cochrane Review evaluated interventions for improving upper limb function after stroke.[31] The overall conclusion was that there are large numbers of overlapping reviews, but there is no high-quality evidence for interventions currently used. Robust randomized controlled trials (RCTs) of clinical interventions are needed.

Constraint-Induced Movement Therapy

Constraint-induced movement therapy (CIMT) or "forced use therapy" is a technique originally studied by Knapp et al in 1958[32] and is now the most investigated intervention for the rehabilitation of patients.[33] CIMT was developed to overcome upper-limb impairments after stroke. It is based on the laboratory observation of learned nonuse in primates. In 1963, Knapp explained learned nonuse in monkeys with a deafferented upper extremity and the positive efficacy after applying a forced-use paradigm.[34]

CIMT forces the use of the paretic side by restraining the unaffected, nonparetic side, usually in a mitt that prevents its use during fine movements. The patient then uses his or her hemiparetic limb repetitively and intensively for a set time. Having the unaffected limb constrained, operant conditioning is used to increase task difficulty for the affected hand in small amounts, so the patient can succeed in using the affected paretic limb. The first translational studies on CIMT in the 1980s examined the efficacy of applying the intervention on one hemiplegic patient or a small group of stroke or traumatic brain injury patients.[35,36] Following these studies were ones that controlled factors, such as severity of hemiparesis and time after onset of symptoms.[37,38] The next trials focused on location of improved function, and it was determined that the hemiparetic hand most benefited from CIMT in their pre-test/post-test analysis.[39]

There are RCTs of CIMT. Taub et al conducted a placebo-controlled trial of CMT versus a fitness, cognition, and relaxation exercise program.[40] Also there was a conventional, intervention-controlled trial of CIMT versus traditional occupational therapy, including strength, range of motion, and activity of daily living (ADL) training.[41] Another RCT by Lin et al showed increased motor function, basic and extended functional abilities, and improved quality of life after a modified CIMT intervention (of intensive training with restraint wear out of clinic) compared with a control group of conventional rehabilitation.[42]

In 2006, Wolf et al published the EXCITE trial, an RCT with 222 patients 3 to 9 months post-stroke.[43] In the study, the patients did repetitive task practice and behavioral shaping for 6 hours per day. CIMT versus conventional care produced statistically significant improvement in arm motor function, which persisted for at least 1 year.

There are now several systematic reviews and meta-analyses related to CIMT. Hakkennes and Keating performed a systematic review of RCTs regarding CIMT in the post-stroke population.[44] In 2010, Corbetta et al published a comprehensive inclusion of relevant trials on two main comparisons: CIMT versus control for arm function and ADL outcomes.[45] The most recent meta-analysis of CIMT in 2014 included 23 trials and concluded that CIMT can improve arm motor function and improve arm motor activities and may have a lasting effect on arm motor activity.[46]

Neuromuscular Electrical Stimulation

Another option for therapeutic approach to motor recovery after stroke is neuromuscular electrical stimulation (NMES) or functional electrical stimulation (FES). NMES bypasses the central nervous system input to the muscles and stimulates the lower motor neuron or its terminal branches. This causes depolarization of the motor neuron and subsequent contraction of the corresponding muscle. In the upper limb, NMES is used to activate the posterior interosseous nerve to extend the wrist; in the lower limb, the deep peroneal nerve is stimulated to cause ankle dorsiflexion.[47] NMES is most appropriate for upper motor neuron injury, such as stroke, because it requires an intact motor unit. Denervated muscle cannot be safely stimulated; therefore, it is not suitable in the presence of lower motor neuron disease, such as peripheral neuropathy or radiculopathy.

NMES can be therapeutic, to promote motor recovery, or functional, which provides functional movement during stimulation only. Functional application of NMES is called neuroprosthesis.[25] In this case, the paralyzed limb undergoes stimulation in a coordinated sequence leading to functional movement. Functional application is mostly used for alleviating foot drop caused by total or partial paresis of the ankle dorsiflexors muscles. Ankle dorsiflexion weakness that impedes walking affects about 30% of people post-stroke.[48] Due to ineffective clearance of the foot during gait, there is increased risk of falls and mortality. Electrical stimulation, orthotic-substitute walking devices facilitate the use of surface electrodes during therapeutic gait training. A Cochrane Review in 2009 reviewed 24 randomized controlled trials of electrostimulation and its effect on the ability to improve voluntary movement and/or use of the affected limb in everyday activities.[49] It concluded that when electrostimulation is compared to no treatment, there might be a small effect on some aspects of function in favor of electrostimulation. Overall, there was insufficient robust data to inform clinical use of electrostimulation for neuromuscular retraining. In another review by Bosch et al, it was noted there was insufficient evidence to conclude that walking with an electrical stimulation, orthotic-substitute device is superior to walking with an ankle foot orthosis (AFO).[48]

The concepts underlying neuroplasticity suggest that extensive use of a neu-roprosthesis may convey the greatest therapeutic benefit in terms of motor recovery. A large randomized controlled trial of 495 subjects with foot drop over a 12-month follow-up compared changes in gait quality and function between FES and AFOs.[50] At 12 months, both FES and AFO continued to demonstrate equivalent gains in gait speed. The FES group did have statistically significant improvements for the 6-minute walk test (6MWT) and the Modified Emory Functional Ambulation Profile (mEFAP) stair-time subscore, suggesting FES use may lead to additional improvements in walking endurance and functional ambulation. Evidence for improved motor function after FES has been proven in randomized controlled trials and a meta-analysis.[51] A double-blind, randomized trial showed similar positive results and demonstrated cortical changes by fMRI in the NMES-treated subjects.[52] In this trial, there were intensive treatments at home (60 hours/3 weeks) with NMES compared with sham. Unlike the treat-ment group, the sham subjects did not improve on any grasp and release measure. NMES remains a practical treatment option for select patients, especially those who are too impaired to participate in the forced-use paradigm, but noncoverage by some insurance providers is a barrier to widespread utilization.

Body-Weight-Supported Treadmill Training and Electromechanical-Assisted Gait Training

Therapeutic approaches to walking are imperative to undertake after stroke. The standard rehabilitation technique for gait training after stroke is to walk over ground. Gains can be limited due to several patient factors, and patients often develop compensatory walking habits, such as hip hiking and circumduction. Body-weight-supported treadmill training (BWSTT) was developed to facili-tate gait retraining in patients with stroke by allowing them to practice gait cycles unweighted (see Figure 9.1). BWSTT is a type of CIMT that allows the patient to practice nearly normal gait patterns and avoid developing those com-pensatory walking habits.[53] BWSTT uses a harness to suspend the patient from an overhead frame over a standard treadmill. The counterweight system is able to unload up to 40% of the patient's weight.[25] This technique is very labor intensive because it requires one or two therapists to provide assistance with advancing the weak limb through a reciprocal stepping pattern, and another may need to stand behind the patient to provide pelvic support.

Gait training on a treadmill was first described by Finch and Barbeau in 1985[54] and first tested in stroke patients for gait restoration by Hesse and colleagues in 1994.[55] Since then, there have been many studies on the topic. The biologic mechanism of BWSTT may be associated with cortical activation changes. Enzinger et al noted bi-hemispheric activation increases with greater

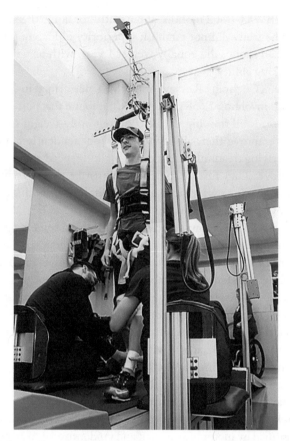

FIGURE 9.1 Body-weight-supported treadmill training

Source: Courtesy of TIRR Memorial Hermann.

recovery in both cortical and subcortical regions with movement of the paretic foot.[56] Furthermore, greater walking endurance was associated with increased brain activity in the primary sensorimotor cortex, the paracentral lobules, the cingulate motor area, the bilateral caudate nuclei, and the lateral thalamus of the affected hemisphere. For gait training, BWSTT has been shown to be superior to neurodevelopmental balance and weight-bearing techniques.[57] In other trials, patients who trained with BWSTT achieved better gait speed, improved balance, and better motor recovery than patients trained with overground walking, resistive leg cycling, or treadmill walking without body-weight support.[58,59] Not all trials established superiority of locomotor training. The LEAPS trial was a large randomized controlled trial done with 408 stroke patients by Duncan and colleagues.[60] The stroke patients were stratified by walking impairment, randomized to BWSTT at 2 months, at 6 months, or home therapy with physical therapy. The study did not establish superiority of locomotor training. It concluded that all groups did equally well at 1 year, with 52% increasing their functional walking ability.

Furthermore, a Cochrane Review of BWSTT performed in 2014 identified 44 relevant trials involving 2,658 participants.[61] It found that post-stroke patients who received treadmill training with or without body-weight support are not more likely to improve their ability to walk independently compared with patients not receiving treadmill training, but walking speed and walking endurance may improve. They further specified that stroke patients who are able to walk (not those unable to walk) appear to benefit most from this type of intervention and have persisting beneficial effects.

Although BWSTT has shown efficacy in improving some aspects of gait, it is limited clinically due to the effort needed by the therapist to set the paretic limbs and control weight shift.[47] Therapists fatigue after 15 to 20 minutes. One solution was the design of a robotic treadmill system that provides the physical assistance previously given by a therapist. Robot-assisted therapies have been used in stroke rehabilitation for more than 20 years. One such gait system is called the Lokomat (Hocoma Ag, Volketswil, SZ), which has a treadmill with counterbalanced harness with a motor-driven leg orthosis that produces a near-normal walking pattern timed with the motion of the treadmill belt. The Lokomat is the most studied robot-assisted, lower-limb device. The study results have been mixed. One randomized controlled trial by Morone and colleagues looked at robotic gait training in 48 patients with subacute stroke.[62] They were stratified by motor impairment and randomized into an equal amount of 20 sessions of robotic-assisted training or conventional floor-based gait training. The results found that at discharge and 2 years after discharge, those with more severe impairments in the robotic group improved in regard to functional ambulation category, using the Barthel Index or Rivermead mobility index. Both conventional and robotic therapies were effective in the high motricity groups. A Cochrane Review of 23 trials with 999 participants was updated in 2013.[63] The review found evidence that electromechanically assisted gait training combined with physiotherapy may improve recovery of independent walking in patients after stroke. Specifically, people in the first 3 months post-stroke and those unable to walk appear to benefit the most from this type of intervention.

Transcranial Magnetic Stimulation

There are several other interventions that can potentially augment motor recovery and are at varying stages of investigation. These include transcranial magnetic stimulation (TMS), cortical brain stimulation, neuronal transplantation, and use of autologous stem cells.[25] TMS and transcranial direct current stimulation (tDCS) are noninvasive methods to stimulate the human brain. They have been investigated as potential tools to modulate motor recovery and influence motor, sensory, language, and cognitive functioning.[64] TMS is delivered by passing a brief, strong magnetic field created by an electric current circulating within a coil on the scalp. This penetrates the skull and induces electrical current in the cortex that depolarizes the axons.[65] (See Figure 9.2.)

TMS has been used since 1985 in several contexts, both therapeutically and diagnostically. As a diagnostic tool, TMS is primarily used for evaluation of excitability of cortical motor areas and motor pathways.[66] As a therapeutic tool, TMS has the potential to be used to induce changes in excitability and modulate behavior. TMS can enhance or reduce activity in cortical regions and influence function based on variables such as pulse frequency, duration and time frame of stimulation, shape of coil, and strength of magnetic field.[65] An absolute contraindication for TMS use is the presence of metallic hardware close to the discharging coil.[67] TMS is becoming more studied in stroke populations. Nineteen trials with 588 participants were included in a Cochrane Review in 2013 that looked at magnetic brain stimulation for improving people's functional ability after stroke.[68] The review concluded that the evidence does not support the routine use of TMS after stroke. Overall, it appeared to be safe, and there were few mild adverse events observed in the TMS groups. The most common side effects

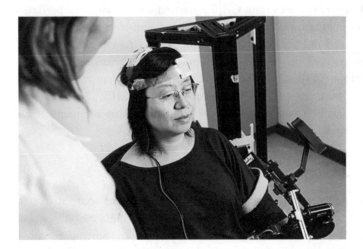

FIGURE 9.2 Transcranial direct current stimulation

Source: Courtesy of the McGovern Medical School at UTHealth Department of Physical Medicine and Rehabilitation NeuroRecovery Lab.

reported were transient or mild headaches (2.4%) and local discomfort at the site of the stimulation.

COGNITION AND LANGUAGE DISORDERS

Up to one-half of stroke survivors experience speech and language disorders.[69] Aphasia is an acquired communication disorder that affects speech and language centers in the dominant hemisphere. Recovery patterns are more variable for language than for motor function, and recovery from aphasia usually occurs at a slower rate and over a more prolonged time course. It is also known that patients with nonfluent aphasia generally have a less favorable prognosis than those with fluent aphasia. Also, language comprehension usually returns earlier and to a greater extent than oral expression.[70] There is a lot of evidence that there is a benefit from speech and language therapy but insufficient evidence for determining the best approach.[71]

A novel treatment approach to treatment of post-stroke aphasia is constraint-induced language therapy (CILT). This approach differs from conventional therapy in that it is more intensive (e.g., 3 hours/day, 5 days a week for 2 weeks), and it integrates techniques preventing gestural communication or shared object regard. The patient is forced to engage solely in verbal communication to execute therapy tasks. An initial study of CILT done by Pulvermuller et al administered at least 30 hours of CILT therapy over 10 days and compared this to patients who received 4 weeks of conventional therapy.[72] Therapists used shaping techniques to stimulate verbal interaction. CILT improved formal language performance and daily life communication activities compared with control therapy. CILT has also been studied in conjunction with memantine. In a randomized, double-blind, placebo-controlled, parallel-group study of both memantine and constraint-induced aphasia therapy on post-stroke aphasia, 28 patients were followed over 48 weeks. Results showed that both memantine and CILT alone improved aphasia severity, but best outcomes were achieved combining memantine with CILT. The beneficial effects persisted on long-term follow-up.[73]

SPATIAL NEGLECT

Spatial neglect after stoke affects more than 50% of acute stroke survivors, adversely affects recovery, and is associated with higher in-hospital and post-hospital care expense.[66] It is defined as asymmetric reporting, response, or orientation to contralesional stimuli. A uniform, patient-centered definition of spatial neglect is more adequately defined by spatial bias causing a functional disability. The deficit cannot be due to primary sensory deficits, such as hemianopia, or due to motor deficits. The stroke survivor with spatial neglect may have spared speech and language, memory, and other mental abilities, but the prognosis for recovery of independent function in patients with persistent spatial neglect is significantly worse than that for deficits in other areas.[74] Additional dysfunctions in stroke patients with spatial neglect include impaired self-monitoring, such as anosognosia or anosodiaphoria; impaired emotional processing, such as affective agnosias and aprosody, hypoarousal; and personal neglect.

Rehabilitation for spatial neglect focuses on visuomotor, cognitive, and behavioral training with specific interventions that target each type of deficit.[75] Caregivers also must be involved in the management to help with alterations in the patient's environment.

Prism adaptation training (PAT) is a promising neglect therapy that targets the motor-intentional aiming systems.[76] PAT is simple and amenable to short, frequent, in-patient rehabilitation sessions. The 20-diopter, 12.4-degree, right-displacing wedge prism lenses are usually worn for 10 short sessions of intensive motor training. During training, patients' views of their own arm movements are partially blocked while they repeatedly point to targets or perform continuous manual tasks.

Perceptual deficit rehabilitation may be performed via environmental modification techniques. The bedside environment (e.g., television, seats, doors) may be placed leftward to make the patients perceive their left side. Other interventions used to attempt to shift the representation of space toward the neglected side include caloric stimulation,[77] trunk rotation treatment,[78] optokinetic stimulation,[79] and vibration of left posterior neck muscles.[78] Cueing can also be used as part of perceptual deficit rehabilitation.[80] Scanning training encourages patients to direct their gaze to the neglected side and to scan their environment with verbal cueing. Other methods used by therapists include cueing patients to find a red line or other stimulus on the left margin of a page.

Other techniques in this field are unawareness rehabilitation performed via environmental modification and family education. Caregivers would modify the bedroom by placing the patient's bed asymmetrically in the room, either in the preferred or neglected space. Another technique would be simplifying the visual environment by setting the table with as few items as possible to help improve attention to the food and utensils. Caregivers can also aid in emotional processing rehabilitation. Finally, if a patient has personal neglect, personal neglect rehabilitation can be utilized. Occupational therapists address this during their treatments for activities of daily living, and it can involve direct verbal, visual, or tactile cueing.

DYSPHAGIA

Swallowing difficulties are common after stroke, with approximately 50% of patients clinically being diagnosed with dysphagia.[81] Dysphagia places the patient at risk of aspiration pneumonia, which is a dangerous medical complication and leads to increased hospital length of stay and, in some cases, death. It has been found that up to 51% of patients have clinical aspiration on admission. Although many swallowing problems resolve over the first 7 days, a small percentage of patients have persistence of dysphagia, and some even develop it later in the history of their stroke.[81] Risk factors for patients who develop long-term dysphagia and placement of a percutaneous gastrostomy tube are high National Institutes of Health Stroke Scale (NIHSS) score and bihemispheric infarcts.[82]

Given the high risk of dysphagia, it is imperative that screening should be performed before any oral intake. Dynamic instrumental assessment with videofluoroscopic swallowing (also known as modified barium swallow) study or fiberoptic endoscopic evaluation of swallowing (FEES) can help guide therapy. The treatment goals of dysphagia are to improve food transfer and prevent aspiration. Speech and language pathologists are specialists in the realm of swallow rehabilitation therapy as this has been a field for 40 years. Evidence is relatively new, with one of the first papers published in 1972.[83] It is important for the clinician to gather information regarding the patient's cognition, physiologic impairments, sensory impairments, and appropriateness of oral intake. An objective assessment should be done with trials of compensatory strategies to provide the patient with the safest and least restrictive diet. See Table 9.1 for information on aspiration precautions. Information from the clinical and objective assessment is used together to create the most appropriate and individualized rehabilitation program.[84]

There are both compensatory and rehabilitative approaches to dysphagia rehabilitation.[85] Compensatory strategies reduce the symptoms of dysphagia without altering the pathophysiology and include the strategies listed in Table 9.2.

TABLE 9.1 Aspiration precautions

- Eat/drink only when alert
- Sit as upright as possible/30 degrees at rest, 90 degrees when eating
- Encourage self-feeding
- Remain upright after meals for at least 30 minutes

Source: Adapted from Reference 84.

TABLE 9.2 Strategies that may be recommended for dysphagia patients

- No straws
- All liquids via cup or spoon
- Allow extra time to swallow
- Eat slowly with small bites and sips
- Chew each bite completely
- Alternate each bite of food with a sip of liquid
- Put fork or spoon down after each bite
- Oral hygiene before and after each meal
- Check and sweep mouth with tongue to clear residual food
- Multiple swallows
- Crushed medications for those who cannot swallow pills
- Head tilt–chin lift

Source: Adapted from Reference 84.

Rehabilitative approaches actually have the aim of recovering swallowing physiology and improving swallow safety. Traditional treatment techniques implemented by speech language pathologists include tongue strengthening exercises, thermal-tactile stimulation, tongue hold exercises, Mendelsohn maneuvers, supraglottic and super-supraglottic swallows, effortful swallows, and the Shaker exercise.[86] Biofeedback methods, such as surface electromyography (sEMG), can also be used with traditional approaches. sEMG allows the patient to increase the awareness of his or her swallowing pattern and is reported to increase the rate of progress seen for patients with chronic dysphagia.[87]

Neuromuscular electrical stimulation was discussed earlier in this chapter, but it is also employed as a treatment for dysphagia. In dysphagia rehabilitation, it is controversial but has been reported to retrain pharyngeal musculature, improve swallow function, and promote reorganization of the motor cortex.[88] There are both positive and neutral trials when it comes to NMES in dysphagia. In 2009, Permsirivanich and colleagues published a trial comparing NMES with rehabilitation swallow therapy. In this randomized controlled trial, both traditional swallow therapy and NMES therapy showed a positive effect in the treatment of persistent dysphagia in stroke patients, with NMES being significantly superior.[89] A trial by Bulow and colleagues also randomized patients to traditional therapy versus electrical stimulation. Findings demonstrated statistically significant positive therapy effects for both NMES and traditional therapy, but there was no statistically significant difference in therapy effect between the groups.[88] Given inconsistencies, it is still controversial whether this therapy is effective.

There is more of an emphasis now on the diagnosis of lingual dysfunction and how lingual strength has serious effects on swallowing. Decreased lingual muscle mass has been found to negatively impact bolus propulsion into the pharynx.[90] Robbins and colleagues have studied the effects of lingual exercises in post-stroke dysphagia. All subjects who participated in the 8-week isometric lingual exercise program increased isometric and swallowing pressures, with some improving airway protection and lingual volume.[91] There is more research needed on these interventions and their effectiveness in combination with traditional therapy in stroke patients with dysphagia.

CONCLUSION

The majority of patients with stroke now survive the initial event. According to the American Stroke Association, more than 7 million Americans are

TABLE 9.3 Prevention of complications

- Prompt evaluation and treatment of healthcare-associated infections (e.g., urinary tract infection, aspiration pneumonia)
- Formal assessment of swallow by a licensed speech and language pathologist
- Nutrition assessment by a licensed dietician
- Prevent contracture with early mobilization, range of motion, proper positioning, and orthotic use
- Treat spasticity with a patient-centered and stepwise approach
- Pharmacologic or mechanical prophylaxis for venous thromboembolism
- Mitigation of shoulder pain via shoulder sling or taping, positioning schedule when supine, avoidance of uncontrolled abduction, and overhead pulley use
- Neurogenic bladder and urinary incontinence management through timed voids, accurate measurement of intake and output, and use of external or intermittent urinary catheterization
- Bowel regimen involving the use of stool softeners, bowel training, and laxatives, if indicated
- A stage I decubitus ulcer can form in 2 hours; judicious use of turning protocols with wedge pillows to position patients, nursing education, barrier sprays, lubricants, and protective dressings
- Central nervous system depressants, such as neuroleptics, benzodiazepines, and barbiturates, should be avoided whenever feasible
- Identification and early treatment of post-stroke depression

Source: Adapted from Reference 95.

stroke survivors.[92] It behooves us to ensure that these survivors live with as little disability as possible through rehabilitation and ensure they are treated with appropriate secondary stroke prophylaxis to prevent a repeat stroke. There are now more human subject data showing mechanisms of recovery from stroke, and this research needs to translate into clinical studies to help stroke survivors.

Post-stroke rehabilitation has focused on therapies to maximize surviving brain function or provide compensatory approaches. As of 2016, there are updated published American Heart Association/American Stroke Association guidelines for stroke rehabilitation and recovery.[93] These guidelines, made by an expert panel, serve as a resource for practitioners to have knowledge of best clinical practices available to them to ensure stroke survivors receive evidenced-based rehabilitative care. We know that stroke rehabilitation requires a coordinated effort from a large team, with the patients and their goals at the center. Communication among team members is essential in ensuring the stroke survivor has an effective and accelerated rehabilitation course. Furthermore, we are in a time of healthcare improvement and quality. The Institute of Healthcare Improvement has developed the triple aim of simultaneously improving population health, improving the patient experience of care, and reducing per capita cost.[94] Systems of care are currently evolving with post-acute rehabilitation care being considered very costly. We must recognize and provide more data that post-stroke rehabilitation treatments are clinically impactful and decrease the risk of downstream medical morbidity[95] (see Table 9.3). Comprehensive rehabilitative programs, where evidenced-based dose, duration, and types of therapy are implemented, are essential in post-stroke care and for the future of population health.

References

1. Mozaffarian D, Go A, Arnett DK, et al. Heart disease and stroke statistics—2015 update. *Circulation*. 2015:e29-e322.
2. Griffin LJ. Considerations and strategies for educating stroke patients with neurological deficits. *J Nurs Educ Pract*. 2013;3:125–137.
3. Luengo-Fernandez R, Gray AM, Pendlebury ST, et al. Population-based study of disability and institutionalization after transient ischemic attack and stroke: 10-year results of the Oxford Vascular Study. *Stroke*. 2013;44:2854–2861.
4. Hachinski V, Gorelick PB, et al. Stroke: working toward a prioritized world agenda. *Cerebrovasc Dis*. 2010;30:127–147.
5. *Chronic Diseases and Health Promotion*. World Health Organization; 2015.
6. Jaunch E, Adams HP Jr, et al. Guidelines for the early management of patients with acute ischemic stroke: a guideline for healthcare professionals from the American Heart Association/American Stroke Association. *Stroke*. 2013;44:870–947.

7. Prvu Bettger J, Reeves MJ, et al. Assessing stroke patients for rehabilitation during the acute hospitalization: findings from the get with the guidelines-stroke program. *Arch Phys Med Rehabil.* 2013;94:38–45.

8. *Get with the Guidelines-Stroke Patient Management Tool.* American Heart Association; 2014.

9. Centers for Medicare and Medicaid Services. Physician quality reporting system 2015.

10. Bagherpour R, Barrett AM, et al. A comprehensive neurorehabilitation program should be an integral part of a comprehensive stroke center. *Front Neurol.* 2014;5:1–5.

11. Inpatient rehabilitation facilities. CMSgov; 2012.

12. Chan L SM, Jette AM, et al. Does postacute care site matter? A longitudinal study assessing functional recovery after a stroke. *Arch Phys Med Rehabil.* 2013;94:622–629.

13. Wang H CM, Terdiman J, Hung Y, Sandel ME. Time to inpatient rehabilitation hospital admission and functional outcomes of stroke patients. *PM R.* 2011;3:296–304.

14. Mayo NE W-DS, Cote R, et al. There's no place like home: an evaluation of early supported discharge for stroke. *Stroke.* 2000;31:1016–1023.

15. Wang H, Terdiman J, et al. Postacute care and ischemic stroke mortality: findings from an integrated health care system in northern California. *PM R.* 2011;3:686–694.

16. Twitchell T. The restoration of motor function following hemiplegia in man. *Brain.* 1951;74:443–480.

17. Brunnstrom S. Motor testing procedures in hemiplegia: based on sequential recovery stages. *Phys Ther.* 1966;46:357–375.

18. Jorgensen HS, Raaschou HO, Vive-Larsen J, et al. Outcome and time course of recovery in stroke. Part II: Time course of recovery. The Copenhagen Stroke Study. *Arch Phys Med Rehabil.* 1995;76:406–412.

19. Vanderbeek JM, van Peppen R, van der Wees PJ, et al. What is the evidence for physical therapy poststroke? A systematic review and meta-analysis. *PLoS ONE.* 2014.

20. Marque P, Castel-Lacanal E, De Boissezon X, Loubinoux I. Post-stroke hemiplegia rehabilitation: evolution of the concepts. *Ann Phys Rehab Med* 2014;57:520–529.

21. Seitz RJ, Knorr U, Binkofski F, et al. The role of diaschisis in stroke recovery. *Stroke.* 1999;30:1844–1850.

22. Flint AC, Wright CB. Ataxic hemiparesis from strategic frontal white matter infarction with crossed cerebellar diaschisis. *Stroke.* 2006;37:e1-e2.

23. Nudo RJ. Reorganization of movement representations in primary motor cortex following focal ischemic infarcts in adult squirrel monkeys. *J Neurophysiol.* 1996;75:2144–2149.

24. Loubinoux I, Pariente J, Dechaumont S, et al. Correlation between cerebral reorganization and motor recovery after subcortical infarcts. *Neuroimage.* 2003;20:2166–2180.

25. Harvey RL, Roth EJ, Yu DT, Celnik P. Stroke syndromes. *Physical Medicine and Rehabilitation.* Philadelphia, PA: Elsevier Saunders; 2011.

26. Voss D, Ionta M, Myers B. *Proprioceptive Neuromuscular Facilitation: Patterns and Techniques.* Philadelphia, PA: Harper & Row; 1985.

27. Bobath B. *Adult Hemiplegia: Evaluation and Treatment.* Oxford, UK: Heinemann; 1990.

28. Brunnstrom S. Associated reactions of the upper extremity in adult patients with hemiplegia: an approach to training. *Phys Ther Rev.* 1956;36:225–236.

29. Stockmeyer S. An interpretation of the approach of Rood to the treatment of neuromuscular dysfunction. *Am J Phys Med.* 1967;6:900–955.

30. Carr J, Shepherd R. *Neurological Rehabilitation: Optimizing Motor Performance.* Oxford, UK: Butterworth Heinemann; 1998.

31. Pollock A, Farmer S, Brady M, et al. Interventions for improving upper limb function after stroke (review). In: Group CS, ed. *The Cochrane Collaboration.* New York: Wiley & Sons; 2014.

32. Knapp H, Taub E, Berman A. Effect of deafferentation on a conditioned avoidance response. *Science.* 1958;128:842–843.

33. Kwakkel G, Veerbeek J, van Wegen E, Wolf S. Constraint-induced movement therapy after stroke. *Lancet Neurol.* 2015;14:224–234.

34. Knapp H, Taub E, Berman A. Movements in monkeys with deafferented forelimbs. *Exp Neurol.* 1963;7:305–315.

35. Ostendorf C, Wolf S. Effect of forced use of the upper extremity of a hemiplegic patient on changes in function. A single-case design. *Phys Ther.* 1981;61:1022–1028.

36. Wolf S, Lecraw D, Barton L, Jann B. Forced use of hemiplegic upper extremities to reverse the effect of learned nonuse among chronic stroke and head-injured patients. *Exp Neurol.* 1989;104:125–132.

37. Boake C, Noser E, Ro T, et al. Constraint induced movement therapy during early stroke rehabilitation. *Neurorehabil Neural Repair.* 2007;21:14–24.

38. Bonifer N, Anderson K. Application of constraint-induced movement therapy for an individual with severe chronic upper-extremity hemiplegia. *Phys Ther.* 2003;83:384–398.

39. Koyama T, Sano K, Tanaka S, et al. Effective targets for constraint induced movement therapy for patients with upper-extremity impairment after stroke. *NeuroRehabilitation.* 2007;22:287–293.

40. Taub E, Uswatte G, King D, et al. A placebo-controlled trial of constraint-induced movement therapy for upper extremity after stroke. *Stroke.* 2006;37:1045–1049.

41. Dromereick A, Edwards D, Hahn M. Does the application of constraint-induced movement therapy during acute rehabilitation reduce arm impairment after ischemic stroke? *Stroke.* 2000;31:2984–2988.

42. Lin K, Chang Y, Wu C, Chen Y. Effects of constraint-induced therapy versus bilateral arm training on motor performance, daily functions, and quality of life in stroke survivors. *Neurorehabil Neural Repair.* 2009;23:441–448.

43. Wolf S, Winstein C, Miller J, et al. Effect of constraint-induced movement therapy on upper extremity function 3 to 9 months after stroke: the EXCITE randomized clinical trial. *JAMA.* 2006;296:2095–2104.

44. Hakkennes S, Keating J. Constraint-induced movement therapy following stroke: a systematic review of randomised controlled trials. *Aust J Physiother.* 2005;51:221–231.

45. Corbetta D, Sirtori V, Moja L, Gatti R. Constraint-induced movement therapy in stroke patients: systematic review and meta analysis. *Eur J Phys Rehabil Med.* 2010;46:537–544.

46. Thrane G, Friborg O, Anke A, Indredavik B. A meta-analysis of constraint-induced movement therapy after stroke. *J Rehabil Med.* 2014;46:833–842.

47. Ifejika-Jones NL, Barrett AM. Rehabilitation—emerging technologies, innovative therapies, and future objectives. *Neurotherapeutics.* 2011;8:452–462.

48. Bosch P, Harris J, Wing K. Review of therapeutic electrical stimulation for dorsiflexion assist and orthotic substitution from the American Congress of Rehabilitation Medicine stroke movement interventions subcommittee. *Arch Phys Med Rehabil.* 2014;95:390–396.

49. Pomeroy V, King L, Pollock A, et al. Electrostimulation for promoting recovery of movement or functional ability after stroke. *Cochrane Sys Rev;* 2009.

50. Bethoux F, Rogers H, Nolan K, et al. Long-term follow-up to a randomized controlled trial comparing peroneal nerve functional electrical stimulation to an ankle foot orthosis for patients with chronic stroke. *Neurorehabil Neural Repair.* 2015;29(10):911–922.

51. Glanz M, Klawansky S, Stason W, et al. Functional electrostimulation in poststroke rehabilitation: a meta-analysis of the randomized controlled trials. *Arch Phys Med Rehabil.* 1996;77:549–553.

52. Kimberley T, Lewis S, Auerbach E, et al. Electrical stimulation driving functional improvements and cortical changes in subjects with stroke. *Exp Brain Res*. 2004;154: 450–460.

53. Chen G, Patten C. Treadmill training with harness support: selection of parameters for individuals with poststroke hemiparesis. *J Rehabil Res Dev*. 2006;43:485–498.

54. Finch L, Barbeau H. Hemiplegic gait: new treatment strategies. *Physiother Can*. 1985; 38:36–41.

55. Hesse S, Bertlet C, Schaffrin A, et al. Restoration of gait in nonambulatory hemiparetic patients by treadmill training with partial body-weight support. *Arch Phys Med Rehabil*. 1994;75:1087–1093.

56. Enzinger C, Dawes H, Johansen-Berg H, et al. Brain activity changes associated with treadmill training after stroke. *Stroke*. 2009;40:2460–2467.

57. Hesse S, Bertelt C, Jahnke M, et al. Treadmill training with partial body weight support compared with physiotherapy in nonambulatory hemiparetic patients. *Stroke*. 1995; 26:976–981.

58. Sullivan K, Brown D, Klassen T, et al. Effects of task-specific locomotor and strength training in adults who were ambulatory after stroke: results of the STEPS randomzied clinical trial. *Phys Ther*. 2007;87:1580–1602.

59. Visintin M, Barbeau H, Korner-Bitensky N, Mayo N. A new approach to retrain gait in stroke patients through body weight support and treadmill stimulation. *Stroke*. 1998; 29:1122–1128.

60. Duncan P, Sullivan K, Behrman A, et al. Body-weight supported treadmill rehabilitation after stroke. *N Engl J Med*. 2011;364:2026–2036.

61. Merholz J, Pohl M, Elsner B. Treadmill training and body weight support for walking after stroke. *Cochrane Database Syst Rev*; 2014.

62. Morone G, Iosa M, Bragoni M, et al. Who may have durable benefit from robotic gait training? A 2-year follow-up randomized controlled trial in patients with subacute stroke. *Stroke*. 2012;43:1140–1142.

63. Mehrholz J, Elsner B, Kugler J, Pohl M. Electromechanical-assisted training for walking after stroke. *Cochrane Database Sys Rev*; 2013 Jan 23;(1):CD002840.

64. Harvey R, Nudo R. Cortical brain stimulation: a potential therapeutic agent for upper limb motor recovery following stroke. *Top Stroke Rehabil*. 2007;14:54–67.

65. Hallett M. Transcranial magnetic stimulation and the human brain. *Nature*. 2000;406: 147–150.

66. Barrett A, Oh-Park M, Chen P, Ifejika N. Neurorehabilitation: five new things. *Neurol Clin Pract*. 2013;3:484–492.

67. Rossi S, Hallett M, Rossini P, Pascual-Leone A. Safety of TMSCG. Safety, ethical considerations, and application guidelines for the use of transcranial magnetic stimulation in clinincal practice and research. *Clin Neurophysiol*. 2009;120:2008–2039.

68. Hao Z, Wang D, Zeng Y, Liu M. Magnetic brain stimulation for improving people's functional ability after stroke. *Cochrane Database Sys Rev*; 2013;(5):CD008862.

69. Wade D, Hewer R, David R, Enderby P. Aphasia after stroke: natural history and associated deficits. *J Neurol Neurosurg Psychiatry*. 1986;49:11–16.

70. Prins R, Snow C, Wagenaar E. Recovery from aphasia. Spontaneous speech versus language comprehension. *Brain Lang*. 1978;6:192–211.

71. Brady M, Kelly H, Godwin J, Enderby P. Speech and language therapy for aphasia following stroke. *Cochrane Database Sys Rev*; 2012. May 16;(5):CD000925.

72. Pulvermuller F, Neininger B, Elbert T, et al. Constraint-induced therapy of chronic aphasia after stroke. *Stroke*. 2001;32:1621–1626.

73. Berthier M, Green C, Lara J, et al. Memantine and constraint-induced aphasia therapy in chronic poststroke aphasia. *Ann Neurol.* 2009;65:577–585.

74. Jehkonen M, Ahonen JP, Dastidar P, et al. Visual neglect as a predictor of functional outcome one year after stroke. *Acta Neurol Scand.* 2000;101(3):195–201.

75. Riestra AR, Barrett AM. Rehabilitation of spatial neglect. *Handb Clin Neurol.* 2013. 110:347–355.

76. Barrett AM, Goedert KM, Basso JC. Prism adaptation for spatial neglect after stroke: translational practice gaps. *Nat Rev Neurol.* 2012;8(10):567–577.

77. Geminiani G, Bottini G. Mental representation and temporary recovery from unilateral neglect after vestibular stimulation. *J Neurol Neurosurg Psychiatry.* 1992;55(4):332–333.

78. Karnath HO, Christ K, Hartie W. Decrease of contralateral neglect by neck muscle vibration and spatial orientation of trunk midline. *Brain.* 1993;116(Pt 2):383–396.

79. Vallar G, Guarglia C, Nico D, Pizzamiglio L. Motor deficits and optokinetic stimulation in patients with left hemineglect. *Neurology.* 1997;49(5):1364–1370.

80. Priftis K, Passarini L, Pilosio C, et al. Visual scanning training, limb activation treatment, and prism adaptation for rehabilitating left neglect: who is the winner? *Front Hum Neurosci.* 2013;7:360.

81. Smithard DG, O'Neill PA, England RE, et al. The natural history of dysphagia following a stroke. *Dysphagia.* 1997;12(4):188–193.

82. Kumar S, Langmore S, Goddeau RP Jr, et al. Predictors of percutaneous endoscopic gastrostomy tube placement in patients with severe dysphagia from an acute-subacute hemispheric infarction. *J Stroke Cerebrovasc Dis.* 2012;21(2):114–120.

83. Larsen GL. Rehabilitation for dysphagia paralytica. *J Speech Hear Disord.* 1972;37(2): 187–194.

84. Gonzalez-Fernandez M, Ottenstein L, Atanelov L, Christain AB. Dysphagia after stroke: an overview. *Curr Phys Med Rehabil Rep.* 2013;1(3):187–196.

85. Huckabee M, Pelletier C. *Management of Adult Neurogenic Dysphagia.* San Diego: Singular Publishing Group; 1999.

86. Kiger M, Brown CS, Watkins L. Dysphagia management: an analysis of patient outcomes using VitalStim therapy compared to traditional swallow therapy. *Dysphagia.* 2006;21(4): 243–253.

87. Crary MA, Carnaby Mann GD, Groher ME, Helseth E. Functional benefits of dysphagia therapy using adjunctive sEMG biofeedback. *Dysphagia.* 2004;19(3):160–164.

88. Bulow M, Speyer R, Baijens L, et al. Neuromuscular electrical stimulation (NMES) in stroke patients with oral and pharyngeal dysfunction. *Dysphagia.* 2008;23(3):302–309.

89. Permsirivanich W, Tipchatyotin S, Wongchai M, et al. Comparing the effects of rehabilitation swallowing therapy vs. neuromuscular electrical stimulation therapy among stroke patients with persistent dysphagia: a randomized controlled study. *J Med Assoc. Thai.* 2009;92(2):259–265.

90. Hewitt A, Hind J, Kays S, et al. Standardized instrument for lingual pressure movement. *Dysphagia.* 2008;23(1):16–25.

91. Robbins J, Kays SA, Gangnon RE, et al. The effects of lingual exercise in stroke patients with dysphagia. *Arch Phys Med Rehabil.* 2007;88(2):150–158.

92. American Stroke Association. http://www.strokeassociation.org/STROKEORG /LifeAfterStroke/Life-After-Stroke_UCM_308546_SubHomePage.jsp. Accessed June 17, 2017.

93. Winstein CJ, Stein J, Ross A, et al. Guidelines for Adult Stroke Rehabilitation and Recovery—A Guideline for Healthcare Professionals from the American Heart Association/American Stroke Association. *Stroke.* 2016;47:e98–e169.

94. Stiefel M, Nolan K. *A Guide to Measuring the Triple Aim: Population Health, Experience of Care, and Per Capita Cost*. IHI Innovation Series white paper. Cambridge, MA: Institute for Healthcare Improvement; 2012.
95. Lindberg RH, Khan M. Cerebrovascular disorders Part 2 (management and treatment, cutting edge concepts in practice, gaps in evidence based practice). *PM&R Knowledge NOW*/American Academy of Physical Medicine and Rehabilitation. https://now.aapmr .org/cerebrovascular-disorders-part-2-management-and-treatment-cutting-edge -concepts-in-practice-gaps-in-evidence-based-practice/. Published October 3, 2012; modified May 5, 2016.

Cardiac Arrhythmias and Stroke 10

Frank Wilklow

Stroke was the second leading cause of death in the world behind heart disease in 2013, and it is a leading cause of serious disability in the United States.[1] Cardiac arrhythmias account for 15% to 20% of ischemic strokes.[1] Strokes associated with cardiac arrhythmias often carry more morbidity than strokes from other etiologies.[2]

The most common cardiac arrhythmia is atrial fibrillation, with 9% of people aged 65 or above affected by atrial fibrillation at some point in their lives.[2] The risk factors for atrial fibrillation include age, hypertension, sleep apnea, congestive heart disease, thyroid disease, alcohol use, coronary artery disease, and structural or valvular heart disease.[2]

The presence of atrial fibrillation increases the risk of stroke more than five-fold over the general population.[2] Atrial fibrillation is often associated with shortness of breath, labile blood pressure, peripheral and pulmonary edema, and tachycardia.[2] Patients presenting to an emergency room or clinic with risk factors for atrial fibrillation without overt electrocardiogram (ECG) findings should have a detailed history and physical performed and be screened for atrial fibrillation, especially if there are any worrisome clinical symptoms such as paroxysmal palpitations, intermittent dizzy spells, or new orthopnea. The history should be directed toward family members with atrial fibrillation because genetic predisposition is a significant risk factor.[3,4]

On physical exam, a patient with paroxysmal atrial fibrillation will often have secondary findings of long-standing hypertension, such as S4 gallop, elevated jugular venous pressure, or laterally displaced point of maximal impulse. Patients may have peripheral edema and bibasilar crackles consistent with expanded intravascular volume.[2]

The electrocardiogram often shows left atrial dilation as evidenced by a biphasic P-wave in V1, or a broad notched P-wave in lead II with duration greater than 120 ms (p-mitrale). The chest X-ray may show cardiomegaly and bilateral pleural effusions.[2]

Atrial flutter is a less common rhythm than atrial fibrillation, but it also carries a risk of thromboembolic stroke. Workup for atrial flutter and atrial fibrillation is similar, with the two disease processes having similar risk factors. Atrial flutter usually has a more organized pathway in one of the atria, with higher left atrial appendage emptying velocities; the stroke potential is similar to atrial fibrillations that usually coexist with occult atrial fibrillation, and patients who undergo definitive therapy for atrial flutter are sometimes left with paroxysmal atrial fibrillation in the aftermath.

ANTITHROMBOTIC THERAPY

The hallmark of atrial fibrillation and atrial flutter therapy is antithrombotic therapy.[2] Often, therapy is complicated by significant bleeding risk, advanced age, or significant concomitant illnesses that make therapy with antithrombotics anxiety-producing for the patient and the healthcare provider. Decisions regarding risk of stroke, risk of bleeding, pharmacologic agent, cost, and side-effect profile make decisions regarding antithrombotic therapy very difficult. To complicate matters, documentation is particularly important during this process because antithrombotic therapy is a particularly litigious area of medicine.

Underprescribing of antithrombotic and anticoagulation medication in the setting of paroxysmal atrial fibrillation has increasingly become a concern, especially in the advancing age population.[5] Studies have shown that up to one-third of patients who are at least at moderate risk of stroke from atrial fibrillation are being treated with aspirin, which is inadequate treatment.[5] The reasons for the undertreatment include perceived inflated risk of bleeding with advancing age, underestimation of risk of stroke, and concern for the safety of the novel oral anticoagulants.[6]

All patients who are being considered for antithrombotic therapy should have a calculation of their CHA2DS2-VASc score.[2,7] CHA2DS2-VASc is preferred over the older CHADS2 scoring system because it identifies vascular disease, myocardial infarct, aortic plaque and peripheral vascular disease (PVD), and the higher risk for stroke in women in the risk calculation.[7] The CHA2DS2-VASc score should be calculated and documented at each visit, as well as the calculated annual risk of stroke, and the score should be explained to the patient and family at each visit. Furthermore, each patient should have a HAS-BLED calculation performed compared to the risk of stroke with CHA2DS2-VASc.[8] Comparing these numbers and documenting the patient's and families' reaction to this information will help maintain transparency in the decision-making process and prevent confusion later should there be a complication with the medication or therapy leading to bleeding or stroke. Asking elderly patients to include family members in the decision-making process can also help mitigate family displeasure should complications arise.

The CHA2DS2-VASc score assigns numerical risk to the stroke risk factors of age (one or two points), female gender, congestive heart failure, hypertension, history of stroke or transient ischemic attack (TIA), vascular disease (as evidenced by arterial plaque or history of myocardial infarction), and diabetes. A score of 0 or 1 is considered "low" or "low-moderate" risk, and antiplatelet therapy alone can be considered; a score of 2 or greater is considered "moderate or high," and anticoagulation is recommended.[7]

The HAS-BLED score assigns a numerical risk to the bleeding risk factors of hypertension, liver disease, renal disease, stroke history, prior bleeding, labile international normalized ratio (INR), age, and high-risk medication (nonsteroidal anti-inflammatory drugs [NSAIDs]/antiplatelet).[8] A patient scoring 3 or higher is determined to be high risk, and consideration should be given to alternatives to anticoagulation. HAS-BLED was derived from the European Heart Survey in 2010 and has been shown to have superior performance to other risk calculators in risk assessment.

OPTIONS FOR ANTICOAGULATION

Dabigatran (Pradaxa) is a direct thrombin inhibitor that acts on free and clot-bound thrombin.[9] Dabigatran has a half-life of 12 to 17 hours; 80% of dabigatran is renally metabolized. The dabigatran package insert includes a black box warning of increased risk of stroke if therapy is temporarily held for reasons other than significant bleeding. Dabigatran is renally dosed according to creatinine clearance (CrCl). The Randomized Evaluation of Long-Term Anticoagulation Therapy (RE-LY) trial randomized more than 18,000 patients with atrial fibrillation to one of two doses of dabigatran or warfarin.[9] The higher dose of dabigatran (150 mg, twice daily) was superior to warfarin in prevention of stroke or systemic embolism (relative risk reduction [RRR] 34%) with a non-significant difference in major bleeding and a lower rate of hemorrhagic stroke. Dabigatran is the only novel oral anticoagulant that currently has a U.S. Food and Drug Administration (FDA)–approved reversal agent in Praxbind (idarucizumab).[10]

Rivaroxaban (Xarelto) is a selective inhibitor of factor Xa (FXa), has a half-life of 5 to 9 hours, and has mixed hepatic and renal metabolism.[11] Rivaroxiban also carries a black box warning regarding increased risk of stroke or TIA when stopped for surgery or other planned elective. Currently, there is no FDA-approved reversal agent for rivaroxiban; and it is not dialyzable. The Rivaroxaban Once Daily Oral Direct Factor Xa Inhibition Compared with Vitamin K Antagonism for Prevention of Stroke and Embolism Trial in Atrial Fibrillation (ROCKET AF trial) randomized more than 14,000 patients with nonvalvular atrial fibrillation to a daily dose of 20 mg rivaroxaban or dose-adjusted warfarin.[11] For the primary endpoint of stroke or system embolism, rivaroxaban was noninferior; no significant differences in adverse events were found.

Apixaban (Eliquis) is a selective inhibitor of FXa free and bound clot.[12] The half-life of apixaban is around 12 hours; it is predominantly hepatically metabolized with only 27% renal clearance. Eliquis also carries a black box warning regarding early termination for any reason other than bleeding. Currently, there is no FDA-approved reversal agent. Apixaban is not dialyzable. In the Apixaban versus Acetylsalicylic Acid to Prevent Stroke in Atrial Fibrillation Patients Who Have Failed or Are Unsuitable for Vitamin K Antagonist Treatment (AVERROES) trial, more than 5,000 patients with atrial fibrillation who had been deemed unsuitable for warfarin were randomized to apixaban (5 mg, twice daily) or aspirin (81–324 mg, daily).[12] The rate of stroke or systemic embolism was significantly lower in patients treated with apixaban, with no significant difference in adverse bleeding events. In the Apixaban for Reduction in Stroke and Other Thromboembolic Events in Atrial Fibrillation (ARISTOTLE) trial, more than 18,000 patients with atrial fibrillation and at least one other stroke risk factor were randomized to apixaban (5 mg, twice daily) or dose-adjusted warfarin.[13] The primary outcome of stroke or systemic embolism occurred less frequently in patients taking apixaban, and major bleeding—specifically, hemorrhagic stroke—occurred less frequently.

Edoxaban (Savaysa) is a selective FXa inhibitor with a half-life of 9–11 hours and 50% renal and 50% hepatic clearance.[14] Edoxaban is contraindicated in patients with normal renal function and can only be used if CrCl is less than 90 ml/min. There is a black box warning regarding early termination of the drug and for use in patients with normal renal function. There is no FDA-approved reversal agent for edoxaban; it is not dialyzable. In the Effective Anticoagulation with Factor Xa Next Generation in Atrial Fibrillation–Thrombolysis in Myocardial Infarction 48 (ENGAGE AF-TIMI) trial, more than 21,000 patients with moderate- to high-risk atrial fibrillation were randomized to one of two doses of edoxaban or to dose-adjusted warfarin.[14] The primary endpoint of stroke or systemic embolization occurred less frequently in the higher dose of edoxaban group compared to the warfarin group; the systemic bleeding rate was also lower in the higher dose group.

Warfarin (Coumadin) is a vitamin K–dependent inhibitor of factors II, VII, IX, and X and proteins C and S. Coumadin is the only anticoagulant indicated for atrial fibrillation in the setting of artificial valves; significant valvular disease, including mitral stenosis; hypercoaguable syndromes; and end-stage renal disease. In 1991, the Stroke Prevention in Atrial Fibrillation (SPAF) study demonstrated that patients randomized to warfarin, dose-adjusted to prothrombin time ratio 1.3 to 1.8/INR 2.0 to 4.5, had a lower rate of stroke than patients randomized to placebo.[15] SPAF II provided a direct comparison of warfarin to aspirin 325 mg, daily, in parallel trials stratified by age (dichotomized at 75 years). Warfarin offered a significant relative risk reduction of 33%, a relationship affected by age and underlying risk for thromboembolism.[16] Meta-analysis of pooled randomized controlled trials demonstrated an overall relative risk reduction of 68% compared with placebo, but the efficacy declines with INR < 2.0.[17,18]

Warfarin reversal can be readily achieved with weight-based 3-factor or 4-factor prothrombin complex concentrate (PCC) in the setting of emergency surgery or life-threatening bleeding along with vitamin K, 10 mg IV, and further correction with fresh frozen plasma (FFP) to limit a prothrombotic state.[19] If PCC is not available, FFP should be given along with vitamin K. In the setting of emergency surgery or life-threatening bleeding within 5 half-lives of dabigatran use or with renal insufficiency and recent use, idarucizumab (5 g IV in two divided doses) can be administered. If idarucizumab is not available, PCC is recommended. Hemodialysis may augment recovery of functional hemostasis. If last ingestion was within 2 hours of presentation with life-threatening hemorrhage, activated charcoal should also be administered. At this time, no specific antidote is available to reverse coagulopathy associated with FXa inhibitors (rivaroxaban, apixaban, edoxaban). Andexanet alfa is FDA approved, but not commercially available at the time of this writing. The current recommendation is to administer activated charcoal for ingestion within 2 hours of presentation and PCC if last use was within 5 half-lives of detection of life-threatening bleeding, such as intracerebral hemorrhage (ICH).

Alternatives to vitamin K agonists and novel oral anticoagulants include aspirin and Plavix. Aspirin (75–100 mg) combined with Plavix (75 mg) was inferior to warfarin therapy in preventing cardiovascular events, specifically stroke, in the Atrial fibrillation Clopidogrel Trial with Irbesartan for prevention of Vascular Events (ACTIVE W) trial, without any significant change in the risk of major bleeding. The number needed to treat with warfarin to prevent one stroke was 84.[20] The Atrial fibrillation Clopidogrel Trial with Irbesartan for prevention of Vascular Events (ACTIVE A) trial evaluated aspirin (75–100 mg) with or without Plavix (75 mg) in patients who were not candidates for long-term anticoagulation. With dual antiplatelet therapy, there was a decrease in stroke (number needed to treat was 34), but this advantage was offset by an increase in life-threatening bleeding (number needed to harm was 42).[21]

The American Heart Association/American Stroke Association (AHA/ASA) Guidelines for the Primary Prevention of Stroke recommend warfarin, targeting INR 2.0 to 3.0 for valvular atrial fibrillation (Class I: Level of Evidence A) for acceptable candidates.[22] For nonvalvular atrial fibrillation, acceptable candidates with a CHADS-VASC score of at least 2 should be treated with warfarin (Level of Evidence A), dabigatran, rivaroxaban, or apixaban (each Level of Evidence B), based on individualized factors. Patients with a CHADS-VASC score of 0 probably do not require an antithrombotic, and patients with a score of 1 should individualize the choice of anticoagulation, antiplatelet, or no therapy.

For secondary stroke prevention, AHA/ASA Guidelines recommendations are similar, yet stronger for warfarin, apixaban, and dabigatran (Class I) than rivaroxaban (Class IIa).[23] Antiplatelet therapy is recommended for patients who are poor candidates for anticoagulation. Careful consideration for risk of early recurrent stroke and hemorrhagic conversion should be made when deciding to initiate anticoagulation. The guidelines support initiation within 14 days unless there is a high risk for hemorrhagic conversion. In a nonrandomized, large (>1,000 patients) cohort of patients with ischemic stroke and atrial fibrillation, initiating anticoagulation (without bridging therapy) between days 4 and 14 post-stroke was associated with significantly reduced risk of a composite endpoint of stroke, TIA, systemic embolism, or symptomatic brain or extracranial bleeding.[24]

Typically, low-dose heparin or low-molecular-weight heparinoids can be started immediately after ischemic stroke and 1 to 4 days after a stabilized intracerebral hemorrhage to prevent venous thrombosis.[23,25]

RHYTHM CONTROL

Atrial fibrillation in the acute setting is often an unstable rhythm. Patients often present hemodynamically unstable with tachycardia and blood pressure instability. Several studies have been done to determine whether it is best to try developing a strategy of rhythm control versus simply rate and blood pressure control.

The Atrial Fibrillation Follow-up Investigation of Rhythm Management (AFFIRM) study was a landmark trial that randomized antiarrhythmic drugs and cardioversion versus rate-limiting medications.[26] The trial showed no survival or stroke prevention benefit of maintaining rhythm and greater potential for adverse drug effects. Rhythm control alone does not adequately reduce the risk of stroke in patients with atrial fibrillation.

The advent of radiofrequency ablation has added another alternative for treatment in atrial fibrillation.[27] Several studies have been done and are currently in progress to evaluate radiofrequency ablation versus rate or rhythm management.[27-29] Small early trials appear promising; however, the outcomes must be weighed against the procedural risks associated with transeptal puncture and the significant risk for stroke, cardiac tamponade, pulmonary vein stenosis, and esophageal fistula.[27-29]

OCCLUSION OF THE LEFT ATRIAL APPENDAGE

Autopsy studies have shown that the left atrial appendage (LAA) is the site of thrombi formation that causes central thromboembolism in up to 90% of patients with atrial fibrillation. Research has been directed toward devices that can be percutaneously placed to exclude the left atrial appendage to prevent stroke and decrease need for systemic anticoagulation.

Currently the Watchman (Boston Scientific) is the only FDA-approved device for LAA closure. It is a device placed through a transeptal puncture from the right atrium into the left atrium under transesophageal or intracardiac echocardiographic guidance. The WATCHMAN Left Atrial Appendage System for Embolic Protection in Patients With Atrial Fibrillation (PROTECT AF) trial showed decreased risk of stroke, systemic embolism, or unexplained cardiovascular death but higher procedural risk.[30,31] Follow-up studies, including Evaluation of the WATCHMAN LAA Closure Device in Patients With Atrial Fibrillation Versus Long Term Warfarin Therapy (PREVAIL), and meta-analyses of PROTECT AF and PREVAIL, show decreased procedural complications and continued benefit in stroke reduction.[32,33]

The Amplatzer (St. Jude) and other LAA closure devices are available in Europe and are currently being tested in trials in the United States. In early European trials, the device has similar efficacy trials with decreased procedural risk and lower risk of dislodgment.[34] Left atrial appendage closure is an option for stroke prevention in patients who are not candidates for long-term anticoagulation.[35] The stroke prevention guidelines recommend consideration of LAA closure for high-risk patients who are poor candidates for long-term anticoagulation, provided the procedure is performed by an experienced proceduralist with a low complication rate and the patient could take anticoagulation for the first 45 days after closure (Class IIb; Level of Evidence B).[23]

ANTICOAGULATION FOR ATRIAL FIBRILLATION
AFTER INTRACEREBRAL HEMORRHAGE

Lastly, the subject of anticoagulation after a hemorrhagic stroke is somewhat controversial. Understandably, there is trepidation by clinicians in restarting anticoagulation to avoid rebleeding or new bleeding and worsening of neurological condition. Most research, though limited in sample sizes, however, supports the early reintroduction of anticoagulation, weighing the risk and benefit analysis for the individual case. A nonrandomized, large (>700 patients) cohort of patients surviving discharge with anticoagulation-associated ICH were followed for 1 year.[36] Oral anticoagulation (all vitamin K antagonists) was resumed in less than 20% of patients who had atrial fibrillation (110 of 566) with median time to resumption of 31 days post-stroke. Atrial fibrillation patients who resumed anticoagulation after ICH had significantly reduced mortality and rate of ischemic complications without an increase in hemorrhagic complications as compared with those who did not resume anticoagulation. Those who resumed anticoagulation were younger, had lower ICH severity, and were less functionally disabled than those who did not resume anticoagulation after ICH. These relationships persisted even in analysis of propensity score–matched groups, suggesting age and ICH severity alone (with accompanying disability) could not explain all of the variance in subsequent ischemic stroke.

Cochrane analyzed randomized controlled trials of antithrombotic therapy after ICH and was able to include 121 patients from two randomized controlled trials, including short-term use of heparin or enoxaparin.[37] No significant difference in any endpoint was found, including growth of ICH. In a propensity score–matched study of patients with atrial fibrillation who had LAA occlusion after ICH compared to patients receiving standard medical therapy (anticoagulation), the risk of all-cause mortality, ischemic stroke, and major bleeding was lower in patients with LAA occlusion than in those managed medically.[38] Lobar ICH associated with amyloid angiopathy poses significant risk to resumption of anticoagulation; anticoagulation is usually withheld permanently in this population.[39,40] Presence of micro-bleeds is also considered a high-risk feature because they suggest diffuse vasculopathy from amyloid.[39,40] Resumption after a hypertensive ICH, however, is probably safe, provided the blood pressure is well controlled and not labile.[40] Other high-risk features include chronic atrial fibrillation, mechanical heart valve, age, comorbidities, and poorly controlled INR after initial stroke.[40]

References

1. Benjamin EJ, Blaha MJ, Chiuve SE, et al. Heart disease and stroke statistics—2017 update: a report from the American Heart Association [published online ahead of print January 25, 2017]. *Circulation*. doi: 10.1161/CIR.0000000000000485.
2. January CT, Wann LS, Alpert JS, et al. 2014 AHA/ACC/HRS guideline for the management of patients with atrial fibrillation. *J Am Coll Cardiol*. 2014;64(21):2246–2280.
3. Lemmens R, Hermans S, Nuyens D, Thijs V. Genetics of atrial fibrillation and possible implications for ischemic stroke. *Stroke Res Treat*. 2011;2011:208694.
4. Ritchie MD, Rowan S, Kucera G, et al. Chromosome 4q25 variants are genetic modifiers of rare ion channel mutations associated with familial atrial fibrillation. *J Am Coll Cardiol*. 2012;60(13):1173–1181.
5. Ogilvie IM, Newton N, Welner SA, et al. Underuse of oral anticoagulants in atrial fibrillation: a systematic review. *Am J Med*. 2010;123:638–645. doi: 10.1016/j.amjmed.2009.11.025.
6. Vallakai A, Lewis WF. Underuse of anticoagulation in patients with atrial fibrillation. *Postgrad Med*. 2016;128(2):191–200.
7. Olesen JB, Lip GY, Hansen ML, et al. Validation of risk stratification schemes for predicting stroke and thromboembolism in patients with atrial fibrillation: nationwide cohort study. *BMJ*. 2011;342:d124.
8. Zhu W, He W, Guo L, et al. The HAS-BLED score for predicting major bleeding risk in anticoagulated patients with atrial fibrillation: a systematic review and meta-analysis. *Clin Cardiol*. 2015;38(9):555–561.
9. Connolly SJ, Ezekowitz MD, Yusuf S, et al. Dabigatran versus warfarin in patients with atrial fibrillation. *N Engl J Med* 2009;361;1139–1151.
10. Pollack CV Jr, Reilly PA, Eikelboom J, et al. Idarucizumab for dabigatran reversal. *N Engl J Med*. 2015;373(6):511–520.
11. Patel MR, Mahaffey KW, Garg J, et al. Rivaroxaban versus warfarin in nonvalvular atrial fibrillation. *N Engl J Med*. 2011;365(10):883–891.
12. Connolly SJ, Eikelboom J, Joyner C, et al. Apixaban in patients with atrial fibrillation. *N Engl J Med*. 2011;364(9):806–817.
13. Granger CB, Alexander JH, McMurray JJ, et al. Apixaban versus warfarin in patients with atrial fibrillation. *N Engl J Med*. 2011;365(11):981–992.
14. Giugliano RP, Rff CT, Braunwald E, et al. Edoxaban versus warfarin in patients with atrial fibrillation. *N Engl J Med*. 2013;369(22):2093–2104.
15. Stroke prevention in atrial fibrillation study. Final results. *Circulation*. 1991;84(2):527–539.
16. Warfarin versus aspirin for prevention of thromboembolism in atrial fibrillation: Stroke Prevention in Atrial Fibrillation II Study. *Lancet*. 1994;343(8899):687–691.
17. Risk factors for stroke and efficacy of antithrombotic therapy in atrial fibrillation: analysis of pooled data from five randomized controlled trials. *Arch Intern Med*. 1994;154:1449–1457.
18. Hylek EM, Skates SJ, Sheehan MA, Singer DE. An analysis of the lowest effective intensity of prophylactic anticoagulation for patients with nonrheumatic atrial fibrillation. *N Engl J Med*. 1996;335:540–546.
19. Frontera JA, Lewin JJ, Rabinstein AA, et al. Guideline for Reversal of Antithrombotics in Intracranial Hemorrhage. A statement for healthcare professionals from the Neurocritical Care Society and Society of Critical Care Medicine. *Neurocrit Care* 2016;24:6–46.
20. Connolly S, Pogue J, Hart R, et al. Clopidogrel plus aspirin versus oral anticoagulation for atrial fibrillation in the Atrial fibrillation Clopidogrel Trial with Irbesartan for prevention of Vascular Events (ACTIVE W): a randomized controlled trial. *Lancet*. 2006;367(9526):1903–1912.

21. Connolly SJ, Pogue J, Hart RG, et al. Effect of clopidogrel added to aspirin in patients with atrial fibrillation. *N Engl J Med.* 2009;360(20):2066–2078.

22. Meschia JF, Bushnell C, Boden-Albala B, et al. Guidelines for the Primary Prevention of Stroke. A statement for healthcare professionals from the American Heart Association/American Stroke Association. *Stroke.* 2014;45:3754–3832.

23. Kernan WN, Ovbiagele B, Black HR, et al. Guidelines for the Prevention of Stroke in Patients with Stroke and Transient Ischemic Attack. A guideline for healthcare professionals from the American Heart Association/American Stroke Association. *Stroke.* 2014; 45:2160–2236.

24. Paciaroni, M, Agnelli G, Falocii N, et al. Early recurrence and cerebral bleeding in patients with acute ischemic stroke and atrial fibrillation: effect of anticoagulation and its timing: the RAF study. *Stroke.* 2015;46(8):2175–2182.

25. Morgenstern LB, Hemphill JC, Anderson C, et al. Guidelines for the Management of Spontaneous Intracerebral Hemorrhage. A guideline for healthcare professionals from the American Heart Association/American Stroke Association. *Stroke. 2010*;41:2108–2129.

26. Sherman DG, Kim SG, Boop BS, et al. Occurrence and characteristics of stroke events in the Atrial Fibrillation Follow-up Investigation of Sinus Rhythm Management (AFFIRM) Study. *Arch Intern Med.* 2005;165(10):1185–1191.

27. Cosedis Nielsen J, Johannessen A, Raatikainen P, et al. Radiofrequency ablation as initial therapy in paroxysmal atrial fibrillation. *N Engl J Med.* 2012;367:1587–1595. doi: 10.1056/NEJMoa1113566.

28. Pappone C, Vicedomini G, Augello G, et al. Radiofrequency catheter ablation and anti-arrhythmic drug therapy: a prospective, randomized, 4-year follow-up trial: the APAF study. *Circ Arrhythm Electrophysiol.* 2011;4:808–814. doi: 10.1161/CIRCEP.111.966408.

29. Jais P, Cauchemez B, Macle L, et al. Catheter ablation versus antiarrhythmic drugs for atrial fibrillation: Rhe A4 study. *Circulation.* 2008;118:2498–2505. doi: 10.1161/CIRCULATIONAHA.108.772582

30. Holmes DR, Reddy VY, Turi ZG, et al. Percutaneous closure of the left atrial appendage versus warfarin therapy for prevention of stroke in patients with atrial fibrillation: a randomised non-inferiority trial. *Lancet.* 2009;374:534–542. See more at: http://www.acc.org/latest-in-cardiology/articles/2016/09/20/06/41/left-atrial-appendage-closure-in-2016.

31. Reddy VY, Sievert H, Halperin J, et al. Percutaneous left atrial appendage closure vs warfarin for atrial fibrillation: a randomized clinical trial. *JAMA.* 2014;312(19):1988–1998.

32. Holmes DR Jr, Kar S, Price MJ, et al. Prospective randomized evaluation of the Watchman Left Atrial Appendage Closure device in patients with atrial fibrillation versus long-term warfarin therapy: the PREVAIL trial. *J Am Coll Cardiol.* 2014;64(1):1–12.

33. Holmes DR Jr, Doshi SK, Kar S, et al. Left atrial appendage closure as an alternative to warfarin for stroke prevention in atrial fibrillation: a patient-level meta-analysis. *J Am Coll Cardiol.* 2015;65(24):2614–2623.

34. Landmesser U, Schmidt B, Nielsen-Kudsk JE, et al. Left atrial appendage occlusion with the AMPLATZER Amulet device: periprocedural and early clinical/echocardiographic data from a global prospective observational study. *EuroIntervention.* 2017. pii: EIJ-D-17-00493. doi: 10.4244/EIJ-D-17-00493.

35. Reddy VY, Möbius-Winkler S, Miller MA, et al. Left atrial appendage closure with the Watchman device in patients with a contraindication for oral anticoagulation: the ASAP study (ASA Plavix Feasibility Study with Watchman Left Atrial Appendage Closure Technology). *J Am Coll Cardiol.* 2013;61:2551–2556. See more at: http://www.acc.org/latest-in-cardiology/articles/2016/09/20/06/41/left-atrial-appendage-closure-in-2016.

36. Kuramatsu JB, Gerner ST, Schellinger PD, et al. Anticoagulant reversal, blood pressure levels, and anticoagulant resumption in patients with anticoagulation-related intracerebral hemorrhage. *JAMA*. 2015;313(8):824–836.

37. Perry LA, Berge E, Bowditch J, et al. Antithrombotic treatment after stroke due to intracerebral hemorrhage. *Cochrane Database Syst Rev*. 2017;5:CD012144.

38. Nielsen-Kudsk JE, Johnsen SP, Wester P, et al. Left atrial appendage occlusion versus standard medical care in patients with atrial fibrillation and intracerebral hemorrhage: a propensity score-matched follow-up study. *EuroIntervention*. 2017;13(3):371–378.

39. Paciaroni M, Agnelli G. Should oral anticoagulants be restarted after warfarin-associated cerebral haemorrhage in patients with atrial fibrillation? *Thromb Haemost*. 2014;111(1): 14–18.

40. Goldstein JN, Greenberg SM. Should anticoagulation be resumed after intracerebral hemorrhage? *Cleve Clin J Med*. 2010;77(11):791–799.

Evaluation and Prevention of Stroke due to Structural Heart Disease

11

Christopher Favilla, James S. McKinney,
and Steven R. Messé

Cardioembolic strokes account for between 14% and 30% of ischemic strokes. The evaluation and work-up of cardiac sources of embolic strokes are previously discussed in detail in Chapter 5, and the most common cause for cardioembolism is atrial fibrillation (discussed in Chapter 10). However, other potential high-risk sources of cardiogenic embolism include left atrial or ventricular thrombus; cardiomyopathies, including global or focal wall motion abnormalities; atrial and septal defects; rheumatic and other valvular heart diseases; and recent myocardial infarctions. Other potential cardiac sources of embolism are likely associated with a lower or unclear risk of stroke (Table 11.1). This chapter will provide an overview of stroke due to structural cardiac abnormalities and current optimal management strategies.

INTRACARDIAC THROMBUS

Left Ventricular Thrombus

Left ventricular (LV) thrombus is an important source of emboli, particularly in patients with acute or recent myocardial infarctions (MIs). LV thrombus may be visualized on transthoracic echocardiography or suspected in "high-risk" patients with a low ejection fraction (<40%) and/or anterior or apical akinesis or left ventricular aneurysms. Mural LV thrombi are presumed to form due to stasis of blood in akinetic segments and endothelial injury and inflammation leading to activation of the clotting cascade.

The incidence of LV thrombus in patients with acute anterior wall MIs ranges from 4% to 17% in patients treated with thrombolysis or percutaneous coronary

158

TABLE 11.1 Cardioembolic sources of stroke

High risk	Atrial fibrillation/flutter
	Left atrial or ventricular thrombus
	Recent MI with ventricular aneurysm
	Infective endocarditis
	Nonbacterial thrombotic endocarditis
	Mechanical heart valves
Intermediate/low risk	Cardiomyopathy
	Mitral annular calcification
	Bioprosthetic heart valves
	Patent foramen ovale
	Atrial septal aneurysm

intervention.[1–3] However, in patients that do not receive timely reperfusion therapy, up to 56% of patients with anterior wall myocardial infarctions may develop LV thrombus.[1,4] Coronary intervention likely reduces the risk of LV thrombus formation and subsequent embolization by reducing infarct volume. A 1993 meta-analysis of patients with an anterior wall MI had a 52% reduction in the odds of developing LV thrombus if treated with thrombolytic therapy.[5]

Anticoagulation may also lower the risk of thrombus formation in the setting of acute anterior wall MI. Dalteparin, a low-molecular-weight heparin (LMWH), was associated with a significant reduction in LV thrombus formation in the Fragmin in Acute Myocardial Infarction (FRAMI) study; however, there was an increased risk of hemorrhagic complications and no observed difference in the rate of embolism.[6] A randomized, open-label study comparing warfarin, aspirin, or a combination in 3,630 patients with acute MI reported significant relative risk reductions in the primary outcome of death, nonfatal recurrent MI, or thromboembolic stroke in subjects randomized to warfarin (19%) and the combination (29%) compared to those receiving aspirin alone.[7] An earlier meta-analysis of outcomes after acute MI reported that anticoagulation with vitamin K antagonists lowered the risk of LV thrombus formation (odds ratio [OR] 0.32, confidence interval [CI] 0.20–0.52) and embolization (OR 0.14, CI 0.04–0.52).[5]

The potential benefits of anticoagulation must be weighed against the risks of hemorrhagic complications. Patients with acute MI, particularly those treated with percutaneous coronary intervention (PCI), are treated with dual antiplatelet therapy (DAPT). Those at risk for LV thrombus may also be anticoagulated.

This "triple therapy" places patients at increased risk of bleeding complications, particularly relevant if thromboembolism to the brain occurs. A statistical analysis published in 2012 by the American College of Chest Physicians (ACCP) estimated risk of stroke (relative risk [RR] 0.56, 95% CI 0.39–0.82) and major systemic bleeding (RR 2.37, 95% CI 1.62–3.47) in patients treated with triple antithrombotic therapy compared to dual antiplatelet therapy.[8]

ACCP guidelines recommend starting systemic anticoagulation with parenteral unfractionated heparin or LMWH in high-risk patients as soon as they are identified and continuing until a therapeutic warfarin dose (INR 2.0–3.0) has been achieved.[8] The length of time that anticoagulation is needed is unknown, but the risk of embolization is highest within the first 1 to 2 weeks and then declines. Current guidelines recommend that warfarin should be continued for up to 3 months.[8] At present, there are no data regarding the safety or efficacy in prevention of LV thrombus formation or embolization for other oral anticoagulant therapies. However, it may be reasonable to consider these agents or LMWH in high-risk patients who are unable to tolerate warfarin therapy.[9]

CARDIOMYOPATHY

There is an association between chronic systolic heart failure (HF) and cardioembolic stroke. The reported annual incidence of stroke in HF patients with an ejection fraction (EF) less than 35% is estimated between 1.5% and 3.5%.[10–12] Studies that have observed an increased risk of embolism in HF have found that older-age, prior stroke/transient ischemic attack (TIA), hypertension, diabetes mellitus, and lower ejection fraction may be independent risk factors for stroke in this patient population.[10,12,13]

Current evidence does not suggest a clear clinical benefit for antiplatelet or anticoagulant therapy for primary stroke prevention in patients with HF without atrial fibrillation (AF). A Cochrane analysis of the Heart failure Long-term Antithrombotic Study (HELAS) and the Warfarin/Aspirin Study in Heart Failure (WASH) showed no significant reduction in nonfatal stroke, MI, or death in HF patients in sinus rhythm treated with warfarin compared to a placebo.[14–16]

Two large clinical trials (WATCH and WARCEF) have also failed to show any significant benefit of anticoagulation with warfarin when compared to antiplatelet therapy in HF patients in sinus rhythm. The Warfarin and Antiplatelet Therapy in Chronic Heart Failure (WATCH) study randomized 1,587 subjects to aspirin (162 mg, daily), clopidogrel (75 mg, daily), or warfarin (goal international normalized ratio [INR] range 2.5–3.0).[17] Warfarin was associated with a significant reduction in nonfatal strokes compared to antiplatelet therapy.

However, when hemorrhagic and fatal strokes were included, there was no difference in outcomes between treatment groups (warfarin 1.7%, clopidogrel 2.5%, aspirin 2.9%).[17]

The Warfarin versus Aspirin in Reduced Cardiac Ejection Fraction (WARCEF) study enrolled 2,305 subjects with an EF < 35% and sinus rhythm to aspirin (325 mg, daily) or warfarin (target INR 2.0–3.5). There was no significant difference in the percentage of subjects reaching the primary endpoint of ischemic stroke, intracerebral hemorrhage, or all-cause mortality (7.5% vs. 7.9%). Anticoagulation was associated with a significant reduction in ischemic stroke compared to aspirin (hazard ratio [HR] 0.52, CI 0.33–0.82). The rates of intracranial bleeding were similar, but warfarin therapy was associated with a significant increase in the adjusted risk of major hemorrhage (RR 2.05, CI 1.36–3.12).[18] These results were confirmed in a meta-analysis of 3,681 subjects enrolled in four clinical trials that observed a 41% reduction in the risk of stroke but a two-fold increase in the risk of major hemorrhage with anticoagulation in HF patients.[19]

Antithrombotic therapy in patients with heart failure should be individualized. ACCP guidelines recommend against antithrombotic (antiplatelet or anticoagulant) therapy for primary cardiovascular protection in HF patients without another coronary artery disease or LV thrombus. For patients with prior systemic or pulmonary emboli, the 2010 Heart Failure Society of America guidelines recommend anticoagulation with a goal INR of 2.5 (range 2.0–3.0); however, this was based on expert opinion. The 2014 American Heart Association/American Stroke Association (AHA/ASA) guidelines note that anticoagulation is of uncertain benefit when compared to antiplatelet therapy and recommend individualized secondary stroke prevention strategies for patients with HF.[9] It is important to note that non–vitamin K antagonist anticoagulants, including direct thrombin inhibitors and factor Xa inhibitors, have demonstrated lower rates of bleeding complications with similar or better rates of ischemic events. However, these have not specifically been tested in patients with cardiomyopathy.

Patients with severe heart failure requiring LV assist devices (LVADs) as a bridge to transplantation or recovery or as final, long-term supportive (destination) therapy without plans for transplantation are at particularly high risk of stroke and arterial embolization. However, LVAD patients are also at increased risks of intracranial and gastrointestinal bleeding. Ischemic stroke rates have been reported to occur in 4% to 13% of cases of continuous-flow LVADs.[20] Hemorrhagic stroke has been observed in between 1% and 8% of cases.[20] Decisions regarding antithrombotic therapy should be made on a case-by-case basis.

VALVULAR HEART DISEASE

Valvular heart disease may be associated with an increased risk of cerebral embolism and stroke. Neither aortic valve stenosis, regurgitation, nor calcification is independently associated with an increased risk of stroke. However, mitral valve disease, infective endocarditis, noninfective thrombotic endocarditis, and prosthetic valves all carry an increased risk of embolic disease. The management of valvular heart disease in terms of stroke prevention is discussed later.

Mitral Valve Stenosis

Mitral stenosis usually results from the progressive fibrosis of mitral valve leaflets following rheumatic fever.[21] However, the symptoms of rheumatic heart disease do not often appear for years or decades after the initial streptococcal infection. Progressive mitral stenosis often leads to left atrial enlargement, impaired atrial emptying, atrial fibrillation, clot formation, and embolization. Stroke and arterial embolization were common prior to antithrombotic treatment, with systemic embolization with rates reported between 30% and 65% of cases.[22,23] No clinical trials evaluating the efficacy of antithrombotic therapy in patients with rheumatic mitral stenosis have been performed. Patients with stroke and mitral stenosis are at increased risk of recurrent embolic events even in the absence of coexisting atrial fibrillation.[24] Therefore, systemic anticoagulation with warfarin (target INR 2.0–3.0) is recommended in patients with rheumatic mitral stenosis with coexisting atrial fibrillation or prior stroke or arterial embolization.[9] The addition of aspirin to warfarin is not routinely recommended but may be considered in patients with rheumatic mitral stenosis who have an arterial embolization despite adequate anticoagulation.

Mitral Valve Regurgitation

Mitral valve regurgitation (MVR) may result from valve dysfunction due to infective endocarditis, rheumatic heart disease, mitral valve prolapse (MVP), or myxomatous degeneration or may occur in the presence of normal heart valves due to ventricular enlargement in patients with cardiomyopathies. Mitral valve regurgitation may be associated with left atrial enlargement and subsequent atrial fibrillation. However, in patients without coexisting atrial fibrillation, mitral regurgitation is not considered a high-risk source of cardioembolism.[9] A community-based observational study showed a small excess in the risk of ischemic stroke in 777 patients with MVR compared to the general population; however, this was largely driven by older patients and those with mitral valve thickening, atrial fibrillation, and the need for cardiac surgery.[25] There was no observed association between stroke and MVR in younger patients.

Mitral Annular Calcification

Calcification of the mitral valve is common in the general population and is associated with common cardiovascular risk factors for atherosclerosis. The risk of stroke in patients with mitral annual calcification (MAC) has been studied in several population-based studies. The Framingham Heart Study reported an adjusted two-fold increased risk of all strokes in patients with MAC (13.8%) compared to those without MAC (5.1%).[26] However, after restricting the analysis to patients with only ischemic strokes and including the presence of atrial fibrillation in the multivariable model, the increased risk of stroke was marginally significant (RR 1.78, CI 1.00–3.16). MAC was also associated with an increased risk of stroke in patients enrolled in the Stroke Heart Study and in the Cardiovascular Health Study.[27,28] It is unclear how MAC affects the risk of recurrent stroke in patients with prior stroke or TIA. No clinical trials have examined the safety or efficacy of specific antithrombotic drugs in prevention of stroke in patients with MAC. The AHA/ASA guidelines on secondary stroke prevention recommend antiplatelet therapy for secondary prevention of stroke in patients with MAC in the absence of atrial fibrillation or other indication for anticoagulation.[9]

Infective Endocarditis

Infective endocarditis (IE) is an important cause of both ischemic and hemorrhagic stroke, particularly in patients with prosthetic valves, recent medical procedures (indwelling catheters, orthopedic implants, or cardiac devices), or intravenous drug use. Timely diagnosis of IE is important because appropriate antimicrobial therapy may prevent embolic events, and antithrombotic therapy may increase the risk of intracerebral hemorrhage. Stroke and other neurological complications have been reported to occur in at least 25% of cases of IE in large retrospective series.[29,30] However, rates of asymptomatic embolic events may be higher if neuroimaging is obtained. The majority of embolic events occur within the first 2 weeks of therapy.[31] The majority of neurological events are ischemic events; however, meningitis, intracerebral or subarachnoid hemorrhage, mycotic aneurysms, and brain abscesses may occur.

The diagnosis of IE is usually made based on the combination of bacteremia with evidence of cardiac valvular vegetations. The modified Duke criteria provide diagnostic criteria for the diagnosis of IE (Table 11.2).[32] A definite diagnosis of IE requires a pathological diagnosis by histology or culture of a cardiac vegetation or the combination of clinical Duke criteria (two major, one major and three minor, or five minor criteria) be met. A possible diagnosis of IE may be made if one major plus one minor or three minor Duke criteria are fulfilled. Echocardiography should be performed in patients suspected of having endocarditis.

TABLE 11.2 Modified Duke criteria for diagnosis of infective endocarditis

Major Criteria	
1. Positive blood culture with typical IE organism from at least 2 separate blood cultures	• Viridians-group streptococci
	• Streptococcus bovis
	• HACEK group
	• *Staphylococcus aureus*
	• Community-acquired enterococci
2. Evidence of endocardial involvement with positive echocardiogram	• Mobile intracardiac mass on valve or supporting structures
	• Abscess
	• New prosthetic valve dehiscence or regurgitation
Minor Criteria	
1. Predisposing factor	• Known cardiac lesion
	• IV drug abuse
2. Fever	• Temperature >38°C
3. Embolism	• Arterial emboli
	• Pulmonary infarcts
	• Janeway lesions
	• Conjunctival hemorrhages
4. Immunological involvement	• Glomerulonephritis
	• Osler's nodes
	• Roth's spots
	• Rheumatoid factor
5. Microembolic evidence	• Positive blood culture that does not meet major criteria
	• Serological evidence of infection

Source: Adapted from Reference 32.

Transthoracic echocardiography (TTE) is highly specific (98%) but has relatively low sensitivity (44%), whereas transesophageal echocardiography (TEE) has great specificity (100%) and sensitivity (94%) for detection of vegetations in patients with suspected IE.[33] TEE should be performed in patients in whom IE is suspected despite a negative or limited TTE, as well as those with prosthetic or known valve lesions.

Treatment of IE should be appropriate antimicrobial therapy targeted to the causative organism. Initiation of therapy can usually wait until an organism is identified on blood culture, unless the patient appears unstable and empiric broad coverage is required. At least three sets of blood cultures should be sent within a short time frame, prior to initiation of therapy. The first and last sets should be obtained at least 60 minutes apart. In acutely ill patients, empiric antibiotic therapy with good gram-positive coverage (e.g., vancomycin) of most common causative organisms may be considered. Once an organism is identified, antibiotic therapy should be tailored based on available sensitivity data. Antibiotic therapy should be continued for up to 6 weeks from the time of documented negative blood cultures.[34] Shorter durations of therapy may be considered for patients with IE caused by particularly sensitive organisms. Infectious disease expert consultation should be obtained to help direct antimicrobial therapy.

Anticoagulation therapy in patients with IE may increase the risk of adverse events due to the high risk of hemorrhage from mycotic emboli. Continuation of anticoagulation in patients with mechanical valves is controversial. However, current guidelines recommend cessation of anticoagulation for at least 2 weeks in patients with IE who experience an embolic central nervous system (CNS) event.[34] A retrospective series of 637 consecutive patients with IE caused by *Staphylococcus aureus* reported a two-fold increase in mortality in patients with prosthetic valve infections compared to those with native valves (71% vs. 37%).[35] While this series found no difference in age, sex, embolic events, or CNS complications between groups, 90% of the prosthetic valve group and none of the native valve group were anticoagulated at the time of diagnosis. A small, randomized trial comparing aspirin to placebo in patients with IE has been conducted.[36] This study found similar rates of embolic phenomena in the aspirin (28%) and placebo (20%) groups (OR 1.62, CI 0.68–3.86) with an excess of bleeding complication in the aspirin group (OR 1.92, CI 0.76–4.86).[36]

Surgical intervention may be necessary in some patients. Clinical indications for consideration for early cardiac surgery may include valvular dysfunction with heart failure, valve perforation or rupture, large (>10 mm) or mobile vegetations, fungal endocarditis or infection caused by highly resistant organisms, and persistent bacteremia or recurrent embolization despite appropriate medical therapy.

When surgical intervention is considered, careful attention should be paid to those patients with neurological complications. Intra-operative anticoagulation with heparin may increase risks of CNS bleeding complications, particularly in those with hemorrhagic stroke and/or mycotic aneurysms. Mycotic aneurysms result from septic embolization with vegetation proliferation within the lumen of the vessel or in the arterial vasa vasorum. For patients with ischemic strokes without hemorrhage, noninvasive vascular imaging with CT or MR angiography to exclude mycotic aneurysm is likely sufficient. IE patients with intracranial hemorrhage should have a conventional catheter cerebral angiogram if noninvasive imaging is unremarkable to fully evaluate the intracranial circulation for mycotic aneurysms, particularly before undergoing cardiac surgery or starting systemic anticoagulation. Mycotic aneurysms may resolve with appropriate antibiotic therapy. However, aneurysms in patients with intracranial bleeding or in those needing urgent cardiac surgery should be treated. Treatment options include endovascular embolization and surgical resection.

Nonbacterial Thrombotic Endocarditis

Nonbacterial thrombotic endocarditis (NBTE) is an infrequent condition but may lead to thromboembolism. NBTE, also known as marantic endocarditis or Libman-Sacks endocarditis, is due to a prothrombotic state, such as can occur in patients with malignancies or systemic lupus erythematosus (SLE). NBTE is characterized by thrombus formation on previously normal heart valves. Thromboembolism may lead to arterial occlusion and stroke. Diagnosis is typically made in the proper clinical setting by echocardiography and by excluding an infective etiology.

NBTE is usually asymptomatic and diagnosed at autopsy in a small minority (1.25%) of cancer patients.[37,38] However, NBTE may occur more frequently in patients with adenocarcinoma, particularly those with pancreatic and mucin-secreting tumors (10%).[38] NBTE is rarely diagnosed in asymptomatic patients. However, it is estimated that approximately 50% of patients with known NBTE will suffer a thromboembolic event.[39,40]

NBTE should be considered in patients with acute ischemic stroke or arterial embolization in the setting of underlying cancer, SLE, antiphospholipid antibody syndrome, or disseminated intravascular coagulopathy. It may also be considered in patients with presumed infective endocarditis that is nonresponsive to antibiotic therapy.

The treatment of NBTE typically includes systemic anticoagulation, in addition to treatment of the underlying cancer or associated condition. Unlike patients with infective endocarditis, in which anticoagulation is contraindicated due to increased risks of intracranial bleeding and valve dysfunction, patients with NBTE should be anticoagulated. Although there are no studies comparing the efficacy of specific anticoagulants, guidelines recommend LMWH or unfractionated heparin.[41] Some series have suggested that warfarin is less effective, and no current data exist for other oral anticoagulant medications.[40,42]

Valve surgery for the treatment of NBTE may be considered in select cases. The indications for valve repair or replacement are similar to those for infective endocarditis and include decompensated heart failure, acute valve rupture, and recurrent embolization despite adequate medical therapy. Anticoagulation should be continued postoperatively due to an increased risk of recurrent disease.[39,43]

Prosthetic Heart Valves

Mechanical heart valves increase the risk of stroke and arterial embolism. Bioprosthetic valves are associated with lower risks of cardioembolism. Antithrombotic strategies for stroke prevention vary based on valve type, position, and associated comorbid conditions.

Prevention of stroke in patients with mechanical aortic valves requires anticoagulation with warfarin. Current consensus guidelines vary in the recommended intensity of anticoagulation. The 2012 ACCP guidelines recommend a goal INR of 2.5 (range 2.0–3.0), whereas the 2007 ACC/AHA and 2014 AHA/ASA guidelines recommend more intensive therapy with a target of 3.0 (range 2.5–3.5).[9,41,44] There are no clinical trials to date that have evaluated the efficacy and safety of more or less intensive anticoagulation in patients with mechanical aortic valves for either primary or secondary stroke prevention. Although, there are no clinical trials to direct the intensity of anticoagulant therapy for patients with mechanic mitral valves, there is a consensus among expert bodies, with all groups recommending more intensive therapy with a target INR of 3.0 (range 2.5–3.5).[9,41,44]

Antiplatelet therapy may be added to warfarin in patients felt to be at low risk of bleeding complications. A meta-analysis of 13 clinical trials that included 4,122 subjects reported the addition of an antiplatelet agent to anticoagulation resulted in a significant reduction in the risk of thromboembolic events (OR 0.43, CI 0.32–0.59) and total mortality (OR 0.57, CI 0.42–0.78) despite an increase in major bleeding (OR 1.58, CI 1.14–2.18).[45]

Non–vitamin K–dependent oral anticoagulant drugs have been shown to be effective in reducing the risk of stroke in patients with non-valvular atrial fibrillation. However, they should not be used in patients with mechanical heart valves until additional studies are performed. The Randomized Phase II Study to Evaluate the Safety and Pharmacokinetics of Oral Dabigatran Etexilate in Patients After Heart Valve Replacement (RE-ALIGN) trial was terminated early after an excess of thromboembolic events and bleeding complications were observed in the dabigatran group.[46]

Bioprosthetic aortic and mitral valves are associated with a lower risk of stroke than mechanical valves. The risk of stroke is highest in the 90 days following valve replacement and then sharply declines. Anticoagulation during this initial postoperative period may lower the risk of stroke.[47] Current ACCP and ACC/AHA guidelines recommend long-term antiplatelet therapy with 75 to 100 mg of aspirin daily for patients with bioprosthetic heart valves in sinus rhythm.[9,41,44]

Anticoagulation may be considered for patients with bioprosthetic valves and prior cardioembolism despite antiplatelet therapy.

PATENT FORAMEN OVALE AND SEPTAL DEFECTS

Patent foramen ovale (PFO) is a common congenital cardiac finding. While in utero, fetal lungs do not participate in gas exchange, and the pulmonary vascular resistance is high. This results in high right-sided cardiac pressures and a consequent right-to-left pressure gradient. This gradient drives right-to-left shunting through the foramen ovale because the positioning of the septum primum and secundum results in a one-way valve.[48] When pulmonary ventilation begins at birth, pulmonary perfusion leads to a quick rise in left atrial pressure, reversing the previous right-to-left gradient. This new left-to-right gradient forces the septum primum in a rightward direction, against the secundum, resulting in functional closure of the foramen ovale.[49] Eventually, anatomical closure will occur over time, but this process fails in ~25% of healthy individuals, resulting in a PFO.[50] The one-way nature of the valve created by the septum primum and secundum is often preserved, so conditions of elevated right-sided cardiac pressures will result in right-to-left shunting, as is generated during Vasalva maneuver or coughing,[51,52] as well as a number of pathologic conditions.[53] Normal right atrial filling may also generate a transient pressure gradient, resulting in a small amount of intermittent right-to-left shunt with each cardiac cycle.[54]

PFO has been implicated in a variety of pathophysiologic processes, most notably cryptogenic stroke. Mechanistically, the potential for right-to-left shunt during times of elevated right-sided cardiac pressure may facilitate paradoxical embolism of venous thrombus into the arterial circulation, which was first proposed in 1877 by Julius Cohnheim, based on autopsy identification of PFO in a young patient with cerebral embolism.[55] Additionally, the theoretical space between the septum primum and secundum may foster stagnant blood, ultimately promoting thrombus formation on the atrial septum. PFO may also increase the risk of atrial arrhythmia and thrombus formation.[56]

The association between PFO and stroke has largely been reported in retrospective case–control studies, and the relatively low event rate has made it difficult to explore in a more robust cohort model. The association is particularly noticeable among younger patients with otherwise cryptogenic stroke and TIA,[57–60] and cohorts of individuals with asymptomatic PFO have failed to demonstrate an increase rate of primary ischemic stroke.[61–63] Consequently, the focus has remained on the subgroup of cryptogenic stroke patients with PFO in order to better understand the potentially causative relationship. The Risk of Paradoxi-

TABLE 11.3 Risk of Paradoxical Embolism (RoPE) score, PFO attributable fraction, and subsequent 2-year risk of stroke

RoPE Score	PFO Attributable fraction (%)	2-Year stroke risk (%)
0–3	0	16 (9–24)
4	38	9 (4–14)
5	34	3 (0–6)
6	62	4 (2–7)
7	72	2 (0–4)
8	84	3 (0–5)
9–10	88	1 (0–2)

Source: Adapted from Reference 65.

Note: The RoPE score is determined by adding one point for each decade under 70, down to 20, and then adding one point for no history of hypertension, diabetes, prior stroke/TIA, not being a smoker, and presence of cortical infarction on imaging. This results in a maximum possible score of 10, suggesting a high likelihood of finding a PFO on work-up, and a minimum possible score of 0, suggesting a very low likelihood that a PFO will be identified on work-up

cal Embolism (RoPE) study merged 12 prior cohorts of cryptogenic stroke patients—2,546 total patients—in order to generate a patient-specific score that indicates the likelihood that a patient's PFO was pathogenically related to the cryptogenic stroke rather than incidental.[64] The components of the RoPE score and attributable risk of the PFO are presented in Table 11.3.[65]

Advances in echocardiography and transcranial Doppler (TCD) ultrasonography have dramatically enhanced clinical detection of PFO.[66] The gold standard for PFO detection is direct visualization of transcardiac shunting during TEE with contrast medium.[67–69] Though less sensitive, a less invasive approach may be pursued with TTE with color-flow Doppler or contrast medium.[70,71] Another commonly employed noninvasive approach utilizes TCD of the cerebral vessels during intravenous injection of agitated saline, monitoring for right-to-left shunting during Valsalva maneuver or cough, which is nearly as sensitive as TEE[72–74] but fails to directly visualize the PFO and cannot differentiate cardiac from non-cardiac right-to-left shunts and does not allow for detection of other mechanisms of stroke and TIA originating in the heart and aorta.

Medical Management of PFO

Secondary stroke prevention in patients with PFO remains a highly controversial management dilemma. Because there is no clear increased risk of stroke in asymptomatic patients with PFO,[61] there is no evidence to support medical therapy for primary stroke prevention. Although there have been a number of studies addressing secondary stroke prevention in patients with PFO, optimal therapy remains uncertain.

Medical management for secondary stroke prevention after PFO includes either antiplatelet therapy or anticoagulation. Meta-analyses of non-randomized studies of antiplatelet and anticoagulant medication have reported a benefit for anticoagulation. However, there are tremendous biases in who receives each medication, and only randomized data can reasonably answer this question. Homma et al explored a subgroup of patients with cryptogenic stroke from the Warfarin versus Aspirin for Recurrent Stroke Study (WARSS).[75,76] Of the 265 patients with cryptogenic stroke, 98 were found to have PFO, but there was no difference in stroke recurrence or death at 2 years between PFO patients treated with aspirin or warfarin, 17.9% and 9.5%, respectively (risk reduction [RR] 8.4%; 95% CI 6.8–23.6). While the point estimate appeared to favor warfarin, it is important to note that patients without PFO had similar event rates on aspirin and warfarin (16.3% and 8.3%, respectively), and thus anticoagulation may be beneficial for any cryptogenic stroke patient. In addition, the recurrent stroke rate after cryptogenic stroke in Patent Foramen Ovale in the Cryptogenic Stroke Study (PICSS) was similar in patients with and without PFO, 20.4% and 16.6% respectively (HR 1.23; 95% CI 0.69–2.20, $p=0.49$). In 2013, Shariat et al completed a randomized trial of 44 patients with cryptogenic stroke in the context of PFO.[77] Patients were assigned to either aspirin 240 mg, daily, or warfarin (goal INR 2.0–3.0), but over 18 months of follow-up, there was no difference in the ischemic events or death between the two treatment arms, 13% and 28%, respectively (HR 0.45; 95% CI 0.1–1.8, $p=0.259$). Given the small size of these two trials and the imprecise nature of the data, as is evident by the broad confidence intervals, it is difficult to exclude a potentially important difference in efficacy between anticoagulation and antiplatelet therapy. However, numerous studies of anticoagulation for secondary stroke prevention have confirmed a higher rate of bleeding complications for the former.[75,78]

PFO Closure

Open surgical closure of PFO is rarely pursued; it is typically reserved for cases where open cardiac surgery is indicated for another reason but subsequent stroke rates remain high.[79] Percutaneous, catheter-based PFO closure was first introduced in 1992,[80] offering a less invasive approach, which is now much more commonly employed. Observational non-randomized data have suggested that percutaneous PFO closure may be superior to medical management after cryptogenic stroke,[81,82] and randomized trials of PFO closure have been very slow to enroll. In 2004, the Food and Drug Administration (FDA) revoked the humanitarian device exemption for the percutaneous PFO occluder, and in 2009, the

AHA/ASA recommended limiting the clinical application of PFO closure for secondary stroke prevention to clinical trials.[83] After long enrollment periods, the results of five randomized clinical trials have been reported in the past few years.

In the CLOSURE I trial,[84] Furlan et al randomized 909 patients to PFO closure with a STARFLEX percutaneous device (NMT Medical) or medical therapy after cryptogenic stroke/TIA. Patients that underwent closure were also treated with clopidogrel 75 mg, daily, for the first 6 months, followed by aspirin 81 mg or 325 mg, daily. Patients assigned to medical therapy were treated at the discretion of the enrolling investigator with aspirin 325 mg, daily, warfarin (goal INR 2.0–3.0), or both. At 2 years, recurrent stroke occurred in 2.9% of patients who underwent closure and 3.1% of patients on medical therapy (HR 0.90; 95% CI 0.41–1.98; $p=0.79$). Three of the 12 strokes in the closure group were ascribed to new-onset AF, two of which had device-associated thrombus. Only one of 13 strokes in the medical therapy group was ascribed to new-onset AF, which only occurred after an off-study device was implanted to close the PFO. During the follow-up period, AF was identified in a larger number of patients who underwent closure, 5.7% as compared to 0.7% of patients assigned to medical therapy ($p<0.001$). Major vascular procedural complications were reported in 3.2% of patients who underwent closure, including cardiac perforation in two patients. It warrants note that the number of patients who either crossed over or were lost to follow-up was nearly three times the number of patients who suffered recurrent strokes, ultimately limiting the strength of any conclusions.

In the PC trial,[85] Meier et al randomized 414 cryptogenic stroke patients to percutaneous closure with the Amplatzer device (St. Jude Medical) or medical therapy. Patients assigned to PFO closure were also treated with aspirin 100–325 mg, daily, for at least the first 5 months in addition to ticlopidine 250–500 mg, daily, or clopidogrel 75–150 mg, daily, for 1–6 months. Patients in the medical therapy arm were treated at the discretion of the enrolling investigator, with either antiplatelet or oral anticoagulation. Over the 4-year follow-up period, there was no significant difference in stroke recurrence, which occurred in 0.5% of patients who underwent closure and 2.4% of patients assigned to medical therapy (HR 0.20; 95% CI 0.02–1.72, $p=0.14$). There was also no difference in the prespecified primary endpoint of composite death, nonfatal stroke, TIA, or peripheral embolism, which occurred in 3.4% of patients who underwent closure and 5.2% of patients assigned to medical therapy (HR 0.70; 95% CI 0.27–1.85, $p=0.48$). New-onset AF was identified in 2.9% of the closure arm and 1.0% of the medical treatment arm ($p=0.16$).

In the RESPECT trial,[86] Carroll et al randomized 980 patients to closure with the Amplatzer device or medical therapy. Patients who underwent PFO closure were also treated with aspirin 81 to 325 mg, daily, plus clopidogrel 75 mg, for 1 month, followed by aspirin monotherapy for 5 additional months, followed by antiplatelet therapy at the discretion of the enrolling investigator. Patients in the medical therapy arm were treated with antiplatelet or oral anticoagulation at the discretion of the enrolling investigator. Over the 2.5-year follow-up period, there was no significant difference in stroke recurrence, which occurred in only 1.8% of patients who underwent closure and 3.3% of patients assigned to medical therapy (HR 0.49, 95% CI 0.22–1.11, $p=0.08$). The per-protocol analysis did identify a significant benefit of closure, with 1.3% recurrent stroke in the closure arm and 3.0% recurrent stroke in the medical therapy arm (HR 0.37; 95% CI 0.14–0.96, $p=0.03$). Importantly, there was an imbalance in the loss to follow-up between the two arms: 9% of the patients in the closure arm dropped out of the study, as compared to 17% of the medical therapy arm. New-onset AF occurred in 3% of the closure arm and 1.5% of the medical therapy arm ($p=0.13$).

The long-term follow-up from the RESPECT trial provides more convincing evidence of a benefit for PFO closure.[87] After following patients for a median of 5.9 years, compared to only 2.3 years in the initial publication, the stroke recurrence HR was 0.55, 95% CI 0.305–0.999, log-rank $p=0.046$. Importantly, there was a fairly high loss to follow-up at the final database lock: 27% overall with 33% lost in medical arm versus 21% in the closure arm. In addition, there was a higher rate of deep vein thrombosis (DVT) (0.16 vs. 0.04 per 100 patient-years, HR 4.44; 95% CI 0.52–38.05, $p=0.14$) and pulmonary embolism (0.41 vs. 0.11 per 100 patient-years, HR 3.48; 95% CI 0.98–12.34, $p=0.04$) in patients who underwent closure, presumably due to the fact that about one-fourth of patients in the medical arm were given anticoagulation, which was rare in the patients who underwent closure. Based on these results, the FDA approved the Amplatzer PFO occluder for use in the United States in young patients with cryptogenic stroke.

Two additional randomized studies were just completed.[88,89] The Gore REDUCE trial also demonstrated a benefit for stroke recurrence reduction in patients who underwent transcatheter closure compared to antiplatelet therapy alone.[88] In this trial, 664 patients were randomized in a 2:1 ratio to closure with a Gore Helex septal occluder or cardioform septal occluder or with antiplatelet therapy with aspirin, clopidogrel, or aspirin plus extended release dipyridamole. After a median follow-up of 3.2 years, there were fewer strokes in the patients who underwent closure (0.39 per 100 person-years vs. 1.70 per 100 person-years; HR 0.23; 95% CI 0.09–0.62; log-rank $p=0.001$). The rate of serious adverse events (SAEs) was similar between groups, though there was a higher rate of atrial fibrillation/flutter in patients who were closed (6.6% vs. 0.4%, $p<0.001$). The vast majority of these events were periprocedural and self-limited. Finally, the French CLOSE trial randomized 663 patients to PFO closure, aspirin, or anticoagulation with warfarin.[89] After a mean follow-up of 5.3 years, recurrent stroke was reduced with PFO closure by a relative 97% compared with antiplatelet therapy alone (HR 0.03; 95% CI 0–0.12). There were no strokes in the closure group and 14 in the controls. There was no significant difference between oral anticoagulation and aspirin therapy (HR 0.43; 95% CI 0.10–1.50).

Taken together, these randomized trials suggest that transcatheter PFO closure can reduce stroke risk in carefully selected patients. Importantly, the absolute risk of stroke was low, and this intervention likely is not needed on an emergent basis for most patients. All of these trials limited inclusion to patients under 60 years of age, and they all required a thorough evaluation to rule out other causes of stroke, making the PFO the most likely etiology. Future medical therapy trials may also prove to be important, particularly with the availability of several novel oral anticoagulants, which have demonstrated efficacy and safety in patients at risk of venous thromboembolism.

Atrial Septal Aneurysm

Atrial septal aneurysm (ASA) is characterized by a saccular deformity of the atrial septum, which is a redundancy of the atrial septum resulting in excessive movement throughout the cardiac cycle. The degree of movement that constitutes an ASA is not agreed upon, though most studies have utilized 10 to 15 mm of excursion as a cutoff.[90] ASA is far less common than PFO, occurring in less than 2% of the general population, but when present, it is often seen in association with PFO.[91,92] When ASA and PFO co-occur, there is some evidence that there may be a higher risk of stroke, but this relationship is controversial and has not been seen in all cohorts.[93–96] The potential mechanism of stroke in these patients remains largely unclear. Left atrial dysfunction has been reported in patients with both ASA and PFO, so one hypothesis is that such dysfunction contributes to thrombus formation and subsequent cardioembolic risk.[97] If ASA is found in isolation, the optimal treatment is unclear.[98,99] The risk of recurrent stroke with isolated ASA is exceptionally low,[98,100] so treatment with antiplatelet therapy is a reasonable course of action. If an ASA and PFO co-occur, which is not infrequent, PFO closure should be considered if no other stroke etiology is apparent, as described earlier.

Atrial Septal Defect

Atrial septal defect (ASD) is less common than PFO, and it consists of several subtypes, all of which are characterized by a failure of atrial septation.[101] While PFO serves as a one-way flap valve for possible right-to-left shunt, ASD represents an open interatrial communication. In a sizable defect, the normal left-to-right pressure gradient results in shunting, which may result in increased pulmonary vascular pressures and right heart strain or failure. Still, a very small ASD may not present with clinical symptoms for several decades, if at all.[102] In fact, the ACC/AHA recommends against closure of a small ASD (<5 mm) that is identified in adulthood without evidence of right heart compromise. If ASD is identified after cryptogenic stroke, the role of closure remains unclear.[102,103] In the absence of cardiopulmonary compromise, closure is often clinically pursued for secondary stroke prevention without substantial evidence to support this practice. Regardless of closure, attention should be paid to cardiac rhythm monitoring, given the significant risk of AF.[104]

Aortic Arch Atheroma

Aortic arch atheromatous (AAA) plaques, which result from atherosclerosis, may be associated with arterial embolism and stroke.[105,106] While there is no clear association with vascular events in the general population, there is likely an association with recurrent ischemic strokes in patients with cerebrovascular disease.[107,108] The risk of recurrent cerebral embolism appears to be directly associated with plaque thickness. Aortic atheromas (AoAs) with an aortic-wall thickness of ≥4 mm are associated with a stroke incidence of 11.9 per 100 person-years; whereas atheromas with 1- to 3.9-mm thickness and <1-mm thickness have a stroke incidence of 3.9 and 2.8 per 100 person-years, respectively.[108] In addition to atheroma thickness ≥4 mm, other complex features, such as mobile, ulcerated, and/or protruding plaques, are associated with an increased risk of stroke and vascular events.[108,109] Stroke and arterial embolization may occur spontaneously in these patients or as a complication of procedures that may manipulate or disrupt aortic endothelium or plaque. Cardiac surgery,[110,111] catheterization/endovascular procedures,[112,113] and intra–aortic balloon counterpulsation[114] all may increase the risk of cerebral embolism in patients with complex thoracic aortic atherosclerotic disease.

Several different imaging techniques may be used to detect AoA, including echocardiography, computed tomography (CT), and magnetic resonance (MR).[115] TEE, which can detect mobile elements in real time, is highly accurate in characterizing aortic plaque morphology with a sensitivity and specificity greater than 90%.[116] CT angiography may be less sensitive in detecting AoA compared to TEE.[115] In a study of 47 patients with stroke/TIA, the sensitivity of CT angiography compared to TEE was reported to be 52.6%.[117] Although not widely available, cardiovascular MR is also a useful technique to diagnose and characterize AoA in the proximal aorta for both small, 1 to 3.9 mm (sensitivity 90%, specificity 100%), and large, ≥4 mm (sensitivity 71%, specificity 93%) plaques.[118]

Treatment of AoA is primarily medical therapy aimed at treatment of modifiable vascular risk factors, including treatment of hypertension, hyperlipidemia, diabetes, and smoking cessation coupled with antithrombotic therapy to lower risk of embolization. The optimal antithrombotic therapy (antiplatelet vs. anticoagulant) for either primary or secondary stroke prevention is not well defined. In a subset of patients enrolled in the Stroke Prevention in Atrial Fibrillation III (SPAF-III) trail with complex aortic plaques (≥4 mm, ulcerated, mobile, or pedunculated), the stroke rate after 1.1 years average follow-up was 16% in the low-dose warfarin (INR 1.2–1.5) plus aspirin group versus 4% in the warfarin (INR 2.0–3.0) group.[119] However, all of these patients had atrial fibrillation, and increased event rates may have been secondary to atrial fibrillation–related cardioembolism rather than AoA. The Aortic Arch Related Cerebral Hazard (ARCH) trial was a prospective randomized, open-label trial that randomized subjects with prior stroke/TIA or arterial embolization and complex aortic plaque to either aspirin (75–150 mg, daily) plus clopidogrel (75 mg, daily) or warfarin (INR 2.0–3.0).[120] The trial was stopped early because of poor enrollment but included 349 subjects who were followed for a median of 3.4 years. In this cohort of enrolled patients, vascular events (stroke, MI, peripheral embolism, death) occurred less often in patients receiving dual antiplatelet therapy (7.6%) than in those receiving warfarin (11.3%), but this was not significant ($p = 0.20$).[120] In a retrospective cohort study of 519 patients with complex thoracic aortic plaques, statin therapy was independently associated with decreased odds of embolic events (OR 0.3, CI 0.2–0.6).[121] Medical management of patients with stroke/TIA and large, complex AoA should include a combination of antiplatelet and statin therapy, as well as modification of vascular risk factors.

References

1. Greaves SC, Zhi G, Lee RT, et al. Incidence and natural history of left ventricular thrombus following anterior wall acute myocardial infarction. *Am J Cardiol.* 1997;80: 442–448.
2. Nayak D, Aronow WS, Sukhija R, et al. Comparison of frequency of left ventricular thrombi in patients with anterior wall versus non-anterior wall acute myocardial infarction treated with antithrombotic and antiplatelet therapy with or without coronary revascularization. *Am J Cardiol.* 2004;93:1529–1530.
3. Kalra A, Jang IK. Prevalence of early left ventricular thrombus after primary coronary intervention for acute myocardial infarction. *J Thromb Thrombolysis.* 2000;10:133–136.
4. Asinger RW, Mikell FL, Elsperger J, Hodges M. Incidence of left-ventricular thrombosis after acute transmural myocardial infarction. Serial evaluation by two-dimensional echocardiography. *N Engl J Med.* 1981;305:297–302.
5. Vaitkus PT, Barnathan ES. Embolic potential, prevention and management of mural thrombus complicating anterior myocardial infarction: a meta-analysis. *J Am Coll Cardiol.* 1993;22:1004–1009.

6. Kontny F, Dale J, Abildgaard U, Pedersen TR. Randomized trial of low molecular weight heparin (dalteparin) in prevention of left ventricular thrombus formation and arterial embolism after acute anterior myocardial infarction: the fragmin in acute myocardial infarction (frami) study. *J Am Coll Cardiol.* 1997;30:962–969.

7. Hurlen M, Abdelnoor M, Smith P, et al. Warfarin, aspirin, or both after myocardial infarction. *N Engl J Med.* 2002;347:969–974.

8. Vandvik PO, Lincoff AM, Gore JM, et al. Primary and secondary prevention of cardiovascular disease: antithrombotic therapy and prevention of thrombosis, 9th ed: American College of Chest Physicians Evidence-Based Clinical Practice Guidelines. *Chest.* 2012; 141:e637S–e668S.

9. Kernan WN, Ovbiagele B, Black HR, et al. Guidelines for the prevention of stroke in patients with stroke and transient ischemic attack: a guideline for healthcare professionals from the American Heart Association/American Stroke Association. *Stroke.* 2014;45: 2160–2236.

10. Abdul-Rahim AH, Perez AC, Fulton RL, et al. Risk of stroke in chronic heart failure patients without atrial fibrillation: analysis of the Controlled Rosuvastatin in Multinational Trial Heart Failure (CORONA) and the Gruppo Italiano per lo Studio della Sopravvivenza nell'insufficienza Cardiaca-Heart Failure (GISSI-HF) trials. *Circulation.* 2015;131:1486–1494; discussion 1494.

11. Mahajan N, Ganguly J, Simegn M, et al. Predictors of stroke in patients with severe systolic dysfunction in sinus rhythm: role of echocardiography. *Int J Cardiol.* 2010;145:87–89.

12. Freudenberger RS, Hellkamp AS, Halperin JL, et al. Risk of thromboembolism in heart failure: an analysis from the Sudden Cardiac Death in Heart Failure Trial (SCD-HEFT). *Circulation.* 2007;115:2637–2641.

13. Loh E, Sutton MS, Wun CC, et al. Ventricular dysfunction and the risk of stroke after myocardial infarction. *N Engl J Med.* 1997;336:251–257.

14. Cokkinos DV, Haralabopoulos GC, Kostis JB, Toutouzas PK. Efficacy of antithrombotic therapy in chronic heart failure: the HELAS study. *Eur J Heart Fail.* 2006;8:428–432.

15. Cleland JG, Findlay I, Jafri S, et al. The Warfarin/Aspirin Study in Heart Failure (WASH): a randomized trial comparing antithrombotic strategies for patients with heart failure. *Am Heart J.* 2004;148:157–164.

16. Lip GY, Shantsila E. Anticoagulation versus placebo for heart failure in sinus rhythm. *Cochrane Database Syst Rev.* 2014;3:CD003336.

17. Massie BM, Collins JF, Ammon SE, et al. Randomized trial of warfarin, aspirin, and clopidogrel in patients with chronic heart failure: the Warfarin and Antiplatelet Therapy in Chronic Heart Failure (WATCH) trial. *Circulation.* 2009;119:1616–1624.

18. Homma S, Thompson JL, Pullicino PM, et al. Warfarin and aspirin in patients with heart failure and sinus rhythm. *N Engl J Med.* 2012;366:1859–1869.

19. Kumar G, Goyal MK. Warfarin versus aspirin for prevention of stroke in heart failure: a meta-analysis of randomized controlled clinical trials. *J Stroke Cerebrovasc Dis.* 2013;22: 1279–1287.

20. Eckman PM, John R. Bleeding and thrombosis in patients with continuous-flow ventricular assist devices. *Circulation.* 2012;125:3038–3047.

21. Chandrashekhar Y, Westaby S, Narula J. Mitral stenosis. *Lancet.* 2009;374:1271–1283.

22. Carter AB. Prognosis of cerebral embolism. *Lancet.* 1965;2:514–519.

23. Daley R, Mattingly TW, Holt CL, et al. Systemic arterial embolism in rheumatic heart disease. *Am Heart J.* 1951;42:566–581.

24. Olesen KH. The natural history of 271 patients with mitral stenosis under medical treatment. *Br Heart J.* 1962;24:349–357.

25. Avierinos JF, Brown RD, Foley DA, et al. Cerebral ischemic events after diagnosis of mitral valve prolapse: a community-based study of incidence and predictive factors. *Stroke.* 2003;34:1339–1344.

26. Benjamin EJ, Plehn JF, D'Agostino RB, et al. Mitral annular calcification and the risk of stroke in an elderly cohort. *N Engl J Med.* 1992;327:374–379.

27. Kizer JR, Wiebers DO, Whisnant JP, et al. Mitral annular calcification, aortic valve sclerosis, and incident stroke in adults free of clinical cardiovascular disease: the Strong Heart Study. *Stroke.* 2005;36:2533–2537.

28. Rodriguez CJ, Bartz TM, Longstreth WT Jr., et al. Association of annular calcification and aortic valve sclerosis with brain findings on magnetic resonance imaging in community dwelling older adults: the Cardiovascular Health Study. *J Am Coll Cardiol.* 2011;57:2172–2180.

29. Garcia-Cabrera E, Fernandez-Hidalgo N, Almirante B, et al. Neurological complications of infective endocarditis: risk factors, outcome, and impact of cardiac surgery: a multicenter observational study. *Circulation.* 2013;127:2272–2284.

30. Heiro M, Nikoskelainen J, Engblom E, et al. Neurologic manifestations of infective endocarditis: a 17-year experience in a teaching hospital in Finland. *Arch Intern Med.* 2000; 160:2781–2787.

31. Vilacosta I, Graupner C, San Roman JA, et al. Risk of embolization after institution of antibiotic therapy for infective endocarditis. *J Am Coll Cardiol.* 2002;39:1489–1495.

32. Li JS, Sexton DJ, Mick N, et al. Proposed modifications to the Duke criteria for the diagnosis of infective endocarditis. *Clin Infect Dis.* 2000;30:633–638.

33. Shively BK, Gurule FT, Roldan CA, et al. Diagnostic value of transesophageal compared with transthoracic echocardiography in infective endocarditis. *J Am Coll Cardiol.* 1991;18:391–397.

34. Baddour LM, Wilson WR, Bayer AS, et al. Infective endocarditis in adults: diagnosis, antimicrobial therapy, and management of complications: a scientific statement for healthcare professionals from the American Heart Association. *Circulation.* 2015;132:1435–1486.

35. Tornos P, Almirante B, Mirabet S, et al. Infective endocarditis due to *Staphylococcus Aureus*: deleterious effect of anticoagulant therapy. *Arch Intern Med.* 1999;159:473–475.

36. Chan KL, Dumesnil JG, Cujec B, et al. A randomized trial of aspirin on the risk of embolic events in patients with infective endocarditis. *J Am Coll Cardiol.* 2003;42:775–780.

37. Rosen P, Armstrong D. Nonbacterial thrombotic endocarditis in patients with malignant neoplastic diseases. *Am J Med.* 1973;54:23–29.

38. Gonzalez Quintela A, Candela MJ, Vidal C, et al. Non-bacterial thrombotic endocarditis in cancer patients. *Acta Cardiol.* 1991;46:1–9.

39. el-Shami K, Griffiths E, Streiff M. Nonbacterial thrombotic endocarditis in cancer patients: pathogenesis, diagnosis, and treatment. *Oncologist.* 2007;12:518–523.

40. Lopez JA, Ross RS, Fishbein MC, Siegel RJ. Nonbacterial thrombotic endocarditis: a review. *Am Heart J.* 1987;113:773–784.

41. Whitlock RP, Sun JC, Fremes SE, et al. Antithrombotic and thrombolytic therapy for valvular disease: antithrombotic therapy and prevention of thrombosis, 9th ed: American College of Chest Physicians Evidence-Based Clinical Practice Guidelines. *Chest.* 2012;141:e576S–e600S.

42. Rogers LR, Cho ES, Kempin S, Posner JB. Cerebral infarction from non-bacterial thrombotic endocarditis. Clinical and pathological study including the effects of anticoagulation. *Am J Med.* 1987;83:746–756.

43. Rabinstein AA, Giovanelli C, Romano JG, et al. Surgical treatment of nonbacterial thrombotic endocarditis presenting with stroke. *J Neurol.* 2005;252:352–355.

44. Wilson W, Taubert KA, Gewitz M, et al. Prevention of infective endocarditis: Guidelines from the American Heart Association: A guideline from the American Heart Association Rheumatic Fever, Endocarditis, and Kawasaki Disease Committee, Council on Cardiovascular Disease in the Young, and the Council on Clinical Cardiology, Council on Cardiovascular Surgery and Anesthesia, and the Quality of Care and outcomes Research Interdisciplinary Working Group. *Circulation.* 2007;116:1736–1754.

45. Massel DR, Little SH. Antiplatelet and anticoagulation for patients with prosthetic heart valves. *Cochrane Database Syst Rev.* 2013;7:CD003464.

46. Eikelboom JW, Connolly SJ, Brueckmann M, et al. Dabigatran versus warfarin in patients with mechanical heart valves. *N Engl J Med.* 2013;369:1206–1214.

47. Heras M, Chesebro JH, Fuster V, et al. High risk of thromboemboli early after bioprosthetic cardiac valve replacement. *J Am Coll Cardiol.* 1995;25:1111–1119.

48. Kumar V, Abbas A. Aster J. *Robbins & Cotran Pathologic Basis of Disease.* Philadelphia, PA: Elsevier Saunders; 2014.

49. van Vonderen JJ, Roest AA, Siew ML, et al. Measuring physiological changes during the transition to life after birth. *Neonatology.* 2014;105:230–242.

50. Hagen PT, Scholz DG, Edwards WD. Incidence and size of patent foramen ovale during the first 10 decades of life: an autopsy study of 965 normal hearts. *Mayo Clin Proc.* 1984;59:17–20.

51. Dubourg O, Bourdarias JP, Farcot JC, et al. Contrast echocardiographic visualization of cough-induced right to left shunt through a patent foramen ovale. *J Am Coll Cardiol.* 1984;4:587–594.

52. Lynch JJ, Schuchard GH, Gross CM, Wann LS. Prevalence of right-to-left atrial shunting in a healthy population: detection by Valsalva maneuver contrast echocardiography. *Am J Cardiol.* 1984;53:1478–1480.

53. Movsowitz C, Podolsky LA, Meyerowitz CB, et al. Patent foramen ovale: a nonfunctional embryological remnant or a potential cause of significant pathology? *J Am Soc Echocardiogr.* 1992;5:259–270.

54. Langholz D, Louie EK, Konstadt SN, et al. Transesophageal echocardiographic demonstration of distinct mechanisms for right to left shunting across a patent foramen ovale in the absence of pulmonary hypertension. *J Am Coll Cardiol.* 1991;18:1112–1117.

55. Cohnheim J. Vorlesungen uber allgemeine Pathologie: ein Handbuch fur Aerzte und Studirende. Berlin: *Hirschwald*; 1877.

56. Berthet K, Lavergne T, Cohen A, et al. Significant association of atrial vulnerability with atrial septal abnormalities in young patients with ischemic stroke of unknown cause. *Stroke.* 2000;31:398–403.

57. Webster MW, Chancellor AM, Smith HJ, et al. Patent foramen ovale in young stroke patients. *Lancet.* 1988;2:11–12.

58. Overell JR, Bone I, Lees KR. Interatrial septal abnormalities and stroke: a meta-analysis of case-control studies. *Neurology.* 2000;55:1172–1179.

59. Handke M, Harloff A, Olschewski M, et al. Patent foramen ovale and cryptogenic stroke in older patients. *N Engl J Med.* 2007;357:2262–2268.

60. Lechat P, Mas JL, Lascault G, et al. Prevalence of patent foramen ovale in patients with stroke. *N Engl J Med.* 1988;318:1148–1152.

61. Di Tullio MR, Sacco RL, Sciacca RR, et al. Patent foramen ovale and the risk of ischemic stroke in a multiethnic population. *J Am Coll Cardiol.* 2007;49:797–802.

62. Meissner I, Khandheria BK, Heit JA, et al. Patent foramen ovale: innocent or guilty? Evidence from a prospective population-based study. *J Am Coll Cardiol.* 2006;47:440–445.

63. Di Tullio MR, Jin Z, Russo C, et al. Patent foramen ovale, subclinical cerebrovascular disease, and ischemic stroke in a population-based cohort. *J Am Coll Cardiol.* 2013;62:35–41.

64. Thaler DE, Di Angelantonio E, Di Tullio MR, et al. The risk of paradoxical embolism (rope) study: initial description of the completed database. *Int J Stroke.* 2013;8:612–619.

65. Kent DM, Ruthazer R, Weimar C, et al. An index to identify stroke-related vs incidental patent foramen ovale in cryptogenic stroke. *Neurology.* 2013;81:619–625.

66. Di Tullio M, Sacco RL, Venketasubramanian N, et al. Comparison of diagnostic techniques for the detection of a patent foramen ovale in stroke patients. *Stroke.* 1993;24: 1020–1024.

67. Seiler C. How should we assess patent foramen ovale? *Heart.* 2004;90:1245–1247.

68. Lee RJ, Bartzokis T, Yeoh TK, et al. Enhanced detection of intracardiac sources of cerebral emboli by transesophageal echocardiography. *Stroke.* 1991;22:734–739.

69. Schneider B, Zienkiewicz T, Jansen V, et al. Diagnosis of patent foramen ovale by transesophageal echocardiography and correlation with autopsy findings. *Am J Cardiol.* 1996; 77:1202–1209.

70. Clarke NR, Timperley J, Kelion AD, Banning AP. Transthoracic echocardiography using second harmonic imaging with Valsalva manoeuvre for the detection of right to left shunts. *Eur J Echocardiogr.* 2004;5:176–181.

71. Daniels C, Weytjens C, Cosyns B, et al. Second harmonic transthoracic echocardiography: the new reference screening method for the detection of patent foramen ovale. *Eur J Echocardiogr.* 2004;5:449–452.

72. Jauss M, Kaps M, Keberle M, et al. A comparison of transesophageal echocardiography and transcranial Doppler sonography with contrast medium for detection of patent foramen ovale. *Stroke.* 1994;25:1265–1267.

73. Klotzsch C, Janssen G, Berlit P. Transesophageal echocardiography and contrast-TCD in the detection of a patent foramen ovale: experiences with 111 patients. *Neurology.* 1994; 44:1603–1606.

74. Job FP, Ringelstein EB, Grafen Y, et al. Comparison of transcranial contrast Doppler sonography and transesophageal contrast echocardiography for the detection of patent foramen ovale in young stroke patients. *Am J Cardiol.* 1994;74:381–384.

75. Mohr JP, Thompson JL, Lazar RM, et al. A comparison of warfarin and aspirin for the prevention of recurrent ischemic stroke. *N Engl J Med.* 2001;345:1444–1451.

76. Homma S, Sacco RL, Di Tullio MR, et al. Effect of medical treatment in stroke patients with patent foramen ovale: patent foramen ovale in cryptogenic stroke study. *Circulation.* 2002;105:2625–2631.

77. Shariat A, Yaghoubi E, Farazdaghi M, et al. Comparison of medical treatments in cryptogenic stroke patients with patent foramen ovale: a randomized clinical trial. *J Res Med Sci.* 2013;18:94–98.

78. Chimowitz MI, Lynn MJ, Howlett-Smith H, et al. Comparison of warfarin and aspirin for symptomatic intracranial arterial stenosis. *N Engl J Med.* 2005;352:1305–1316.

79. Homma S, Di Tullio MR, Sacco RL, et al. Surgical closure of patent foramen ovale in cryptogenic stroke patients. *Stroke.* 1997;28:2376–2381.

80. Bridges ND, Hellenbrand W, Latson L, et al. Transcatheter closure of patent foramen ovale after presumed paradoxical embolism. *Circulation.* 1992;86:1902–1908.

81. Schuchlenz HW, Weihs W, Berghold A, et al. Secondary prevention after cryptogenic cerebrovascular events in patients with patent foramen ovale. *Int J Cardiol.* 2005;101:77–82.

82. Wahl A, Juni P, Mono ML, et al. Long-term propensity score-matched comparison of percutaneous closure of patent foramen ovale with medical treatment after paradoxical embolism. *Circulation.* 2012;125:803–812.

83. O'Gara PT, Messe SR, Tuzcu EM, et al. Percutaneous device closure of patent foramen ovale for secondary stroke prevention: a call for completion of randomized clinical trials: a science advisory from the American Heart Association/American Stroke Association and the American College of Cardiology Foundation. *Circulation.* 2009;119:2743–2747.

84. Furlan AJ, Reisman M, Massaro J, et al. Closure or medical therapy for cryptogenic stroke with patent foramen ovale. *N Engl J Med.* 2012;366:991–999.

85. Meier B, Kalesan B, Mattle HP, et al. Percutaneous closure of patent foramen ovale in cryptogenic embolism. *N Engl J Med.* 2013;368:1083–1091.

86. Carroll JD, Saver JL, Thaler DE, et al. Closure of patent foramen ovale versus medical therapy after cryptogenic stroke. *N Engl J Med.* 2013;368:1092–1100.

87. Saver JL, Carroll JD, Thaler DE, et al. Long-term outcomes of patent foramen ovale closure or medical therapy after stroke. *N Engl J Med.* 2017;377:1022–1032.

88. Sondergaard L, Kasner SE, Rhodes JF, et al. Patent foramen ovale closure or antiplatelet therapy for cryptogenic stroke. *N Engl J Med.* 2017;377:1033–1042.

89. Mas JL, Derumeaux G, Guillon B, et al. Patent foramen ovale closure or anticoagulation vs. Antiplatelets after stroke. *N Engl J Med.* 2017;377:1011–1021.

90. Silver MD, Dorsey JS. Aneurysms of the septum primum in adults. *Arch Pathol Lab Med.* 1978;102:62–65.

91. Burger AJ, Jadhav P, Kamalesh M. Low incidence of cerebrovascular events in patients with incidental atrial septal aneurysm. *Echocardiography.* 1997;14:589–596.

92. Hanley PC, Tajik AJ, Hynes JK, et al. Diagnosis and classification of atrial septal aneurysm by two-dimensional echocardiography: Report of 80 consecutive cases. *J Am Coll Cardiol.* 1985;6:1370–1382.

93. Mas JL, Zuber M. Recurrent cerebrovascular events in patients with patent foramen ovale, atrial septal aneurysm, or both and cryptogenic stroke or transient ischemic attack. French study group on patent foramen ovale and atrial septal aneurysm. *Am Heart J.* 1995;130:1083–1088.

94. Cabanes L, Mas JL, Cohen A, et al. Atrial septal aneurysm and patent foramen ovale as risk factors for cryptogenic stroke in patients less than 55 years of age. A study using transesophageal echocardiography. *Stroke.* 1993;24:1865–1873.

95. Weimar C, Holle DN, Benemann J, et al. Current management and risk of recurrent stroke in cerebrovascular patients with right-to-left cardiac shunt. *Cerebrovasc Dis.* 2009;28:349–356.

96. Marti-Fabregas J, Borrell M, Cocho D, et al. Change in hemostatic markers after recombinant tissue-type plasminogen activator is not associated with the chance of recanalization. *Stroke.* 2008;39:234–236.

97. Rigatelli G, Aggio S, Cardaioli P, et al. Left atrial dysfunction in patients with patent foramen ovale and atrial septal aneurysm: an alternative concurrent mechanism for arterial embolism? *JACC Cardiovasc Interv.* 2009;2:655–662.

98. Mas JL, Arquizan C, Lamy C, et al. Recurrent cerebrovascular events associated with patent foramen ovale, atrial septal aneurysm, or both. *N Engl J Med.* 2001;345:1740–1746.

99. Mugge A, Daniel WG, Angermann C, et al. Atrial septal aneurysm in adult patients. A multicenter study using transthoracic and transesophageal echocardiography. *Circulation.* 1995;91:2785–2792.

100. Burger AJ, Sherman HB, Charlamb MJ. Low incidence of embolic strokes with atrial septal aneurysms: a prospective, long-term study. *Am Heart J.* 2000;139:149–152.

101. Webb G, Gatzoulis MA. Atrial septal defects in the adult: recent progress and overview. *Circulation.* 2006;114:1645–1653.

102. Warnes CA, Williams RG, Bashore TM, et al. ACC/AHA 2008 Guidelines for the Management of adults with Congenital Heart Disease: a report of the American College of Cardiology/American Heart Association Task Force on Practice Guidelines (writing committee to develop guidelines on the management of adults with congenital heart disease). Developed in collaboration with the American Society of Echocardiography, Heart Rhythm Society, International Society for Adult Congenital Heart Disease, Society for Cardiovascular Angiography and interventions, and Society of Thoracic Surgeons. *J Am Coll Cardiol.* 2008;52:e143–e263.

103. Khositseth A, Cabalka AK, Sweeney JP, et al. Transcatheter amplatzer device closure of atrial septal defect and patent foramen ovale in patients with presumed paradoxical embolism. *Mayo Clin Proc.* 2004;79:35–41.

104. Gatzoulis MA, Freeman MA, Siu SC, et al. Atrial arrhythmia after surgical closure of atrial septal defects in adults. *N Engl J Med.* 1999;340:839–846.

105. Amarenco P, Duyckaerts C, Tzourio C, et al. The prevalence of ulcerated plaques in the aortic arch in patients with stroke. *N Engl J Med.* 1992;326:221–225.

106. Amarenco P, Cohen A, Tzourio C, et al. Atheroslcerotic disease of the aortic arch and the risk of ischemic stroke. *N Engl J Med.* 1994;331:1474–1479.

107. Russo C, Jin Z, Rundek T, et al. Atherosclerotic disease of the proximal aorta and the risk of vascular events in a population-based cohort: the Aortic Plaques and Risk of Ischemic Stroke (APRIS) study. *Stroke.* 2009;40:2313–2318.

108. Amarenco P, Cohen A, Hommel M, et al. Atherosclerotic disease of the aortic arch as a risk factor for recurrent ischemic stroke. *N Engl J Med.* 1996;334:1216–1221.

109. Tunick PA, Rosenzweig BP, Katz ES, et al. High risk for vascular events in patients with protruding aortic atheromas: a prospective study. *J Am Coll Cardiol.* 1994;23:1085–1090.

110. Van der Linden JD, Hadjinikolaou L, Bergman P, Lindblom D. Postoperative stroke in cardiac surgery is related to the location and extent of atherosclerotic disease in the ascending aorta. *J Am Coll Cardiol.* 2001;38:131–135.

111. Dittrich R, Fedorko L, Borger M, et al. Mild to moderate atherosclerotic disease of the thoracic aorta and new ischemic brain lesions after conventional coronary artery bypass graft surgery. *Stroke.* 2004;35:e356-e358.

112. Karalis DG, Quinn V, Victor MF, et al. Risk of catheter-related emboli in patients with atherosclerotic debris in the thoracic aorta. *Am J Heart.* 1996;131:1149–1155.

113. Büsing KA, Schulte-Sasse C, Flüchter S, et al. Cerebral infarction: incidence and risk factors after diagnostic and interventional cardiac catheterization—prospective evaluation at diffusion-weighted MR imaging. *Radiology.* 2005;235:177–183.

114. Ho AC, Hong CL, Yang MW, et al. Stroke after intraaortic balloon counterpulsation associated with mobile atheroma in thoracic aorta diagnosed using transesophageal echocardiography. *Chang Gung Med J.* 2002;25:612–616.

115. Jansen Klomp WW, Brandon Bravo Bruinsma GJ, van 't Hof AW, et al. Imaging techniques for diagnosis of thoracic aortic atherosclerosis. *Int J Vasc Med.* 2016;2016:4726094.

116. Vaduganathan P, Ewton A, Nagueh SF, et al. Pathologic correlates of aortic plaques, thrombi and mobile "aortic debris" imaged in vivo with transesophageal echocardiography. *J Am Coll Cardiol.* 1997;30:357–363.

117. Benyounes N, Lang S, Savatovsky J, et al. Diagnostic performance of computed tomography angiography compared with transesophageal echocardiography for the detection and analysis of aortic arch atheroma. *Int J Stroke.* 2013;8:E22.

118. Faber T, Rippy A, Hyslop WB, et al. Cardiovascular MRI in detection and measurement of aortic atheroma in Stroke/TIA patients. *J Neurol Disord.* 2013;1:139.

119. Transesophageal echocardiographic correlates of thromboembolism in high-risk patients with nonvalvular atrial fibrillation. *Ann Intern Med*. 1998;128:639–647.

120. Amarenco P, Davis S, Jones EF, et al. Clopidogrel plus aspirin versus warfarin in patients with stroke and aortic arch plaques. *Stroke*. 2014;45:1248–1257.

121. Tunick PA, Nayar AC, Goodkin GM, et al. Effect of treatment on the incidence of stroke and other emboli in 519 patients with severe thoracic aortic plaque. *Am J Cardiol*. 2002; 90:1320–1325.

Treatment of Symptomatic Carotid Stenosis

12

Albert D. Sam II, Kira Long, and Ashlie White

EPIDEMIOLOGY OF CAROTID DISEASE AND STROKE

The percentage of ischemic strokes resulting from atherosclerotic debris that embolizes from the extracranial carotid artery into the cerebral circulation is 20% to 30%.[1,2] Atherosclerosis results from the adverse impact of modifiable risk factors, resulting in inflammation within the circulatory system that causes endothelial injury whose end result is calcium deposition within the arterial wall. These risk factors for developing carotid atherosclerotic disease include smoking, hypertension, hypercholesterolemia, and diabetes.

Smoking is well established to be strongly associated with the development of carotid atherosclerotic disease. In the comparison of age-matched non-smokers, former smokers, and current smokers, the prevalence of clinically significant carotid disease (>50%) was seen in 4.4%, 7.3%, and 9.5% ($p < 0.0001$), respectively.[3] For every 20 mm Hg increase in systolic blood pressure, the odds ratio of developing moderate carotid stenosis is 2.11. Additionally, every 10 mg/dL increase in serum cholesterol level was associated with an odds ratio of 1.10 for developing hemodynamically significant carotid stenosis.[3]

The prevalence of carotid stenosis varies with geographic location due to cultural, genetic, and socioeconomic differences. The southeastern part of the United States has been coined the "stroke belt" because adjusted stroke rates have been shown to be 10% higher than the national average.[4] Nevertheless, the contribution of carotid artery disease to this increased stroke incidence has not been well defined.[5]

CAROTID ARTERY IMAGING IN THE DIAGNOSIS OF CAROTID DISEASE

The diagnostic tools used to image the carotid arteries are duplex ultrasonography (DUS), computed tomography angiography (CTA), magnetic resonance angiography (MRA), and digital subtraction angiography (DSA). The majority of vascular surgeons perform carotid surgery solely from the information provided by the DUS if the performing lab has demonstrated duplex accuracy commensurate with the accrediting bodies that oversee noninvasive vascular laboratories. In the vast majority of cases, this is reasonable and appropriate, and further imaging would not add useful information to the treatment algorithm. In certain instances of discordant information (e.g., significant visualized internal carotid stenosis without velocity elevation or global velocity reductions), or if the planned procedure is carotid stenting, a noninvasive imaging procedure should be performed—either CTA or MRA, depending upon the institution-specific accuracy of the respective modality. Although invasive, DSA remains the gold standard for carotid imaging, but it should rarely be required solely for diagnostic purposes. Prior to carotid stenting, CTA and MRA allow assessment of the carotid artery from the aortic arch to the carotid siphon and intracranially and thus are recommended to be performed prior to all procedures.

CAROTID REVASCULARIZATION FOR STROKE PREVENTION

Carotid Endarterectomy

Carotid endarterectomy (CEA) is arguably the most successful and most rigorously studied surgical procedure in the history of American surgery. First performed in the 1950s, it ranks as one of the most commonly performed peripheral arterial procedures performed in the United States. The initial success in surgical revascularization of the carotid bifurcation was performed by Carrera, Eastcott, Pickering, and Robb in 1954. Controversially, DeBakey reported that he performed the first CEA in 1953, yet it was not published at the time.[6] In the aftermath of several early clinic trials, CEA became extremely popular, despite criticism from the neurology community, because superiority of surgery over medical therapy had not been definitively established. Rates of CEA appropriately diminished throughout the vascular community after the publication of several studies demonstrating that the rates of complications of carotid endarterectomy were excessive.[7] These concerns resulted in the design and execution of several landmark randomized trials in the 1990s under an independent neurological audit that established the role of CEA versus medical treatment for stroke prevention in symptomatic patients (e.g., those presenting with carotid stenosis and an ipsilateral stroke, transient ischemic attack [TIA] or amarosis fugax). These trials—primarily, North American Symptomatic Carotid End-arterectomy Trial (NASCET) and European Carotid Surgery Trial (ECST)—showing benefit from carotid endarterectomy were associated with a dramatic resurgence in the rates of the procedure.

The ECST and NASCET trials were the first to show that CEA was highly beneficial in those with ≥70% stenosis (absolute risk reduction of 16.0%, $p < 0.001$) and a slight but significant benefit in those with 50% to 69% stenosis (absolute risk reduction of 4.6%, $p = 0.04$); the results are summarized in Table 12.1.[8] Criti-cally, the benefit in stroke reduction from CEA relates to the complication rate of the procedure. Reported benefits for NASCET and ECST were predicated on the perioperative risks of stroke or death of 7.5% in the ECST and 6.5% in the NASCET. If major stroke and death rates exceed this by any degree, all benefit from carotid revascularization with CEA is lost.[9] The best outcome to date regarding the efficacy of CEA in symptomatic patients was seen in the Carotid Revascularization Endarterectomy Versus Stent Trial (CREST), where at 30 days, the rate of stroke and death rate was 3.2%.[10]

Despite these admirable results for CEA in the symptomatic cohort, a major criticism centered on how the rigorous selection of patients included in these trials did not represent a "real-world" population of those individuals largely undergoing CEA. The coexistence of coronary artery disease and/or congestive heart failure (CHF) increases mortality after any vascular surgical procedure.

TABLE 12.1 Comparison of the results of the ECST and NASCET trials stratified by degree of stenosis for symptomatic patients

Degree stenosis	Number of patients	Medical risk (%) at 2 years	Surgical risk (%) at 2 years	Risk difference (%)	Relative risk reduction (%)	No need to treat*	Perioperative stroke and death rate (%)
70%–99% NASCET	659	21.4	8.6	12.8	60	8	5.8
70%–99% ECST	501	19.9	7.0	12.9	65	8	5.6
50%–69% NASCET	858	14.2	9.2	5.0	35	20	7.1
50%–69% ECST	684	9.7	11.1	−1.4	−14	—	9.8
<50% NASCET	1368	11.6	10.1	1.5	13	67	6.5
<50% ECST	1882	4.3	9.5	−5.2	−109	—	6.1

Source: Adapted from Reference 8.

The aforementioned trials excluded patients with unstable angina, myocardial infarction in the prior 6 months, CHF, and active coronary disease requiring revascularization.[11] Other factors resulting in exclusion from these CEA trials centered on factors related to the actual surgical site: prior endarterectomy, prior neck dissection or radiation, and surgically inaccessible high or low lesions. Patients with contralateral carotid occlusions were also thought to be problematic because they were felt to have an increased the risk of stroke with CEA. Individuals with one or more of these commonly present conditions would have been denied entry into trial; thus, information regarding the outcome with carotid revascularization via CEA in this "high-risk" population was lacking, resulting in the evolution of the less invasive, non-surgical technique of carotid angioplasty and stenting (CAS).[12]

Carotid Angioplasty and Stenting

First performed by Matthias in 1994, CAS as treatment for carotid stenosis has witnessed a historical progression very similar to CEA, with subsequent trials producing improved results as more knowledge is acquired regarding patient selection and as technological improvements are made (see Figure 12.1). Although currently approved by the U.S. Food and Drug Administration (FDA) for treatment of moderate-risk patients with carotid disease, the Centers for Medicare and Medicaid Services (CMS) has maintained approval of reimbursement only for those individuals with symptomatic, >70% lesions with a "high-risk" qualifying condition. The high-risk criteria are Class III/IV congestive heart failure, left ventricular ejection fraction <30%, open heart surgery within 6 weeks, recent myocardial infarction (>24 hours to <30 days), unstable angina: Class III/IV, concurrent requirement for coronary revascularization, severe pulmonary disease, contralateral carotid occlusion, previous radiation to head/neck, previous CEA, age >80 years, and surgically inaccessible lesions.[13]

The primary limitation for performing CAS is unfavorable anatomy.[14] Unfavorable aortic arch types, vascular anomalies such as bovine anatomy, proximal and distal tortuosity, and other specific arterial lesions can reduce success with this approach, leading to an increase in adverse outcomes.[15,16] Although most CEAs are performed with duplex ultrasound alone, pre-procedure imaging such as CTA or MRA should be performed on all patients being considered for CAS to establish favorable anatomy prior to invasive angiography, to improve patient selection, and to avoid the risks of angiography in those who are poor candidates for CAS.

The initial major trials regarding the efficacy of carotid stenting were performed in a patient population that would not have met the entry criteria for NASCET or ECST due to one of the preceding disqualifying conditions. Both

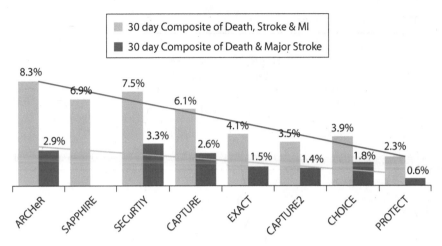

FIGURE 12.1 Carotid stenting outcome improvement over time

Source: Adapted from Dr. Thomas Brott and the CREST investigators.

the ACCULINK for Revascularization of Carotids in High Risk Patient (ARCHER) and the Stenting and Angioplasty with Protection in Patients at High Risk for Endarterectomy (SAPPHIRE) trials established carotid stenting as a feasible revascularization modality for carotid disease in a selected minority of patients deemed high risk for CEA. The two major studies comparing CEA and CAS in the low- to moderate-risk population are the International Carotid Stenting Study (ICSS) and the CREST trial. Both trials compared carotid end-arterectomy with stenting in patients eligible for either procedure.

ICSS was a multicenter, international, randomized controlled trial comparing carotid artery stenting with carotid endarterectomy in patients with recently symptomatic carotid stenosis; the results are summarized in Table 12.2.[8] The trial enrolled 1,713 patients, with 855 randomized to stenting and 858 randomized to surgery. The incidence of stroke, death, or procedural myocardial infarction was 8.5% in the stenting group compared with 5.2% in the endarterectomy group (HR 1.69, 1.16–2.45, $p = 0.006$). Risks of any stroke and all-cause death were higher in the stenting group than in the endarterectomy group. The difference was driven largely by minor strokes yet was offset by a higher frequency of cranial nerve palsy with endarterectomy. The authors concluded that carotid endarterectomy should be the treatment of choice for suitable patients with recently symptomatic carotid artery stenosis. Although ICSS concluded that endarterectomy should be the treatment of choice, there was an inference that some individuals may be better suited for carotid stenting. This inference was substantiated and supported by CREST.[10]

TABLE 12.2 ICSS: 120-day interim safety results

Endpoint	Stenting group, number (%)	Carotid endarterectomy group, number (%)	Hazard ratio (95% CI)	*p*-Value
Disabling stroke or death	34 (4.0)	27 (3.2)	1.28 (0.77–2.11)	0.34
Stroke, death, or procedural MI	72 (8.5)	44 (5.2)	1.69 (1.16–2.45)	0.006
Any stroke	65 (7.7)	35 (4.1)	1.92 (1.27–2.89)	0.002
All-cause death	19 (2.3)	7 (0.8)	2.76 (1.16–6.56)	0.017

Source: Adapted from Reference 8.

Note: CI = confidence interval; ICSS = International Carotid Stenting Study; MI = myocardial infarction

CREST was a multicenter trial supported by the National Institutes of Health. The study included symptomatic (>50% stenosis) and asymptomatic (>70% stenosis) patients. As the largest study on carotid revascularization, which enrolled 2,500 patients from 126 sites throughout North America, a major hallmark of CREST was the most rigorous operator/surgeon entry criteria to date. Sites could not enroll in the trial until the operators performing carotid artery stenting and carotid endarterectomy had been approved and certified by the interventional and surgical management committees, respectively. Certification was achieved by 477 surgeons, whose clinical outcomes were audited by means of a detailed, rigorous selection process documenting that they performed more than 12 procedures per year with rates of complications and death less than 3% among asymptomatic patients and less than 5% among symptomatic patients. A total of 225 interventionists were approved after satisfactory evaluation of their endovascular experience and carotid-stenting results, participation in hands-on training, and participation in a lead-in phase of training.[10] All centers were required to have a team consisting of a neurologist, a surgeon, and an interventionist.

The results demonstrated no significant differences with regard to the combined primary endpoints of stroke, death, and myocardial infarction (MI) with CAS or CEA (7.2% vs. 6.8%, $p=0.51$) (see Table 12.3). Notwithstanding, periprocedural strokes in the CAS group were significantly greater than the CEA group (4.1 vs. 2.3, $p=0.01$), yet this was at the expense of a greater number of MIs in the CEA group compared to the CAS group (2.3 vs. 1.1, $p=0.03$). Quality-of-life assessment data performed indicated a significant negative impact was associated with periprocedural stroke rather than with MI.[17]

TABLE 12.3 CREST primary endpoint results (stroke/MI/death)

CAS	7.2%
CEA	6.8%
Hazard ratio	1.11
95% CI	0.81–1.51
p-value	0.51

Cranial nerve injury occurred in 4.6% of those undergoing CEA, but residual effects were largely nonexistent at 1 year.[18]

Another important finding from CREST was derived from the hazard ratios for the primary endpoint, as calculated for the CAS group versus the CEA group according to age at the time of the procedure. These ratios were estimated from the proportional-hazards model with adjustment for sex and symptomatic status. Graphing of these data revealed that CAS is likely safer in the younger population and that CEA is likely safer in the older patient, with roughly 70 years representing that age demarcation (Figure 12.2).[10] This mirrors the clinical realm where older patients are more likely to have both elongation and a higher calcified plaque burden of the thoracic aortic arch.[19] Additionally, elderly patients have a reduced cerebral vascular reserve, rendering them more susceptible to the effects of embolization.[20]

This important finding of the cohort likely to perform better with the respective procedure helped to clarify the inference established in the ICSS trial. The results of CREST were palatable for both the surgical and intervention communities. Surgeons were encouraged that CEA resulted in lower stroke rates, and interventionists were content that the primary endpoint (stroke/death/MI) was similar between the two methods.

Although carotid revascularization for symptomatic, >50% lesions is not debatable, significant discord exists regarding the treatment of asymptomatic, noncritical carotid lesions. With data extrapolated from randomized trials assessing treatment for intracranial arterial stenosis,[21,22] some may argue that contemporary pharmacologic treatments (including intensively monitored treatments for hypertension, hyperlipidemia, diabetes, and smoking cessation) are acceptable in stroke reduction in those with asymptomatic moderate carotid disease.

There has been no adequately powered assessment of "modern-day" medical management of asymptomatic carotid disease since the ACAS trial 2 decades ago. CREST-2 will assess CEA and CAS, respectively, to the best medical therapy

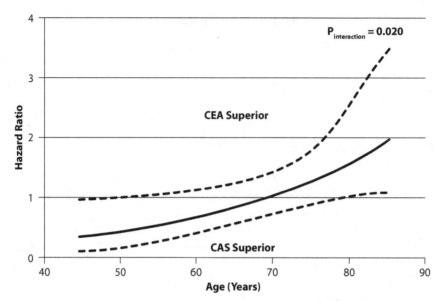

FIGURE 12.2 CREST 4-year primary outcomes

in the asymptomatic cohort. The primary objectives of the trial are (a) to determine if intensive medical therapy alone (mirrored after the aggressive medical management arm of the SAMMPRIS trial, reviewed in Chapter 13) is different from CAS plus intensive medical therapy and (b) to determine if intensive medical therapy is different from CEA plus intensive medical therapy. The primary endpoint will be any stroke or death during the periprocedural period and ipsilateral stroke thereafter, out to 4 years of follow-up. Eligibility criteria include asymptomatic status for less than 180 days from the time of the baseline assessment, carotid stenosis ≥70% as determined by duplex ultrasound, and one confirmatory study (MR or CT angiography). Patients will be randomized to only one of two trials within CREST-2: either CAS plus medical management compared to medical management alone or CEA plus medical management compared to medical management alone.[23] Notably, 50% of patients will be randomized to intensive medical therapy.

COMPLICATIONS OF CEA

Stroke

Neurological complications after CEA are one of the most devastating postoperative complications in the entire field of surgery—particularly if the indication for endarterectomy is asymptomatic disease. An important factor paramount to acceptably low postoperative stroke rates is the CEA case volume of the surgeon.[24–26]

Surgical factors contributing to postoperative neurological events are plaque embolism, carotid occlusion due to platelet aggregation, and inadequate cerebral protection intraoperatively. Trailing only MI, stroke is the second most common cause of death following CEA. Acceptable postoperative stroke rates are <3% for asymptomatic patients and 5% to 7% for symptomatic patients. Any neurologic change in the patient after CEA is a technical problem at the endarterectomy site, until proven otherwise, and warrants expeditious return to the operating room (OR) for evaluation and angiography. If no technical issue is present at reexploration and angiography reveals embolic occlusion of an intracerebral artery, neuro-rescue techniques with intracranial thrombolysis and/or plaque or clot retrieval devices may be employed, if available.

Carotid artery stenting may also be effective for managing perioperative stroke after CEA. In the setting of an anatomically high lesion that proved technically difficult surgically, carotid stenting may provide an adjunctive method to address a flow-limiting lesion that was difficult to address intraoperatively.[27] Carotid stenting, however, is not considered standard for treatment of acute complications of carotid endarterectomy. Because the majority of postoperative events occur in the immediate time period after CEA, our convention is to have all post-op CEA patients remain in the recovery room for 2 hours prior to disposition to either the surgical ward or the intensive care unit. This affords both frequent and continuous neurological assessment by the same attendant and the ability to quickly return to the OR for reexploration if necessary. If there are no blood pressure issues postoperatively, we disposition patients to the surgical floor with neurological and vital assessments every 2 hours with planned discharge for the following day. If there are any hyper- or hypotension issues requiring continuous intravenous pharmacological manipulation, we maintain the arterial line monitoring and disposition patients to the intensive care unit for observation.

Cranial Nerve Injury

Cranial nerve injuries occur in roughly 5% of patients following CEA, with the vast majority resolving completely by 6 months post-surgery.[26–28] This was corroborated in both the ECST and CREST trials. In ECST, the rate of cranial nerve injury postoperatively was 5.1% with resolution of slightly less than half of these injuries by hospital discharge.[28] Typically, the hypoglossal nerve was most frequently involved, occurring in 3% post-CEA, followed by the marginal mandibular branch of the facial nerve at 2%. Vagus and glossopharyngeal nerve injuries occur rarely because they are not encountered in a clinically relevant manner during CEA dissection, yet they may occur at a higher rate during difficult exposures. Factors that increase the risk of cranial nerve injury include urgent procedures, immediate reexploration, and return to the OR for a neurologic event or bleeding. Interestingly, and contrary to conventional teachings, redoing CEA or prior cervical radiation were *not* associated with an increased risk.[26]

Cerebral Hyperperfusion Syndrome

The cerebral hyperperfusion syndrome (CHS) can be a devastating post-carotid revascularization complication that occurs in a small percentage of patients (0.05%–3%). CHS can result in intracerebral hemorrhage post–carotid revascularization and is associated with typical clinical hallmarks[28–34] (see Table 12.4). Despite an unclear mechanism, it is thought that the cause is related to loss of intracerebral autoregulation of perfusion in the previously ischemic carotid vascular bed. To maintain sufficient cerebral blood flow, small vessels compensate with chronic arteriolar maximal dilatation. After correction of the carotid stenosis, blood flow is restored to a normal or elevated perfusion pressure within the previously hypoperfused hemisphere. The dilated vessels are thought to be unable to assume normal tone or to vasoconstrict sufficiently to protect the capillary bed from excess flow, resulting in edema and hemorrhage, which in turn results in the clinical manifestations. Besides the initial presence of critical unilateral or bilateral carotid lesions, post-revascularization hypertension frequently is an associated predecessor of the syndrome, underscoring the importance of good perioperative blood pressure control.[8] Some evidence suggests that this syndrome may be more likely when revascularization is performed after recent stroke.[35–37] This is particularly important because contemporary practitioners now tend to perform post-stroke carotid revascularization without delay due to data refuting the previous practice of a several-week delay.[38,39]

TABLE 12.4 Hyperperfusion features

- Headache ipsilateral to the revascularized internal carotid, typically improved in upright posture; may herald the syndrome in the first week after endarterectomy.
- Focal motor seizures are common, sometimes with post-ictal Todd's paralysis mimicking post-endarterectomy stroke from carotid thrombosis.
- Intracerebral hemorrhage is the most feared complication, occurring in about 0.6% of patients after CEA, usually within 2 weeks of surgery.

Source: Adapted from Reference 34.

The prevention of this complication is aided with fastidious control of post-operative hypertension. Blood pressure parameters depend on the initial severity of stenosis and presumed or known degree of capillary dilatation before surgery. For severe stenosis (>90%), our convention is to maintain systolic blood pressure below 150 mm Hg as aggressively as required with the liberal use of continuous-drip intravenous antihypertensives in short order if bolus intravenous methods fail. Theoretically, patients with less severe stenosis require less conservative parameters than those with severe stenosis; however, it may be more complicated than this because patients have varying sources and flow contribution from collaterals likely contributing to the cerebrovascular reserve. The vast majority of patients do not require sustained antihypertensive infusion and are restarted on their home oral regimen in the first 12 hours after the procedure. Any complaint of severe headache following revascularization is the syndrome, unless proven otherwise, and should be evaluated expeditiously with head CT. All antithrombotics should be discontinued if hemorrhage is confirmed, and platelet transfusion to reverse their effect should be considered. Seizures related to hyperperfusion are usually successfully treated with standard antiepileptic drugs.[39]

Restenosis

Restenosis of the carotid artery after CEA occurs in 3% to 10% of patients and underscores the importance of yearly duplex assessment, even though the majority have little indication for repeat revascularization.[40,41] It is also not uncommon to observe mild restenosis in the initial months after CEA that normalizes after a year, likely the result of carotid remodeling. Although not definitively proven, statin drugs may be protective against restenosis.[42] Additionally, patch angioplasty during CEA has been associated with a decreased risk of long-term recurrent stenosis compared with primary closure.[43]

The mechanism of the restenotic lesion has a direct relationship to the time point of presentation after initial surgery.[44,45] Restenosis occurring within 2 to 3 years after CEA is thought to be attributed to intimal hyperplasia that creates a smooth, tapered lesion with a low likelihood of embolization. Conversely, restenosis after 2 to 3 years is thought to be from the progression of atherosclerotic disease process and thus presents as an irregular plaque that may serve as an embolic source. The former typically does not require intervention unless a near-occlusive lesion results, whereas the latter requires correction if symptoms develop in association with critical restenosis (>70%). Restenosis of post-CEA carotid lesions is increasingly (and appropriately) treated via carotid stenting, when feasible, thus avoiding the potential risks inherent with redo surgical neck exploration.

COMPLICATIONS OF CAROTID STENTING

Carotid artery stenting (CAS) has certain advantages compared to CEA, primarily as it pertains to the avoidance of both an incision and general anesthesia. Resultantly cranial nerve injuries, neck hematomas, and anesthetic/intubation complications are not encountered. However, similar complications of stroke, including cerebral hyperperfusion syndrome and restenosis, likewise occur to some degree with CAS. Additionally, CAS has the unique complications related to access not present in those undergoing CEA.

Stroke

The most serious acute complication associated with CAS is stroke. Periprocedural stroke may develop from several mechanisms: thromboembolism, hemodynamic alteration–induced hypoperfusion, cerebral hyperperfusion, and intracerebral hemorrhage. In addition, filter embolic protection devices—the most common device type used currently—may result in an angiographic "slow-flow phenomenon," appearing as reduced or absent anterograde flow in the internal carotid artery caused by occlusion of the filter membrane pores by microemboli and debris. Occurring in 9% of cases in one study, patients with the slow-flow phenomenon had an increased 30-day risk of stroke compared with those who did not (9.5% vs. 1.7%).[46] Protection devices may also cause arterial spasm and dissection that may lead to periprocedural cerebral events.

Carotid plaque morphology and characteristics also contribute to increased stroke rates with carotid stenting. Ulcerated carotid plaque, increasing degree of carotid stenosis, and longer carotid lesions are aspects of carotid disease associated with an increased risk for stroke.[47] Retrospective studies also suggest that long carotid lesions (>10 mm) or tandem carotid lesions with more than one lesion separated by normal vessel wall have also been associated with a higher stroke risk.[48,49] Appropriate patient selection is the most important factor in minimizing post-CAS stroke. Adequate pre-procedural planning that assesses arch anatomy, carotid tortuosity, and lesion characteristics can minimize the occurrence of this potentially devastating complication.

Hemodynamic Instability

Hemodynamic lability, such as bradycardia and hypotension, occurs frequently after carotid artery stenting; however, associated morbidity has not been established. Occurring in an estimated 20% to 30% of cases, in most patients post-procedural hypotension resolves within 12 hours.[50] The clinical manifestations are thought to be due to the effects of balloon inflation on the carotid baroreceptors during CAS. Carotid sinus baroreceptors are located within the adventitia of the origin of the internal carotid artery and are innervated by a branch of the glossopharyngeal nerve (the sinus nerve of Hering). In response to low blood pressure, the nerve fibers decrease their firing rates, stimulating the sympathetic nervous system and inhibiting the parasympathetic nervous system via a centrally acting mechanism. Hemodynamic instability following CAS is significantly associated with age, >10-mm distance between the carotid bifurcation and the site of minimum lumen diameter, and prior ipsilateral carotid endarterectomy and recent stroke.[50] Neither hypotension nor bradycardia has been predictive of myocardial infarction, stroke, or death.[51]

Access-Related Complications

Access-related issues are grouped into two categories: complications involving the arterial puncture or due to distal embolization. Arterial puncture complication includes hematoma and pseudoaneurysm formation. Distal embolization complications may be due to atheroembolization as a result of a diseased femoral artery or closure device misadventure. Arterial puncture issues may be nearly completely eliminated if care is taken to puncture the common femoral artery in a fluoroscopically confirmed segment overlying the femoral head. The risk factors for pseudoaneurysm development include inadequate post-procedure compression of the puncture site, post-procedural anticoagulation, antiplatelet therapy during the intervention, age >65 years, obesity, hypertension, peripheral artery disease, and hemodialysis.[52]

During any transfemoral catheterization procedure, plaque may become dislodged either from a diseased femoral artery or from more proximal aortic or iliac disease, with occasional limb-threatening ischemia in some instances. Care should be taken to ensure that the targeted femoral artery is suitable for puncture. Fluoroscopic visualization prior to arterial puncture can often demonstrate plaque burden, leading to selection of the contralateral femoral site for puncture.

Restenosis

Restenosis rates after CAS vary, yet overall the durability compares favorably to CEA.[53-55] Meta-analysis of multiple studies shows that restenosis occurs in about 6% of arteries after 1 year. Historical restenosis rates for CEA ranges in the 5% to 10% range.[53] CREST reported no difference in restenosis at 24 months for carotid artery stenting compared with carotid endarterectomy.[10] Secondary analysis revealed that female sex, dyslipidemia, and diabetes were independent predictors of restenosis for both procedures. Interestingly, smoking increased the CEA rate of restenosis but not after CAS.

CONCLUSION

In summary, carotid disease's contribution to stroke remains significant. Despite advances in the surgical and interventional approaches to treatment, carotid disease–related stroke continues to remain an important source of morbidity and mortality. Carotid endarterectomy remains the gold standard for treatment of significant disease. Carotid angioplasty and stenting has been a welcomed addition to the treatment armamentarium; however, there remain strict guidelines for patient inclusion and significant obstacles for practitioners to obtain and maintain expertise. Current studies are under way to assess the efficacy of pharmacologic agents in the treatment of carotid disease, which will provide valuable information as we continue to improve our total approach for those afflicted.

References

1. Roger VL, Go AS, Lloyd-Jones DM, et al. Heart disease and stroke statistics—2012 update: a report from the American Heart Association. *Circulation.* 2012;125(1):E2–E220.
2. Hall HA, Bassiouny HS. Pathophysiology of carotid atherosclerosis. In: Nicolaides A, Beach KW, Kyriacou E, Pattichis CS, eds. *Ultrasound and Carotid Bifurcation Atherosclerosis.* London: Springer; 2011:27–39.
3. Fazel P, Johnson K. Current role of medical treatment and invasive management in carotid atherosclerotic disease. *Bayl Univ Med Cent Proc.* 2008;21(2):133–138.
4. Stroke Belt Initiative: Project accomplishments and lessons learned. National Heart, Lung, and Blood Institute, National Institutes of Health, 1996. https://www.nhlbi.nih.gov/files /docs/resources/heart/sb_spec.pdf.
5. Lloyd-Jones D, Adams RJ, Brown TM, et al. Executive summary: heart disease and stroke statistics—2010 update: a report from the American Heart Association. *Circulation.* 2010;23;121(7):948–954.
6. Robertson JT. Carotid endarterectomy: a saga of clinical science, personalities, and evolving technology: the Willis lecture. *Stroke.* 1998;29(11):2435–2441.
7. Tu JV, Hannan EL, Anderson GM, et al. The fall and rise of carotid endarterectomy in the United States and Canada. *N Engl J Med.* 1998;339(20):1441–1447.
8. Kassem HH, Abd-Allah F, Wasay M. Update on carotid revascularization: evidence from large clinical trials. *INTECH Open Science.* http://www.intechopen.com/books/carotid -artery-disease-from-bench-to-bedside-and-beyond/update-on-carotid-revascularization -evidence-from-large-clinical-trials#B2.
9. Barnett, HJM, Eliasziw M, Meldrum HE. Prevention of ischaemic stroke. *BMJ.* 1999;318:1539–1543.
10. Brott TG, Hobson RW 2nd, Howard G, et al. Stenting versus endarterectomy for treatment of carotid-artery stenosis. *N Engl J Med.* 2010;363(1):11–23.
11. North American Symptomatic Carotid Endarterectomy Trial Collaborators. Beneficial effect of carotid endarterectomy in symptomatic patients with high-grade carotid stenosis. *N Engl J Med.* 1991;325(7):445–453.
12 Katzen BT, Laird, JR Jr, Takao Ohki T. The SAPPHIRE and ARCHER updates: a report on the early progress of two trials critical to our understanding of carotid artery stenting. *Endovascular Today.* Sept 2003:77–78.

13. Decision Memo for Carotid Artery Stenting. https://www.cms.gov/medicare-coverage-database/details/nca-decision.

14. Maldonado TS. What are current preprocedure imaging requirements for carotid artery stenting and carotid endarterectomy: have magnetic resonance angiography and computed tomographic angiography made a difference? *Semin Vasc Surg.* 2007;20:205–215.

15. Ouriel K, Hertzer NR, Beven EG, et al. Preprocedural risk stratification: identifying an appropriate population for carotid stenting. *J Vasc Surg.* 2001;33:728–732.

16. Yadav JS, Roubin GS, King P, et al. Angioplasty and stenting for restenosis after carotid endarterectomy. Initial experience. *Stroke.* 1996;27:2075–2079.

17. Cohen DJ, et al. Health-related quality of life after carotid stenting versus carotid endarterectomy: results from CREST (Carotid Revascularization Endarterectomy versus Stenting Trial). *J Am Coll Cardiol.* 2011;58(15):1557–1565.

18. Hye RJ, Mackey A, Hill MD, et al. Incidence, outcomes, and effect on quality of life of cranial nerve injury in the Carotid Revascularization Endarterectomy versus Stenting Trial. *J Vasc Surg.* 2015;61(5):1208–1214.

19. Redheuil A, Yu W-C, Mousseaux E, et al. Age-related changes in aortic arch geometry: relationship with proximal aortic function and left ventricular mass and remodeling. *J Am Coll Cardiol.* 2011 Sep 13; 58(12): 1262–1270.

20. Ito H, Kanno I, Ibaraki M, Hatazawa J. Effect of aging on cerebral vascular response to Paco2 changes in humans as measured by positron emission tomography. *J Cereb Blood Flow Metab.* 2002;22:997–1003.

21. Wu TY, Anderson NE, Barber PA. Neurological complications of carotid revascularisation. *J Neurol Neurosurg Psychiatry.* 2012;83(5):543–550.

22. Heyer EJ, Mergeche JL, Bruce SS, et al. Statins reduce neurologic injury in asymptomatic carotid endarterectomy patients. *Stroke.* 2013;44(4):1150–1152.

23. Faggioli G, Pini R, Mauro R, et al. Perioperative outcome of carotid endarterectomy according to type and timing of neurologic symptoms and computed tomography findings. *Ann Vasc Surg.* 2013;27(7):874–882.

24. Goldberg JB, Goodney PP, Kumbhani SR, et al. Brain injury after carotid revascularization: outcomes, mechanisms, and opportunities for improvement. *Ann Vasc Surg.* 2011;25(2):270–286.

25. Anzuini A, Briguori C, Roubin GS, et al A. Emergency stenting to treat neurological complications occurring after carotid endarterectomy. *J Am Coll Cardiol.* 2001;37(8):2074.

26. Fokkema M, de Borst GJ, Nolan BW, et al. Clinical relevance of cranial nerve injury following carotid endarterectomy. *Eur J Vasc Endovasc Surg.* 2014;47(1):2–7.

27. Cunningham EJ, Bond R, Mayberg MR, et al. Risk of persistent cranial nerve injury after carotid endarterectomy. *J Neurosurg.* 2004;101(3):445.

28. Youkey JR, Clagett GP, Jaffin JH, et al. Focal motor seizures complicating carotid endarterectomy *Arch Surg.* 1984;119(9):1080.

29. Reigel MM, Hollier LH, Sundt TM Jr, et al. Cerebral hyperperfusion syndrome: a cause of neurologic dysfunction after carotid endarterectomy. *J Vasc Surg.* 1987;5(4):628.

30. Naylor AR, Ruckley CV. The post-carotid endarterectomy hyperperfusion syndrome. *Eur J Vasc Endovasc Surg.* 1995;9(4):365.

31. Coutts SB, Hill MD, Hu WY. Hyperperfusion syndrome: toward a stricter definition. *Neurosurgery.* 2003;53(5):1053.

32. Kablak-Ziembicka A, Przewlocki T, Pieniazek P, et al. Predictors of cerebral reperfusion injury after carotid stenting: the role of transcranial color-coded Doppler ultrasonography. *J Endovasc Ther.* 2010;17(4):556.

33. Bouri S, Thapar A, Shalhoub J, et al. Hypertension and the post-carotid endarterectomy cerebral hyperperfusion syndrome. *Eur J Vasc Endovasc Surg.* 2011;41(2):229–237.

34. Pennekamp CW, Tromp SC, Ackerstaff RG, et al. Prediction of cerebral hyperperfusion after carotid endarterectomy with transcranial Doppler. *Eur J Vasc Endovasc Surg.* 2012; 43(4):371–376.

35. Clagett, GP, Robertson, JT. Surgical considerations in symptomatic disease. In: Barnett, HJM, Mohr, JP, Stein, BM, Yatsu, FM, eds. *Stroke: Pathophysiology, Diagnosis and Management.* New York: Churchill Livingstone; 1998:1209.

36. Gasecki AP, Eliasziw M, Pritz MB, Timing of carotid endarterectomy after stroke. *Stroke.* 1998;29(12):2667–2668.

37. Crozier JE, Reid J, Welch GH, et al, Early carotid endarterectomy following thrombolysis in the hyperacute treatment of stroke. *Br J Surg.* 2011;98(2):235–238.

38. Kieburtz K, Ricotta JJ, Moxley RT 3rd. Seizures following carotid endarterectomy. *Arch Neurol.* 1990;47(5):568.

39. Counsell CE, Salinas R, Naylor R, Warlow CP. A systematic review of the randomised trials of carotid patch angioplasty in carotid endarterectomy. *Eur J Vasc Endovasc Surg.* 1997;13(4):345.

40. Goodney PP, Nolan BW, Eldrup-Jorgensen J, et al. Restenosis after carotid endarterectomy in a multicenter regional registry. *J Vasc Surg.* 2010;52(4):897–904, 905.e1–2; discussion 904–905.

41. LaMuraglia GM, Stoner MC, Brewster DC, et al. Determinants of carotid endarterectomy anatomic durability: effects of serum lipids and lipid-lowering drugs. *J Vasc Surg.* 2005; 41(5):762.

42. Bond R, Rerkasem K, Naylor AR, et al. Systematic review of randomized controlled trials of patch angioplasty versus primary closure and different types of patch materials during carotid endarterectomy. *J Vasc Surg.* 2004;40(6):1126.

43. Sadideen H, Taylor PR, Padayachee TS. Restenosis after carotid endarterectomy. *TS Int J Clin Pract.* 2006;60(12):1625.

44. Fokkema M, de Borst GJ, Nolan BW, et al. Carotid stenting versus endarterectomy in patients undergoing reintervention after prior carotid endarterectomy. *J Vasc Surg.* 2014;59(1):8–15.

45. Casserly IP, Abou-Chebl A, Fathi RB, et al. Slow-flow phenomenon during carotid artery intervention with embolic protection devices: predictors and clinical outcome. *J Am Coll Cardiol.* 2005;46(8):1466.

46. Hofmann R, Niessner A, Kypta A, et al. Risk score for peri-interventional complications of carotid artery stenting. *Stroke.* 2006;37(10):2557.

47. Mathur A, Roubin GS, Iyer SS, et al. Predictors of stroke complicating carotid artery stenting. *Circulation.* 1998;97 (13):1239.

48. Qureshi AI, Luft AR, Janardhan V, et al. Identification of patients at risk for periprocedural neurological deficits associated with carotid angioplasty and stenting. *Stroke.* 2000;31(2):376.

49. Qureshi AI, Luft AR, Sharma M, et al. Frequency and determinants of postprocedural hemodynamic instability after carotid angioplasty and stenting. *Stroke.* 1999;30(10): 2086.

50. Ullery BW, Nathan DP, Shang EK, et al. Incidence, predictors, and outcomes of hemodynamic instability following carotid angioplasty and stenting. *J Vasc Surg.* 2013 Oct;58(4):917–25. Epub 2013 May 10.

51. Wu TY, Ham SW, Katz SG. Predictors and consequences of hemodynamic instability after carotid artery stenting. *Ann Vasc Surg.* 2015;29(6):1281–1285.

52. Ates ML, Sahin S, Konuralp C, et al. Evaluation of risk factors associated with femoral pseudoaneurysms after cardiac catheterization. *Vasc Surg.* 2006;43(3):520–524.

53. Gröschel K, Riecker A, Schulz JB, et al. Systematic review of early recurrent stenosis after carotid angioplasty and stenting. *Stroke.* 2005;36(2):367.

54. Frericks H, Kievit J, van Baalen JM, van Bockel JH. Carotid recurrent stenosis and risk of ipsilateral stroke: a systematic review of the literature. *Stroke.* 1998;29(1):244.

55. Moore WS, Kempczinski RF, Nelson JJ, Toole JF. Recurrent carotid stenosis: results of the asymptomatic carotid atherosclerosis study. *Stroke.* 1998;29(10):2018–2025.

Intracranial Large-Vessel Disease 13

Rajbeer Singh Sangha and Toby I. Gropen

INTRODUCTION

Intracranial atherosclerotic disease (ICAD) is a major subtype of ischemic stroke and represents the most common cause of stroke in the world.[1] It is most prevalent in groups of black, Asian, Hispanic, and Indian populations, with it accounting for approximately 30% to 50% of ischemic stroke in the Asian population[2] compared to approximately 8% to 10% of ischemic stroke in North American Caucasians.[3]

This disease is characterized by a high risk of recurrent stroke, with the Warfarin-Aspirin for Symptomatic Intracranial Disease (WASID) study showing that patients with ICAD have a risk of recurrent stroke as high as 20% in the first 2 years, despite medical therapy.[4] Further evidence of its high risk of recurrence was shown in the Groupe d'Etude des Stenosis Intra-Craniennes Atheromateuses Symptomatiques (GESICA) study that followed 122 symptomatic ICAD patients over a mean period of 23.4 months.[5] It was found that 38.2% of patients developed ischemic stroke or had a transient ischemic attack (TIA) with a rate of 8.8% vascular death during the follow-up period.

In view of the significant morbidity and mortality associated with ICAD, it is important to understand its epidemiology, associated risk factors, pathophysiology, diagnosis, and treatment.

EPIDEMIOLOGY

The distribution of intracranial atherosclerosis has been extensively analyzed, and race/ethnic differences have been well documented, with one of the first major studies being the Northern Manhattan Stroke Study.[3] The authors found ICAD to be more prevalent in African American and Hispanic patients than in white patients.[3] Further analysis and follow-up revealed the prevalence of ischemic stroke in patients with ICAD to be greater in African American and Hispanic individuals (15 and 13 per 100,000 persons, respectively) when compared to white individuals (3 per 100,000 persons).[6] A recent analysis by the German Stroke Study Collaboration found symptomatic ICAD lesions to be the cause in just 2.2% of patients with ischemic stroke.[7] Further racial differences exist in the distribution of ICAD, with cerebral angiographic studies showing African Americans to have a predilection of severe disease in the middle cerebral artery (MCA) stem, supraclinoid internal carotid artery, and basilar artery, whereas Caucasian patients had more severe disease in the cervical region of the carotid and vertebral arteries.[8,9]

Looking at the Asian population, we see a stark contrast in the prevalence of ICAD. One study of 1,167 Korean stroke patients demonstrated via magnetic resonance angiography (MRA) that symptomatic ICAD was more common than symptomatic extracranial atherosclerosis, with an approximate ratio of 7:3.[10] Further studies have demonstrated the high burden of ICAD in the Asian population, with ultrasonography showing that while only 19% of patients with TIA had extracranial disease, approximately 51% had ICAD out of a sample size of 96 patients.[11]

The prevalence of ICAD in ischemic stroke patients has not been well characterized, and its effects on stroke recovery and pathogenesis have yet to be well understood. French investigators looked at 339 consecutive autopsies of patients with fatal stroke and found that 62.2% of the patients had intracranial plaques and 43.2% had stenosis.[12] The study showed that the prevalence and detection of ICAD may be underestimated in the stroke population and also showed the limitations of current imaging modalities. Furthermore, as we continue to elucidate the pathophysiology of the process, underdiagnosis may also be related to an underappreciation of the role of less severe degrees of ICAD leading to stroke.

A paucity of data exists on the prevalence of asymptomatic ICAD in the general population. In an MRA evaluation of 425 asymptomatic Japanese subjects, 3.5% had ICAD.[13]

RISK FACTORS

Risk factors associated with intracranial atherosclerosis include modifiable and non-modifiable risk factors. Modifiable risk factors include hypertension, smoking, diabetes mellitus, and dyslipidemia.[14–16] Metabolic syndrome has been more recently associated with ICAD, with multiple studies and analysis confirming the association.[17,18] A subgroup analysis of the WASID study showed that dyslipidemia was independently associated with severity of intracranial stenosis (odds ratio [OR] 1.62, 95% confidence interval [CI] 1.09–2.42).[19] Furthermore, the analysis of demographic and vascular risk factors showed metabolic syndrome and diabetes to also be associated with severity of vessel stenosis in patients with ICAD. Increased apolipoprotein B/A-I from baseline was associated with progression of stenosis on MRA, whereas increased high-density lipoproteins (HDL) concentrations were associated with stable stenosis.[20] Other biomarkers and factors that have been implicated with the increased risk of progression of ICAD, as well as risk of recurrent stroke, include reduced adiponectin,[21] increased lipoprotein-associated phospholipase A2,[22] C-reactive protein, E-selectin, and lipoprotein (a).[23]

Non-modifiable risk factors include the presence of collaterals in patients with robust collaterals being associated with decreased risk of recurrent stroke.[24] Race is an important non-modifiable risk factor as demonstrated by a study that showed Asians to have intracranial atherosclerosis earlier and more extensively than Caucasian Americans and Europeans.[25] Other non-modifiable risk factors include sex: males have been found to develop intracranial lesions in the fourth and fifth decade with steady progression thereafter; however, females show rapid progression from the sixth decade onward.[26]

PATHOPHYSIOLOGY

Intracranial atherosclerosis is characterized by two features: (a) atherosis caused by deposition of cholesterol and oxidative stress and (b) endothelial dysfunction leading to sclerosis and subsequent arterial stiffness.[27] Changes to the vascular wall lead to difficulties in the ability of the large vessels of the cerebrum to maintain cerebral blood perfusion and thus make the patient susceptible to ischemic stroke.[28]

There are three mechanisms by which stroke occurs in ICAD; in-situ thromboembolism leading to artery-to-artery embolism, plaque extension over penetrating artery ostia (also known as branch disease), and finally, hypoperfusion leading to a watershed pattern of ischemia.[24,29] While each mechanism may occur independently, the combination of factors may also lead to multiple ischemic infarcts or increase the burden of infarct that is present on admission.[30,31] However, it has been observed that plaque extension over a penetrating artery ostia may occur in the absence of significant stenosis.

DIAGNOSIS

Diagnostic imaging is the primary modality by which patients are identified with ICAD. Recent advances in imaging techniques have allowed for more accurate information regarding the degree of stenosis, the location of stenosis, and even identification in changes in perfusion in the brain secondary to occlusion. The noninvasive methods utilized to diagnose ICAD include transcranial Doppler (TCD) ultrasound, MRA, computed tomography angiography (CTA), and high-resolution MRI. These procedures are often preferred because they are less invasive and less expensive than catheter angiography. The gold standard for diagnosis of ICAD is conventional cerebral angiography (CCA), but due to the combination of recent advances in imaging techniques and the risk of stroke from the procedure itself (as high as 1.2% in the Asymptomatic Carotid Atherosclerosis Study [ACAS]),[32] CCA is being utilized less often.

Use of CTA has become one of the main standards for vessel imaging following ischemic stroke. In a single-center study, a comparison of MRA with CTA, in which the standard reference was CCA, showed CTA to be more accurate.[33] Furthermore, CTA has been shown to have a high sensitivity and specificity for detection for ICAD in patients where the vessel stenosis is greater than 50%.[34] The Stroke Outcomes and Neuroimaging of Intracranial Atherosclerosis (SONIA) trial compared the accuracy of TCD and MRA with CCA and showed that while both TCD and MRA have high negative predictive values (86%–91%), they have low positive predictive values (36%–59%).[35]

DIFFERENTIAL DIAGNOSIS

The differential diagnosis of patients presenting with ICAD include nonatherosclerotic disease processes that lead to vessel stenosis and occlusive disease, including moyamoya syndrome, arterial dissection, fibromuscular dysplasia, primary central nervous system (CNS) angiitis, secondary vasculitis processes, and other focal vasculopathies. Often, medical diagnosis of such conditions requires a careful consideration of the patient's risk factors, clinical presentation, examination, and radiologic and laboratory information. For example, primary CNS angiitis (PACNS) is characterized by headaches, cognitive impairment, and ischemic events affecting multiple vascular territories; the onset of such a constellation of symptoms is often subacute and radiographically characterized by a string of beads appearance in the distal small vessels. These patients may not have the extensive vascular risk factors or fit the age/racial profile that is present in patients with ICAD.

Further, conditions such as arterial vessel dissection are often characterized by a history of trauma or neck manipulation; however, they may also occur spontaneously. These patients will present with neck pain or with symptoms secondary to an ischemic stroke. Radiographic imaging will show a tapering off appearance of the vessel and will characteristically occur in the cervical region. Intracranial vessel dissection is difficult to diagnose and is uncommon.

TREATMENT

The treatment of ICAD has evolved along with the understanding of the disease itself. Treatment includes acute treatment of ischemic stroke with tissue plasminogen activator (tPA) and the use of mechanical thrombectomy where appropriate. Recently completed randomized clinical trials have demonstrated the efficacy of mechanical thrombectomy with stent retrievers versus IV tPA alone in patients with large-vessel occlusion of the internal carotid artery or proximal MCA and salvageable tissue, generally in patients presenting with a National Institute of Health Stroke Scale (NIHSS) ≥6 with groin puncture less than 6 hours after ischemic stroke onset.[36–41] We feel it is reasonable to consider mechanical thrombectomy for patients less than 6 hours after symptom onset who have causative occlusion of the M2 or M3 portion of the MCAs, anterior cerebral arteries, vertebral arteries, basilar artery, or posterior cerebral arteries. A recent meta-analysis of individual patient data from the stent retriever trials suggested a benefit of mechanical thrombectomy for patients from 6 to 8 hours after acute ischemic stroke onset.[42]

The second and equally critical aspect of treatment includes the prevention of recurrent stroke. Given the fact that ICAD has such a high rate of recurrence, patients are required to have regular follow-up, close monitoring, and excellent adherence to the medication and lifestyle regimen that is prescribed by the physician. Originally, it was thought that anticoagulation would be the best treatment option for patients presenting with symptoms secondary to ICAD. Early retrospective analyses suggested the use of warfarin to be more effective than aspirin in symptomatic patients.[43] Two multicenter, randomized trials showed that treatment via anticoagulation was proven to be nonsuperior and with greater risk for harm. The first trial was the comparison of warfarin and aspirin for the prevention of recurrent ischemic stroke (WARSS) and found warfarin to be similar in efficacy for the endpoints of ischemic stroke, death, or major hemorrhage in prevention of non-cardioembolic stroke.[44] Investigators next looked at a comparison of warfarin and aspirin for symptomatic intracranial arterial stenosis, also known as the WASID trial. They looked specifically at patients with ICAD and compared aspirin (1,300 mg) with warfarin (target international normalized ratio [INR] 2–3) and found no difference in efficacy for prevention of ischemic stroke or vascular death.[4] Furthermore, they found aspirin to be safer with a lower mortality rate and lower rate of major hemorrhage when compared to warfarin. Subgroup analysis also found that patients with severe stenosis (70%–99%), vertebrobasilar stenosis, or patients who had failed antiplatelet therapy did not benefit from anticoagulation—groups that were previously felt to benefit from warfarin.[45]

Following the failure of anticoagulation as a modality of therapy, investigators looked to data from cardiovascular cohorts for further treatment options. Data supporting the use of antiplatelet agents in artery-to-artery embolism were provided via two randomized trials. One study of patients with symptomatic ICAD utilized TCD to detect the rates of microembolic signals following loading with clopidogrel and being started on aspirin. The patients were found to have significantly lower rates of signals when compared to patients on aspirin alone.[46] The second study was the Clopidogrel and Aspirin for Reduction of Emboli in Symptomatic Carotid Stenosis (CARESS) study, which showed that patients on monotherapy of aspirin had significantly more recurrent stroke events compared to dual antiplatelet therapy of aspirin plus clopidogrel.[47]

Other antiplatelet agents that have been studied include cilostazol, which is a phosphodiesterase-3 inhibitor and was thought to decrease progression of atherosclerosis in patients with symptomatic middle cerebral and basilar artery stenosis. The first study compared cilostazol plus aspirin to aspirin and placebo, randomizing 135 patients, and followed for disease progression via MRA and TCD at 6 months. The cilostazol group had significantly lower disease progression than the placebo group; however, no individuals in either group had strokes or transient ischemic attacks.[48] These data prompted a second trial in which 457 patients were randomly assigned to cilostazol plus aspirin versus clopidogrel plus aspirin. The primary outcome was the number of ischemic lesions measured on MRI at a follow-up period of 7 months. The data showed no difference in both ischemic lesions and hemorrhagic events between the cilostazol and clopidogrel groups.[49]

Investigators also looked to angioplasty as a method of treating intracranial large artery disease. However, data were limited to case reports and retrospective single-center observational reports, most of which had fewer than 30 patients.[50,51] The main complication of this treatment was periprocedural complications of stroke or death, with the highest rate occurring in patients who were symptomatic and unstable. Further systematic review of all open–label case series with three or more cases showed a stroke perioperative complication rate of 7.9%, with a stroke or death rate of 9.5%.[52] A number of drawbacks of intracranial angioplasty have been highlighted since then, including risk of dissection, acute vessel closure, residual stenosis >50% following the procedure, and high restenosis rates. Further data from cardiovascular literature indicating the success of stenting in coronary circulation led to a preference for the use of stent deployment for the restoration of flow in patients with ICAD.

The first randomized, multicenter trial that analyzed balloon angioplasty and stenting and provided support for the use of dual antiplatelet therapy (DAPT) also came from the Stenting and Aggressive Medical Management for Preventing Recurrent Stroke in Intracranial Stenosis (SAMMPRIS) trial, which was a multicenter, randomized trial comparing angioplasty and stenting (percutaneous transluminal angioplasty and stenting—PTAS) and aggressive medical management versus medical management alone in patients with symptomatic ICAD.[53] Aggressive medical management (AMM) was characterized as the DAPT (325 mg aspirin+75 mg clopidogrel), protocol-driven, intensive reduction of blood pressure to below systolic 140 (<130 mm Hg in patients with diabetes) and low–density lipoprotein (LDL) concentration lower than 1.81 mmol/L. Also included in the AMM component was a lifestyle coach who aggressively counseled patients on diet and exercise regimens. The trial was halted prior to completion due to a high rate of complications in the stenting arm with patients having periprocedural strokes. Patients in the AMM arm had a substantially lower rate of stroke or death at 30 days (5.8%) when compared to patients in the PTAS plus AMM group (14.7%). Even in subgroup analysis, investigators of the trial were unable to find a signal that supported the use of PTAS when compared to the AMM regimen.[54] At study end, with a median follow–up of 32 months, the rates of the primary outcome events remained significantly higher for the angioplasty and stenting group in comparison with the medical management group (19.7% vs. 12.6% at 2 year, and 23.9% vs. 14.9% at 3 years). It should be noted, however, that these long-term differences were largely due to the effects of the 30-day outcomes because the rates of stroke and death beyond 30 days were similar for the two groups.

The VISSIT trial was the second trial that examined angioplasty with stenting, but it was terminated early following the results of SAMMPRIS.[55] The trial randomized 112 patients with symptomatic ICAD to treatment with a balloon-expandable stent plus medical therapy or medical therapy alone and found the primary outcome of stroke, intracranial hemorrhage, or death to be significantly higher in the stenting arm (24%) compared to medical therapy alone (9%) at 30 days. At 12 months, the rate continued to be significantly higher in the stent group (36%) when compared to the medical therapy group (15%).

Since these trials, standard accepted practice for patients presenting with isch-emic stroke secondary to ICAD has been to prescribe DAPT for a period of 90 days along with aggressive blood pressure lowering and targeting LDL levels below 1.81 mmol/L. The recommendation of having patients on DAPT only for a period of 90 days comes from data from the Molecular Analysis for Therapy Choice (MATCH) and Clopidogrel for High Atherothrombotic Risk and Isch-emic Stabilization, Management, and Avoidance (CHARISMA) trials, which demonstrated that use of DAPT for a period of greater than 90 days leads to a risk of major hemorrhage.[56,57]

RISK FACTOR CONTROL

Risk factor management is a critical aspect for patients with ICAD. Data col-lected from secondary stroke prevention trials (WASID and SAMMPRIS) have focused on lowering of LDL concentrations and looking at reductions in blood pressure; through the use of statins and angiotensin-converting enzyme (ACE) inhibitors, investigators have looked at their effects in the reduction of stroke. Post hoc analysis of the WASID trial showed that both poorly controlled systolic blood pressure (>140 mm Hg) and cholesterol (>5.20 mmol/L) at follow-up had the highest rates of major vascular events.[58] One of the common practices in patients who present with symptomatic ICAD is to maintain the blood pres-sure at slightly higher levels to prevent ischemia secondary to distal hypoperfu-sion. However, secondary analysis of WASID showed that maintenance of mean high blood pressures at follow-up did not reduce the risk of ischemic stroke but, in fact, increased it.[59]

FUTURE

Current research on ICAD has two focuses: (a) prevention/reduction of sec-ondary stroke in patients who are symptomatic and (b) identification of lesions in the blood vessels that may help point toward future stroke risk. Identifica-tion of high-risk lesions/patients is being done via noninvasive imaging modalities such as quantitative MRA, which gives investigators vessel-specific volumet-ric flow rates. The recently completed Vertebrobasilar Flow Evaluation and Risk of Transient Ischaemic Attack and Stroke (VERiTAS) study examined whether patients with compromised flow distal to the symptomatic vessel helps in prediction of ischemic events.[60] The ongoing Mechanisms of Early Recurrence in Intracranial Atherosclerotic Disease (MyRIAD) study is using noninvasive imaging to determine the mechanisms of stroke and stratify stroke risk in patients with symptomatic high-grade IAD.[61] Advanced neuroimaging techniques that are being utilized include quantitative magnetic resonance imaging (QMRA) to assess volumetric flow rate through stenotic artery, magnetic resonance perfusion weighted imaging (PWI-MRI) to determine distal tissue perfusion, and TCD to assess vasomotor reactivity using breath-holding technique (BHI-TCD), as well as embolic signal monitoring to evaluate artery-to-artery embolism.

Other promising imaging modalities include high-resolution MRI through utilization of 3-Tesla MRI for imaging plaque and vessel wall characteristics. The high-resolution MRI enables assessment of the underlying vessel pathology and identification of atherosclerosis, inflammation, and vasospasm.[62]

Finally, the advent of new pharmacological treatments, including direct thrombin and Xa inhibitors, has provided alternative methods of treating atrial fibrillation, and consideration may be given to their use in patients with symptomatic ICAD.

CONCLUSION

For patients presenting with ischemic stroke or TIA secondary to ICAD, the accepted standard practice is to start the patient on aspirin and clopidogrel for a period of 90 days along with blood pressure control (target systolic <140 mm Hg), hemoglobin A1C target below 7.0, and LDL below 70 mg/dL. Lifestyle changes are stressed for these patients with active cardiovascular exercise and changes to their diets.

With promising imaging, improved understanding of the pathophysiology behind it, and new treatments being investigated, ICAD continues to remain an area of great interest and research in the stroke community given its high burden of recurrent stroke and prevalence in the global population.

References

1. Gorelick PB, Wong KS, Bae HJ, Pandey DK. Large artery intracranial occlusive disease: a large worldwide burden but a relatively neglected frontier. *Stroke*. 2008;39:2396–2399.
2. Wong LK. Global burden of intracranial atherosclerosis. *Int J Stroke*. 2006;1:158–159.
3. Sacco RL, Kargman DE, Gu Q, Zamanillo MC. Race-ethnicity and determinants of intracranial atherosclerotic cerebral infarction. The Northern Manhattan Stroke Study. *Stroke*. 1995;26:14–20.
4. Chimowitz MI, Lynn MJ, Howlett-Smith H, et al. Comparison of warfarin and aspirin for symptomatic intracranial arterial stenosis. *N Eng J Med*. 2005;352:1305–1316.

5. Mazighi M, Tanasescu R, Ducrocq X, et al. Prospective study of symptomatic athero-thrombotic intracranial stenoses: the GESICA study. *Neurology.* 2006;66:1187–1191.

6. White H, Boden-Albala B, Wang C, et al. Ischemic stroke subtype incidence among whites, blacks, and Hispanics: the Northern Manhattan Study. *Circulation.* 2005;111: 1327–1331.

7. Weber R, Kraywinkel K, Diener HC, Weimar C. Symptomatic intracranial atheroscle-rotic stenoses: prevalence and prognosis in patients with acute cerebral ischemia. *Cere-brovasc Dis.* 2010;30:188–193.

8. Gorelick PB, Caplan LR, Hier DB, et al. Racial differences in the distribution of anterior circulation occlusive disease. *Neurology.* 1984;34:54–59.

9. Gorelick PB, Caplan LR, Hier DB, et al. Racial differences in the distribution of poste-rior circulation occlusive disease. *Stroke.* 1985;16:785–790.

10. Kim JT, Yoo SH, Kwon JH, et al. Subtyping of ischemic stroke based on vascular imag-ing: analysis of 1,167 acute, consecutive patients. *J Clin Neurol.* (Seoul, Korea) 2006; 2:225–230.

11. Huang YN, Gao S, Li SW, et al. Vascular lesions in Chinese patients with transient ischemic attacks. *Neurology.* 1997;48:524–525.

12. Mazighi M, Labreuche J, Gongora-Rivera F, et al. Autopsy prevalence of intracranial atherosclerosis in patients with fatal stroke. *Stroke.* 2008;39:1142–1147.

13. Uehara T, Tabuchi M, Mori E. Risk factors for occlusive lesions of intracranial arteries in stroke-free Japanese. *Eur J Neurol.* 2005;12:218–222.

14. Rincon F, Sacco RL, Kranwinkel G, et al. Incidence and risk factors of intracranial ath-erosclerotic stroke: the Northern Manhattan Stroke Study. *Cerebrovasc Dis.* 2009;28: 65–71.

15. Ingall TJ, Homer D, Baker HL Jr., et al. Predictors of intracranial carotid artery athero-sclerosis. Duration of cigarette smoking and hypertension are more powerful than serum lipid levels. *Arch Neurol.* 1991;48:687–691.

16. Wityk RJ, Lehman D, Klag M, et al. Race and sex differences in the distribution of cere-bral atherosclerosis. *Stroke.* 1996;27:1974–1980.

17. Park JH, Kwon HM, Roh JK. Metabolic syndrome is more associated with intracranial atherosclerosis than extracranial atherosclerosis. *Eur J Neurol.* 2007;14:379–386.

18. Mi D, Zhang L, Wang C, et al. Impact of metabolic syndrome on the prognosis of isch-emic stroke secondary to symptomatic intracranial atherosclerosis in Chinese patients. *PloS ONE* 2012;7:e51421.

19. Turan TN, Makki AA, Tsappidi S, et al. Risk factors associated with severity and loca-tion of intracranial arterial stenosis. *Stroke.* 2010;41:1636–40.

20. Kim DE, Kim JY, Jeong SW, et al. Association between changes in lipid profiles and progression of symptomatic intracranial atherosclerotic stenosis: a prospective multicenter study. *Stroke.* 2012;43:1824–1830.

21. Bang OY, Saver JL, Ovbiagele B, et al. Adiponectin levels in patients with intracranial atherosclerosis. *Neurology.* 2007;68:1931–1937.

22. Massot A, Pelegri D, Penalba A, et al. Lipoprotein-associated phospholipase A2 testing usefulness among patients with symptomatic intracranial atherosclerotic disease. *Athero-sclerosis.* 2011;218:181–187.

23. Arenillas JF, Alvarez-Sabin J, Molina CA, et al. Progression of symptomatic intracranial large artery atherosclerosis is associated with a proinflammatory state and impaired fibri-nolysis. *Stroke.* 2008;39:1456–1463.

24. Liebeskind DS, Cotsonis GA, Saver JL, et al. Collaterals dramatically alter stroke risk in intracranial atherosclerosis. *Ann Neurol.* 2011;69:963–974.

25. Resch JA, Okabe N, Loewenson RB, et al. Pattern of vessel involvement in cerebral atherosclerosis. A comparative study between a Japanese and Minnesota population. *J Atheroscl Res* 1969;9:239–250.

26. Pu Y, Liu L, Wang Y, et al. Geographic and sex difference in the distribution of intracranial atherosclerosis in China. *Stroke*. 2013;44:2109–2114.

27. Gomez CR, Qureshi AI. Medical treatment of patients with intracranial atherosclerotic disease. *J Neuroimaging*. 2009;19(Suppl 1):25s–29s.

28. Ritz K, Denswil NP, Stam OC, et al. Cause and mechanisms of intracranial atherosclerosis. *Circulation*. 2014;130:1407–1414.

29. Caplan LR. Intracranial branch atheromatous disease: a neglected, understudied, and underused concept. *Neurology*. 1989;39:1246–1250.

30. Schreiber S, Serdaroglu M, Schreiber F, et al. Simultaneous occurrence and interaction of hypoperfusion and embolism in a patient with severe middle cerebral artery stenosis. *Stroke*. 2009;40:e478–e480.

31. Caplan LR, Wong KS, Gao S, Hennerici MG. Is hypoperfusion an important cause of strokes? If so, how? *Cerebrovasc Dis*. 2006;21:145–153.

32. Endarterectomy for asymptomatic carotid artery stenosis. Executive Committee for the Asymptomatic Carotid Atherosclerosis Study. *JAMA*. 1995;273:1421–1428.

33. Bash S, Villablanca JP, Jahan R, et al. Intracranial vascular stenosis and occlusive disease: evaluation with CT angiography, MR angiography, and digital subtraction angiography. *Am J Neuroradiol*. 2005;26:1012–21.

34. Nguyen-Huynh MN, Wintermark M, English J, et al. How accurate is CT angiography in evaluating intracranial atherosclerotic disease? *Stroke*. 2008;39:1184–1188.

35. Feldmann E, Wilterdink JL, Kosinski A, et al. The Stroke Outcomes and Neuroimaging of Intracranial Atherosclerosis (SONIA) trial. *Neurology*. 2007;68:2099–2106.

36. Berkhemer OA, Fransen PS, Beumer D, et al. A randomized trial of intraarterial treatment for acute ischemic stroke. *N Eng J Med*. 2015;372:11–20.

37. Campbell BC, Mitchell PJ, Kleinig TJ, et al. Endovascular therapy for ischemic stroke with perfusion-imaging selection. *N Eng J Med*. 2015;372:1009–1018.

38. Goyal M, Demchuk AM, Menon BK, et al. Randomized assessment of rapid endovascular treatment of ischemic stroke. *N Eng J Med*. 2015;372:1019–1030.

39. Saver JL, Goyal M, Bonafe A, et al. Stent-retriever thrombectomy after intravenous t-PA vs. t-PA alone in stroke. *N Eng J Med*. 2015;372:2285–2295.

40. Jovin TG, Chamorro A, Cobo E, et al. Thrombectomy within 8 hours after symptom onset in ischemic stroke. *N Eng J Med*. 2015;372:2296–2306.

41. Powers WJ, Derdeyn CP, Biller J, et al. 2015 AHA/ASA Focused Update of the 2013 Guidelines for the Early Management of Patients with Acute Ischemic Stroke Regarding Endovascular Treatment: A Guideline for Healthcare Professionals from the American Heart Association/American Stroke Association. *Stroke*. 2015;46:3020–3035.

42. Goyal M, Menon BK, van Zwam WH, et al. Endovascular thrombectomy after large-vessel ischaemic stroke: a meta-analysis of individual patient data from five randomised trials. *Lancet*. 2016;387:1723–1731.

43. Chimowitz MI, Kokkinos J, Strong J, et al. The Warfarin-Aspirin Symptomatic Intracranial Disease Study. *Neurology*. 1995;45:1488–1493.

44. Mohr JP, Thompson JL, Lazar RM, et al. A comparison of warfarin and aspirin for the prevention of recurrent ischemic stroke. *N Eng J Med*. 2001;345:1444–1451.

45. Kasner SE, Lynn MJ, Chimowitz MI, et al. Warfarin vs aspirin for symptomatic intracranial stenosis: subgroup analyses from WASID. *Neurology*. 2006;67:1275–1278.

46. Wong KS, Chen C, Fu J, et al. Clopidogrel plus aspirin versus aspirin alone for reducing embolisation in patients with acute symptomatic cerebral or carotid artery stenosis (CLAIR study): a randomised, open-label, blinded-endpoint trial. *Lancet Neurol.* 2010;9: 489–497.

47. Markus HS, Droste DW, Kaps M, et al. Dual antiplatelet therapy with clopidogrel and aspirin in symptomatic carotid stenosis evaluated using doppler embolic signal detection: the Clopidogrel and Aspirin for Reduction of Emboli in Symptomatic Carotid Stenosis (CARESS) trial. *Circulation.* 2005;111:2233–2240.

48. Kwon SU, Cho YJ, Koo JS, et al. Cilostazol prevents the progression of the symptomatic intracranial arterial stenosis: the multicenter double-blind placebo-controlled trial of cilostazol in symptomatic intracranial arterial stenosis. *Stroke.* 2005;36:782–786.

49. Kwon SU, Hong KS, Kang DW, et al. Efficacy and safety of combination antiplatelet therapies in patients with symptomatic intracranial atherosclerotic stenosis. *Stroke.* 2011;42:2883–2890.

50. Gupta R, Schumacher HC, Mangla S, et al. Urgent endovascular revascularization for symptomatic intracranial atherosclerotic stenosis. *Neurology.* 2003;61:1729–1735.

51. Gress DR, Smith WS, Dowd CF, et al. Angioplasty for intracranial symptomatic vertebrobasilar ischemia. *Neurosurgery.* 2002;51:23–27; discussion 27–29.

52. Cruz-Flores S, Diamond AL. Angioplasty for intracranial artery stenosis. *Cochrane Database Syst Rev.* 2006:Cd004133.

53. Chimowitz MI, Lynn MJ, Derdeyn CP, et al. Stenting versus aggressive medical therapy for intracranial arterial stenosis. *N Eng J Med.* 2011;365:993–1003.

54. Lutsep HL, Lynn MJ, Cotsonis GA, et al. Does the stenting versus aggressive medical therapy trial support stenting for subgroups with intracranial stenosis? *Stroke.* 2015;46: 3282–3284.

55. Zaidat OO, Fitzsimmons BF, Woodward BK, et al. Effect of a balloon-expandable intracranial stent vs medical therapy on risk of stroke in patients with symptomatic intracranial stenosis: the VISSIT randomized clinical trial. *JAMA.* 2015;313:1240–1248.

56. Diener HC, Bogousslavsky J, Brass LM, et al. Aspirin and clopidogrel compared with clopidogrel alone after recent ischaemic stroke or transient ischaemic attack in high-risk patients (MATCH): randomised, double-blind, placebo-controlled trial. *Lancet.* 2004; 364:331–337.

57. Bhatt DL, Fox KA, Hacke W, et al. Clopidogrel and aspirin versus aspirin alone for the prevention of atherothrombotic events. *N Eng J Med.* 2006;354:1706–1717.

58. Chaturvedi S, Turan TN, Lynn MJ, et al. Risk factor status and vascular events in patients with symptomatic intracranial stenosis. *Neurology.* 2007;69:2063–2068.

59. Turan TN, Cotsonis G, Lynn MJ, et al. Relationship between blood pressure and stroke recurrence in patients with intracranial arterial stenosis. *Circulation.* 2007;115:2969–2975.

60. Amin-Hanjani S, Rose-Finnell L, Richardson D, et al. Vertebrobasilar Flow Evaluation and Risk of Transient Ischaemic Attack and Stroke study (VERiTAS): rationale and design. *Int J Stroke.* 2010;5:499–505.

61. Mechanisms of Early Recurrence in Intracranial Atherosclerotic Disease (MyRIAD). Accessed October 3, 2016, at https://clinicaltrials.gov/show/NCT02121028.

62. Swartz RH, Bhuta SS, Farb RI, et al. Intracranial arterial wall imaging using high-resolution 3-tesla contrast-enhanced MRI. *Neurology.* 2009;72:627–634.

Small-Vessel Disease 14

Joseph Tarsia and Magdy Selim

INTRODUCTION

Definition of Small Vessel Disease

Cerebral small vessel disease (SVD) encompasses a vast spectrum of brain injury due to pathology primarily within the small arteries and arterioles of the brain. The clinical and radiographic spectrum of SVD contains entities that are both ischemic (e.g., small subcortical infarcts and lacunes, which represent approximately 20% of all ischemic strokes) and hemorrhagic (e.g., cerebral microbleeds, intracerebral hemorrhage).

Anatomy of SVD

The small cerebral vessels originate from two distinct locations. First, deep perforators extend from the circle of Willis and proximal segments of large cerebral arteries (e.g., middle cerebral artery [MCA], anterior cerebral artery, posterior cerebral artery, basilar artery). Second, the terminal vessels of long penetrating medullary arteries originate from leptomeningeal vessels found at the surface of the brain in the subarachnoid space. These two systems converge toward each other from opposite directions to supply deep subcortical structures, including the basal ganglia, brainstem, and subcortical white matter.

Spectrum of SVD

The clinical presentations of SVD have been classically described as lacunar syndromes. However, it is not unusual to discover clinically silent lacunes or microbleeds on routine imaging. In addition, white matter hyperintensities, either isolated or diffuse, have come to the forefront in the context of vascular cognitive impairment (VCI) and subcortical vascular dementia. The etiological scope of SVD also includes entities such as cerebral amyloid angiopathy (CAA), monogenetic conditions such as CADASIL (cerebral autosomal-dominant arteriopathy with subcortical infarcts and leukoencephalopathy), inflammatory changes secondary to autoimmune and infectious processes, and post-radiation vasculopathy.[1] We focus our review on sporadic small vessel disease, historically related to hypertension, age, and other vascular risk factors.

EPIDEMIOLOGY AND RISK FACTORS

Small vessel infarcts (i.e., lacunar infarcts) represent approximately 20% to 25% of all ischemic strokes in the United States, with an annual incidence of 27 per 100,000 people.[2] Risk factors for sporadic SVD have traditionally included hypertension (HTN), hyperlipidemia, diabetes mellitus (DM), smoking, and age. The earliest association with these risk factors stemmed from the initial pathological evaluation of small vessel infarcts by C.M. Fisher, in which the involved vessels showed signs of atheromatous changes as well as fibrinoid necrosis and hyalinosis—both of which can be seen elsewhere in the body as a consequence of HTN.[3] The SPS3 (Secondary Prevention of Small Subcortical Strokes) study evaluated 3,020 patients with small-vessel infarcts (SVIs) and found that the mean age was 63; 63% were men, 75% had a history of HTN, 49% had hyperlipidemia, 37% were diabetic, and >50% were previous smokers.[4] Recent studies suggest that microembolism from thromboembolic sources such as atrial fibrillation and severe carotid disease and may be associated with approximately 10%–15% of SVI.[5,6]

One large prospective cohort study did find that SVIs differed from non-SVIs in that they tended to recur less early, dispelling a proximal emboli source, and were followed more often by further lacunar strokes—suggesting that lacunar pathology is indeed distinct.[7] A systematic review suggests that HTN and DM are risk factors for ischemic stroke in general but do not help distinguish SVI from that of large-vessel etiology.[5] A case-control study comparing lacunar stroke ($n = 414$) against large-vessel stroke ($n = 471$) with the elimination of classification bias found HTN to be more common in SVD (odds ratio [OR] 3.43), whereas hypercholesterolemia, smoking, myocardial infarction (MI), and peripheral vascular disease (PVD) were more common in large-vessel disease (LVD).[8]

Aside from the identified rare monogenetic conditions mentioned earlier, genetic studies have been underwhelming at identifying specific loci associated with the development of sporadic SVD. Genome-wide association studies (GWASs) have identified a single nucleotide polymorphism (SNP) (rs2230500), a member of protein kinase C family *PRKCH*, that has a significant associa-tion with SVI (OR 1.40) as well as silent SVI and increases the overall risk of both ischemic and hemorrhagic stroke in Chinese patients. European GWASs have identified two SNPs (rs3744208 and rs1055129) associated with cerebral white matter hyperintensities. Candidate gene studies have identified several poly-morphisms associated with ischemic stroke but only the angiotensin-converting enzyme (ACE) insertion deletion (I/D) has a high affinity for SVI and, possi-bly, white matter hyperintensities.[9–11]

VESSEL PATHOLOGY

The first major process of small vessel pathology consists of thickening of the vessel wall and subsequent structural changes leading to obliteration and com-promise of the lumen.[12] This disruption is characterized by loss of smooth mus-cle cells from the tunica media and deposits of fibro-hyaline material within the vessel wall, as detailed later. Overall, these disease processes intrinsic to the vessel wall can lead to varying degrees of downstream ischemic or hemorrhagic consequences.

The underlying lesions of sporadic SVD were classically described by the seminal necropsy studies performed by Fisher in the 1950s–1970s, prior to CT. He studied the perforating arteries and arterioles that coincided with the presence of lacunes, the latter of which he attributed to the presence of SVD.[3,13,14] He found *fibrinoid necrosis*, the deposition of exudated plasma fibrin and fibrinogen and necrotic smooth muscle cells segmentally along the course of a vessel within the media. Downstream sequelae of fibrinoid necrosis include microaneurysm formation associated with thrombi, leakage of blood components, and segmental arterial disorganization—a complete loss of arte-rial architecture leading to obliteration of the vessel. *Microaneurysms* are miliary saccular aneurysms <1000 μm in size. They are typically lined internally with fibrinoid necrosis and thrombi and surrounded by either extruded red blood cells or hemosiderin-laden macrophages, reflecting either fresh or remote hemor-rhage, respectively. Rupture of these microaneurysms may lead to the formation of a *bleeding globe* or *pseudoaneurysm* and development of macroscopic intracere-bral hemorrhage.[15,16]

Fisher coined the term *lipohyalinosis* when he found this process coinciding with lipid-laden macrophages, a term today that connotes both hypertensive and atherosclerotic changes. Unfortunately, this term is misleading because he used the terms *hyalinosis* and *fibrinoid* interchangeably.[17] *Hyalinosis* describes changes to the vessel wall due to hypertension consisting of degenerated collagen, smooth muscle cells, and amorphous structures that contribute to compromise

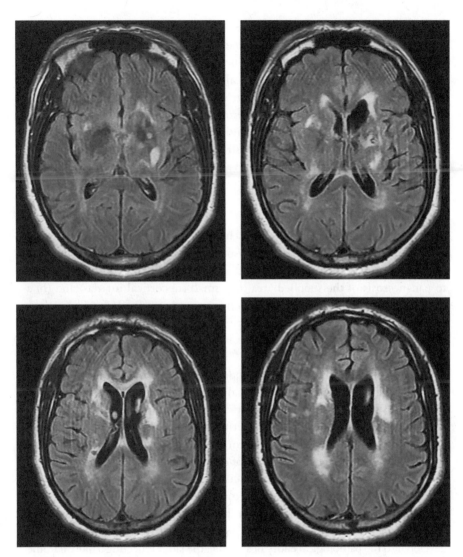

FIGURE 14.1 Patient with small-vessel subcortical white matter disease with evidence of both diffuse white matter changes, including a left basal ganglia lacune, and chronic left basal ganglia small-vessel infarct

of the lumen. Regardless of the semantics, both fibrinoid necrosis and lipohyalinosis remain the hallmark findings of sporadic small vessel disease.

The second major category of small vessel pathology is that of intracranial branch atheromatous disease (Figure 14.1) A *microatheroma* describes atherosclerotic plaque obstruction intrinsic to the penetrating artery itself. This should be distinguished from large, parent artery atherosclerotic disease leading to occlusion of the small vessel orifice either entirely stationed within the parent artery or in a junctional fashion.[12,18,19] These latter entities typically lead to larger and more superficial infarcts and typically involve multiple small penetrators simultaneously at their origin. The large striatocapsular infarct exemplifies this pathology, with either embolic or atherothrombotic occlusion of the M1 segment of the MCA involving multiple lenticulostriate arteries, resulting in infarct of a large territory involving both the striatum and the internal capsule.[20,21]

BRAIN PATHOLOGY AND PATHOPHYSIOLOGY

Ischemic Lesions

The relationship between SVD and ischemic consequences on the brain can be explained by two processes along a spectrum: (a) focal severe ischemia secondary to decreased perfusion in the territory of a penetrating artery leading to pan-necrosis of the supplied area (i.e., small subcortical infarcts) and (b) a less severe, chronic ischemia with selective necrosis, particularly of oligodendrocytes and myelin (i.e., white matter hyperintensities).[1,12]

Small subcortical infarcts (i.e., lacunar infarcts) are found at the deep, terminal territories supplied by perforator vessels. These are most commonly located in the putamen, globus pallidus, thalamus, caudate, internal capsule, pons, and corona radiata. Rarely involved are the cerebral peduncles, medullary pyramids, and subcortical white matter.[12] Asymptomatic lesions occur more often in the internal capsule or caudate nucleus.[22] The term *lacune* describes a specific pathological entity of a discrete, small (3- to 15-mm) cavitary lesion filled with cerebrospinal fluid (CSF) and cobweb-like strands of connective tissue as residual of postinfarction macrophage activity. As discussed earlier, entities such as fibrinoid necrosis, lipohyalinosis, and atherosclerosis have been found concurrently with lacunar pathology; however, thrombosis has not been confirmed pathologically in this setting.[23,24] It is also important to note that not all small subcortical infarcts develop into the pathological entity of a lacune, the latter reflecting a more chronic or completed entity of pathology. Also, the terms *lacunar infarct* and *lacunar stroke* are used interchangeably with *small subcortical infarct* within the literature.

White matter hyperintensities secondary to SVD can occur in isolation or develop into severe confluent disease. The underlying pathophysiology is uncertain. One hypothesis suggests subclinical ischemia secondary to chronic hypoperfusion of white matter. This process, presumably secondary to obliterative disease of small vessels, leads to selective necrosis and degeneration of myelin and loss of oligodendrocytes.[1] This ischemic hypothesis is supported by the fact that a majority occur in border zone vascular areas susceptible to ischemia,[25] are associated clinically with vascular risk factors and both lacunar stroke and intracererbral hemorrhage,[26] reflect the existence of intralesional histological markers of an hypoxic environment,[27] and exhibit white matter components (e.g., oligodendrocytes and myelin) that have a high susceptibility to ischemia.[28] PET studies show an ischemic component to these areas as well, with a decreased cerebral metabolic rate of oxygen and a higher oxygen extraction fraction,[29] and despite varying results across studies, impaired vaso-reactivity and autoregulation are also noted.

Another proposed theory on white matter hyperintensity origin suggests the role of primary endothelial dysfunction and disruption of the blood-brain barrier (BBB)—namely, tight junctions between endothelial cells of the small vessels. This disruption leads to toxic substance leakage (e.g., proteins, inflammatory cells, red blood cells) into the perivascular space, upregulation of matrix metalloproteinases, and perivascular edema. The perivascular edema causes a toxic environment to neurons, glia, and astrocytes, leading to insidious perivascular cumulative tissue damage and demyelination.[12,30–32] The extension of this theory to incorporate the entire spectrum of SVD—from lacune development to hemorrhagic manifestations via direct damage to the vessels—has gained attention and significant evidence over the past few decades.[30–32]

Hemorrhagic Lesions of SVD

Cerebral microbleeds (CMBs) are often detected radiographically and can serve as a marker of small vessel disease. CMBs occur due to increased vessel wall permeability and leakage of blood products with perivascular accumulation of hemosiderin and hemosiderin-laden macrophages.[33] They are found in 6.5% in persons 45 to 50 years old and up to 36% in those 80 years and older, with hypertension and diabetes as associated risk factors. The presence of lacunes and white matter disease are also associated with the presence of microbleeds.[34,35] Use of Coumadin anticoagulation has been associated with an increased risk of developing CMBs, directly proportional to international normalized ratio (INR) level.[36] Antiplatelet use has also been shown to be associated with their development.[37,38] Topographically distinct areas occur depending upon underlying SVD pathology. In keeping with the focus of our discussion, sporadic small vessel, disease-related CMBs are found in deep brain regions, such as the basal ganglia, thalamus, brainstem, and cerebellum. CMBs of cerebral amyloid angiopathy (CAA) are almost exclusively cortico-subcortical and lobar in location, particularly the occipital, but also parieto-temporal distribution and, rarely, the cerebellum.[39,40]

Rupture of small perforating vessels damaged by SVD, commonly in the setting of hypertension, can lead to spontaneous intracerebral hemorrhages. Locations include perforating arteries of the basal ganglia, thalamus, pons, and cerebellum.[41] Studies do show a high frequency of asymptomatic CMBs in the setting of parenchymal intracerebral hemorrhage (ICH).[42] The risk of CMB transition into symptomatic ICH (i.e., macrobleeds) has also been established. A recent systematic review reported the presence of CMBs to have an odds ratio as high as 8.5 for risk of future ICH.[43]

RADIOGRAPHIC SPECTRUM AND DEFINITIONS

Given the size of the vessels related to SVD, direct visualization via magnetic resonance angiography (MRA) or computerized tomography angiography (CTA) is quite limited if not often impossible. Even conventional cerebral angiography may allow visualization of vessels up to 0.5 mm in size; however, a majority of perforator vessels, particularly in the deep white matter are less than 0.1 mm in diameter.[44] This inability to image small vessels has put most of the focus on interpreting the parenchymal changes secondary to that of SVD. Seven tesla (7T) MRA has shown remarkable resolution of these vessels and has been used to study the lenticulostriate arteries and their changes in the setting of hypertension. Unfortunately, 7T MRA is not currently approved for general clinical use but does provide promise for future imaging of these small vessels in the context of patient care.[45–48]

Limitations to using CT as an imaging modality to investigate SVD changes has led to using MRI almost exclusively in characterizing the disease both clinically and for research purposes. Early studies with CT showed significant lack of sensitivity in imaging subcortical infarcts particularly in the hyperacute phase and lesions located in the posterior fossa. Sensitivity ranged from 30% to 50% in these studies, higher in lesions involving the internal capsule.[49–51] The ability to determine chronicity of lacunar infarcts on CT also lacks precision.

A position paper published in 2013 summarized an international effort to standardize the definitions and reporting of vascular changes on neuroimaging secondary to SVD.[52] These definitions pertain to MRI brain findings. The result of this effort defined six neuroradiological entities: (a) recent small subcortical infarcts (SSIs), (b) lacune of presumed vascular origin, (c) white matter hyperintensity of presumed vascular origin, (d) perivascular spaces, (e) cerebral microbleeds, and (f) brain atrophy.

Recent small subcortical infarcts are defined as neuroimaging evidence of recent infarction in the territory of one perforating arteriole with imaging characteristics of a lesion occurring within the past few weeks. Lesion size is limited to <20 mm in maximal diameter in axial plane and should be hyperintense on

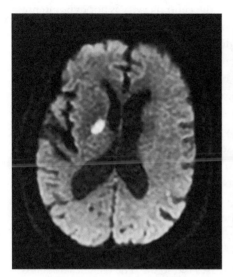 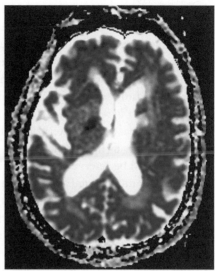

FIGURE 14.2 Small-vessel infarct of right internal capsule, with hyperintensity on diffusion-weighted imaging (left) and corresponding hypointensity on apparent diffusion coefficient sequence

diffusion-weighted imaging (DWI) and hypointense on apparent diffusion coefficient (ADC) (Figure 14.2); beyond the hyperacute phase, they are also hyperintense on fluid-attenuated inversion recovery (FLAIR) and T2 sequences (see Figure 14.1). This term should replace the commonly used terms of *lacunar stroke* and *lacunar infarctions*. Small subcortical infarcts typically transition into cavitary lacunes (76% on FLAIR; 94% on T1 after 90 days), white matter hyperintensities, or may disappear altogether.[53–55] The term *large subcortical infarcts* refers to that of the striatocapsular variety discussed earlier and does not involve SVD pathology but, rather, an atherothrombotic or embolic occlusion of the parent artery. These may be difficult to distinguish early in the hyperacute setting based upon DWI alone because large striatocapsular infarcts due to cardioembolism or large artery disease may initially appear much smaller than their final infarct size. Studies using PWI (perfusion-weighted imaging) have shown this mismatch and are able to identify these non-SVI lesions.[56]

A *lacune of presumed vascular origin* is defined as a round or ovoid, subcortical, fluid-filled cavity with similar signal as CSF and ranges in size between 3 and 15 mm in diameter in the territory of one perforating arteriole. These lesions are best characterized on FLAIR imaging as hypointense with possibly a hyperintense rim reflective of surrounding gliosis—an important distinction from large dilated perivascular spaces. At times, the central cavity is not hypointense on FLAIR despite being hypointense on T1 imaging. These lesions can be either isointense or hypointense on gradient echo (GRE) reflecting intracavity hemosiderin or hemosiderin-laden macrophages. They are the result of earlier small subcortical infarcts but rarely can be the result of healed large striatocapsular infarct (stuttering lacune) or even small deep hemorrhages.[57]

White matter hyperintensities (WMHs) of presumed vascular origin are lesions of variable size that are characteristically hyperintense on T2-weighted sequences and can be iso- or hypointense on T1 sequences. The term *subcortical hyperintensities* should be reserved for lesions in the deep grey matter (i.e., basal ganglia and thalamus) as well as brainstem (see Figure 14.1). These WMHs are the sequelae of small subcortical infarcts or chronic ischemia but have a controversial pathophysiology as mentioned earlier. The nomenclature to describe this entity throughout the literature over the last few decades is plentiful: leukoaraiosis, white matter lesions, white matter changes, leukoencephalopathy, white matter disease, ischemic white matter disease, and so on. The term *leukoaraiosis* is most common in the literature and originated as a term used to describe reduced attenuation (hypodensity) on CT that reflects the rarefied white matter seen in diffuse confluent disease (see Figure 14.1).

Several characteristic features can help distinguish vascular white matter hyperintensities from those of other common mimics, such as multiple sclerosis (MS), migraine, and vasculitis. In clinical practice, this can remain a challenge even for experts. If located peripherally, a vascular pattern of hyperintensities tend to be localized in the sub-"U fiber" zones and spare the juxtacortical area. Overall, they are more common in the deep border zones of the centrum semiovale and can involve the basal ganglia. The periventricular lesions tend to be small and either round or irregular and do not contrast enhance. Lesions in MS (Figure 14.3) tend to be juxtacortical in nature, and the periventricular lesions are ovoid and larger, often extending from the inferior aspect of the corpus callosum as Dawson's fingers. Migraine hyperintensities, more common in those with aura, are predominantly frontal and bilateral (Figure 14.4).[58,59]

Perivascular spaces are defined as fluid-filled spaces that follow the course of a vessel as it penetrates from the extracerebral subarachnoid space through the gray or white matter and is enveloped in leptomeninges. Their enlargement occurs with age and is found concurrently with other entities of SVD, but their true clinical significance remains unknown. These spaces have been referred to previously in the literature as Virchow–Robin spaces, type 3 lacunes, and *etat crible* or perivascular atrophy of brain tissue.

Cerebral microbleeds (CMBs) are defined as small (2–5 mm; can be as large as 10 mm) areas of signal void or hypointensity on T2*/GRE (gradient echo) or

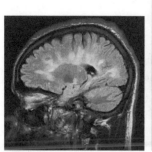
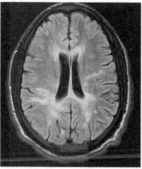
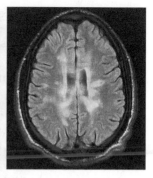

FIGURE 14.3 FLAIR imaging showing white matter hyperintensities in a patient with multiple sclerosis

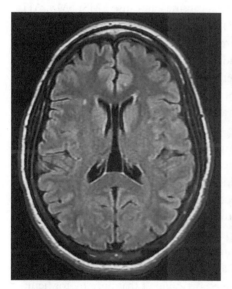
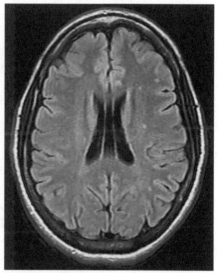

FIGURE 14.4 FLAIR imaging with small frontal white matter hyperintensities in a patient with migraine headaches

SWI (susceptibility-weighted imaging). They are well defined and homogeneous, round or oval in shape. Their pathophysiology and topography specific to their underlying SVD (hypertensive vs. CAA) is discussed earlier.

Brain atrophy secondary to SVD can be global but also focal, affecting corpus callosum, mesencephalon, hippocampus, and focal cortical thinning. The underlying pathological correlates reveal neuronal loss, cortical thinning, and rarefaction and shrinkage of the white matter.

CLINICAL SYNDROMES

Acute Stroke Syndromes

Fisher described up to 21 distinct lacunar syndromes that can be present in the setting of a small vessel infarct or lacunar infarct.[60] The five most common syndromes are discussed here. In order of frequency, these are pure motor stroke (PMS), ataxic hemiparesis (AH), sensorimotor stroke (SMS), dysarthria-clumsy hand syndrome (DCHS), and pure sensory stroke (PSS) (Table 14.1). The most essential unifying clinical theme is that these syndromes are absent of cortical signs (i.e., aphasia, neglect, apraxia, etc.) reflecting their subcortical location.

An important established principle to keep in mind is that a single lacunar syndrome can be caused by lesions in a variety of locations, and lesions in a specific location may cause a variety of lacunar syndromes.[61] For example, lesions in the posterior limb of the internal capsule can cause PMS, SMS, AH, and DCH syndromes. Pure motor stroke may be caused by lesions in the posterior limb of the internal capsule, pons, corona radiate, and medial medulla.[61] In addition, a lot of interest has been paid to the validity or predictive value of these clinical syndromes for true, underlying, small vessel infarcts rather than other stroke subtypes (i.e., cardioembolism, large vessel) as well as the presence of misinterpreted cortical lesions rather than subcortical lesions discovered after imaging is obtained.[56,62,63]

The *capsular warning syndrome* is a description used to describe repeated bursts of transient ischemic attacks (TIAs) in a crescendo pattern that ultimately result in subcortical SVI. This dramatic presentation of repeated transient symptoms that ultimately leads to sustained deficit occurs usually within 72 hours prior to infarction. Episodes range from minutes to several hours in duration prior to remission and can occur up to several times per hour. Early studies suggested this was due to hemodynamic fluctuations within a single small vessel perforator prior to complete infarction. Essentially all of the lacunar syndromes could present in this fashion, but a majority of case reports suggest that pure motor hemiparesis and sensorimotor syndromes are most common, likely given their high predilection for the internal capsule.[64] A similar *pontine warning syndrome* has been reported as a pre-cursor TIA of the brainstem. Population-based studies recently conducted suggest that, overall, the capsular warning syndrome is rare, representing approximately 1.5% of all TIA presentations. However, this presentation of TIA has the highest predictive value of developing into completed ischemic stroke when compared with repeated TIAs of cardioembolic or large-vessel etiology.[65]

Brainstem stroke syndromes are less common than lacunar syndromes. They can be a result of diseased perforator arteries that stem from branches of the

TABLE 14.1 Lacunar syndromes

	Clinical presentation	Associated lesions	Other information
Pure motor stroke	Weakness of face, arm, and leg contralateral to lesion in the absence of additional symptoms	• Posterior limb of internal capsule • Ventral pons • Corona radiata • Medial medulla • Cerebral peduncle	• ~40%–55% of all SVIs • Least-specific syndrome for SVD etiology (~10%–15% cardioembolic, large vessel, hemorrhagic)
Pure sensory stroke	Sensory loss involving face, arm, and leg contralateral to lesion in the absence of additional symptoms	• Ventral posterior lateral (VPL) nucleus of the thalamus • Anterior limb of Internal capsule • Corona radiata • Pontine tegmentum	• ~5%–15% of SVIs • Highly predictive of SVD) etiology (90%–100% with associated lacunar lesion; PPV ranges 88%–100%
Sensorimotor stroke	Weakness and sensory loss involving face, arm, and leg contralateral to lesion	• Posterior limb of internal capsule • Thalamocapsular region • Lateral medulla	• ~20%–30% of SVI
Ataxic hemiparesis	Weakness and incoordination/ataxia (out of proportion to the weakness), contralateral to lesion	• Internal capsule • Pons • Corona radiata • Frontal-subcortical • Thalamus (rare)	• ~10% of SVI • ~50%–90% specificity of syndrome to SVD etiology
Dysarthria-clumsy hand syndrome	Dysarthria (slurred speech) and poor dexterity of the hand contralateral to lesion	• Posterior limb of internal capsule • Pons • Corona radiata • Caudate nucleus • Thalamus	• Least common syndrome • 94% specificity for SVD

Source: Adapted from References 12 and 16.

vertebral, basilar, PICA, AICA, SCA, and PCAs. Overall, compared with lacunar syndromes, brainstem syndromes are much less commonly due to SVD and more commonly due to large-vessel etiologies, especially that of parent artery atheromatous disease, and cardioembolism. This varies by location, with intrinsic SVD being the etiology of midbrain syndromes approximately 10% to 15% of the time, pontine syndromes approximately 20% to 30% of the time, and medullary syndromes approximately 20% of the time.[16] The presentation of these particular syndromes will depend upon the infarct and anatomical structures involved.

Thalamic stroke syndromes secondary to perforators from the posterior communicating arteries and proximal segments of the PCA can lead to a wide array of clinical symptoms, most importantly those that mimic cortical syndromes—aphasia, agnosia, amnesia, neglect, and so on. This is due to its densely packed nuclei and role as the relay center for ascending and descending tracts of the brain involving virtually any function. Along those lines, different syndromes can be expected with right- versus left-sided lesions due to connections with their respective hemisphere's cortical function. Occlusion of the artery of Percheron, characterized as a variant thalamoperforator arising from a proximal posterior cerebral artery, is associated with bilateral mesial thalamic infarction and is attributed to small vessel, large-vessel, or cardioembolic mechanism.[66] The Percheron artery syndrome may include alterations in sensation, consciousness, cognition/memory, and oculomotor and/or pupillary activity.

Vascular Cognitive Impairment

Vascular cognitive impairment (VCI) is the preferred term when discussing the full clinical spectrum of cognitive disorders secondary to vascular disease of the brain. VCI spans in severity from vascular mild cognitive impairment (VMCI) on one end to vascular dementia (VaD) on the other end. These clinical presentations are not exclusive to underlying small vessel etiologies, and most traditional classifications rely upon morphology or location of lesion, which include (a) *multi-infarct dementia (MID)* with gross large territorial infarcts, watershed or borderzone infarcts, and multifocal microinfarcts affecting the cortex; (b) *strategic infarct dementia* with SVIs in important, deep cognitive structures such as the hippocampal formation, basal forebrain, or paramedian nucleus of the thalamus; and (c) *subcortical vascular encephalopathy* (SVE) with confluent white matter disease with or without the addition of superimposed SVIs in subcortical brain regions. While strategic infarct dementia may seem to lend itself to SVD, large-vessel or cardioembolic infarcts affecting these areas and others (i.e., mesial temporal, caudate and thalamic, fronto-cingulate, etc.) would produce cognitive deficits as well.[67,68]

Binswanger's disease (BD), also known as *subcortical arteriosclerotic leukoencephalopathy* or *subcortical vascular encephalopathy*, is exclusive to sporadic SVD etiology. It consists pathologically of severe diffuse white matter disease *with* multiple deep subcortical infarcts and lacunes encompassing the vessel pathophysiology discussed earlier, including atheromatous changes of various degrees within the large vessels at the base of the brain. This process has a predilection for the occipital lobes and anterior periventricular area. Commonly involved structures include the anterior thalamus, frontal subcortical circuits, and structures involved in basolateral limbic circuitry.[69–71]

BD most commonly presents as a subacute to chronic accumulation of focal signs over weeks to months with interspersed plateaus and possible improvement that can span for months to years, although this latter finding may be rare. The course can also be gradual with no acute or obvious individual events. Clinically, these patients have impaired attention, memory, and executive function leading to significant dependence late in the course. Findings such as abulia, euphoria, and disinhibition are common as well as other focally related entities such a vascular parkinsonism, pseudobulbar palsy, or incontinence. A study comparing BD against purely multi-lacunar state and a purely white matter disease did show that those with BD perform worse cognitively, particularly in executive functioning, and have a poorer prognosis.[68–71]

The genetic disease, CADASIL (cerebral autosomal dominant arteriopathy with subcortical infarcts and leukoencephalopathy), associated with lacunar infarcts and progressive confluent white matter ischemic changes was covered in Chapter 3 in Other Mechanisms.

ACUTE TREATMENT

IV tPA (intravenous tissue plasminogen activator) given within the first 3 hours from symptom onset is considered standard of care and a Class IA recommendation by the American Heart Association/American Stroke Association (AHA/ASA) for the treatment of acute ischemic stroke. This time window has been extended to 4.5 hours by recent evidence from the ECASS III trial, although the published results did not specify stroke subtype, and is a Class 1B AHA/ASA recommendation.[72,73] These recommendations apply to all stroke subtypes and do not exclude patients based on presumed etiology.

However, some stroke experts argue against the use of IV tPA in treating acute small vessel infarcts, largely because of the paucity of pathological evidence supporting thrombosis as an inciting factor and also a general notion that SVIs are benign and have favorable recovery. The most valuable study evaluating the efficacy of IV tPA would be one that compares IV tPA vs. placebo. This is represented by the National Institute of Neurological Disorders and Stroke (NINDS) trial in 1995.[74] This trial did show that all subtypes of ischemic stroke improved with IV tPA compared with placebo. Small vessel stroke was represented by 17% of the participants, of which 63% of patients in the tPA group had a favorable outcome (vs. 40% in the placebo group).[74] A smaller, retrospective follow-up study using more stringent clinical and imaging subtyping confirmed similar results from this original NINDS trial.[75] Several subsequent comparisons of outcome between lacunar and non-lacunar ischemic stroke subtypes treated with IV tPA show that lacunar strokes do benefit from IV tPA, but these are not without selection bias and likely reflect the natural history of subcortical small vessel infarcts.[24]

SECONDARY PREVENTION

Secondary prevention for SVIs is important in preventing a high rate of long-term mortality, cognitive impairment, dementia, and further disabling strokes.[76–78] The SPS3 (Secondary Prevention of Small Subcortical Strokes) is the only randomized controlled trial to date that included a large homogeneous population of recent small vessel infarcts of greater than 3,000 patients that were followed over an average of 4 years.[79]

Antiplatelet agents such as aspirin (75–325 mg per day), clopidogrel (75 mg per day), or ASA/dipyridamole (25/200 mg, twice daily) are all considered standard-of-care options for long-term secondary prevention of ischemic stroke.[72,80] When looking at their use specifically in secondary prevention of SVI, a recent pooled analysis included 17 randomized controlled trials that reported outcomes based on stroke subtypes. For SVI, any single antiplatelet agent compared with placebo was associated with a significant reduction in recurrence of ischemic stroke (RR 0.48). There was also no clear benefit of one specific monotherapy agent over another.[81] The question of efficacy for dual antiplatelet therapy (DAPT) versus monotherapy with these agents showed no significant advantage of DAPT.[81] In the SPS3 Trial, similar results showed that the addition of clopidogrel to aspirin did not lead to a significant reduction in stroke compared with aspirin alone but did confer a significant increased risk of bleeding (hazard ratio [HR] 1.97) and all-cause mortality (HR 1.52).[82]

The use of early, limited DAPT for aggressive secondary prevention was evaluated in the recently conducted CHANCE (Clopidogrel with Aspirin in Acute Minor Stroke or Transient Ischemic Attack) trial. This study found this strategy to be beneficial and safe in those with minor strokes (i.e., NIHSS ≤3) or TIA but unfortunately did not specify outcome based upon stroke etiology subtype.[83] Results showed that those with DAPT (clopidogrel 300-mg load followed by 75 mg daily in addition to aspirin 75 mg daily) for the duration of 21 days with aspirin 75-mg monotherapy thereafter proved to significantly reduce the stroke recurrence rate at 90-day follow-up (HR 0.68) compared with aspirin monotherapy alone.[83] Despite its lack of specificity for small vessel infarcts, short-term DAPT as outlined in this trial may prove efficacious in this setting and is a Class IIB AHA recommendation.[80] The bleeding risks during this short-term antiplatelet regimen were equal between the two groups.[83] The currently ongoing POINT (Platelet-Oriented Inhibition in New TIA and Minor Ischemic Stroke) trial (NCT00991029) may prove to shed some light on specific answers regarding secondary prevention in small vessel subtypes.[84]

Statins are considered standard of care for secondary prevention of recurrent stroke. Therapy with intensive lipid-lowering therapy (~50% reduction in low-desnsity lipoprotein cholesterol [LDL-C]) level is recommended (Class IB) to reduce the risk of stroke and cardiovascular events among patients with ischemic stroke or TIA presumed to be of atherosclerotic origin and an LDL-C level ≥100 mg/dL with or without evidence of other clinical ASCVD (atherosclerotic cardiovascular disease); the role for this intervention in groups with LDL-C < 100 is a Class IC recommendation.[80,85] This applies to all stroke subtypes. A meta-analysis looking at both primary and secondary prevention for ischemic stroke showed that a reduction of LDL-C levels has a 21% relative risk reduction in stroke for every 39 mg/dL reduction in LDL-C level.[86] The SPARCL (Stroke Prevention by Aggressive Reduction in Cholesterol Levels) trial showed that high-dose atorvastatin 80 mg daily had a significant reduction in fatal and nonfatal stroke (HR 0.84; absolute risk reduction 2.2%).[87] When looking specifically at subtypes of ischemic stroke in this trial, the risk reduction between atorvastatin and placebo for SVI was 13.1% and 15.5%, respectively (HR 0.85), a similar finding across all subtypes.[88]

Blood pressure reduction would seem to be essential in both primary and secondary prevention in SVD given its prominent role as a risk factor for the development of many of the underlying arterial changes described earlier. Several trials do show a benefit of blood pressure (BP) control for stroke prevention, but optimal targets are not clearly specified. For example, in PROGRESS (Perindopril Protection aGainst Recurrent Stroke Study), a mean reduction of 9/4 mm Hg showed a 28% risk reduction in further stroke.[89] In the PRoFESS study, of which 52% of patients had SVD, the relative risk reduction was 5%.[90] The SPS3 trial also looked at this modifiable risk factor, specifically in the SVI population, and compared two groups: a higher range of 130–149 mm Hg systolic versus a lower range of <130 mm Hg systolic. A nonsignificant risk reduction was seen for all stroke in the lower target group (HR 0.81; $p = 0.08$), but the rate of ICH was reduced significantly (HR 0.37; $p = 0.03$).[91] Recommendations from this trial suggest a target SBP <130 mm Hg as secondary prevention in those with SVI.[91,92] No evidence suggests the use of one particular BP agent over another in the secondary prevention of stroke in those with SVI.

The Safety of Thrombolysis, Anticoagulation, and Antiplatelet Agents in Setting of SVD

Aside from spontaneous ICH, iatrogenic causes of symptomatic intracerebral hemorrhage (sICH) in those with varying degrees of SVD severity have been extensively studied. Important questions remain regarding the safety of using anticoagulants, thrombolytics, and antiplatelet agents in those with known severe SVD and the risk of sICH. The presence of diffuse white matter disease severity as well as multiple lacunes have also been shown to be risk factors for sICH in these particular settings.[93–96]

Asymptomatic CMBs may be a sizable risk factor for the development of symptomatic ICH after thrombolysis with a reported odds ratio (OR) of 2.29 [confidence interval (CI) 1.01–5.17; $p=0.05$]. This risk increased significantly with the number of CMBs, especially greater than 10.[97] The risk was also found to be higher in those with lobar locations, suggesting the underlying SVD to be of CAA in origin and not of sporadic SVD. Increased risk of sICH associated with CMBs has also been found with use of antiplatelet and anticoagulant agents.[98,99] Prospective studies addressing whether or not antithrombotic agents increase the risk of bleeding in those with ischemic stroke or atrial fibrillation with CMBs at baseline, are currently under way (i.e., CROMIS-2, IPAAC, IPAAC-NOAC).

The severity of white matter hyperintensities is important because this may reflect not only clinical burden of disease but severity of white matter disease and has been shown to be an independent risk factor for the development of symptomatic ICH in the setting of both anticoagulant use as well as thrombolytic therapy.[93–96]

References

1. Pantoni L. Cerebral small vessel disease: from pathogenesis and clinical characteristics to therapeutic challenges. *Lancet Neurol.* 2010;9(7):689–701.
2. Sacco S, Marini C, Totaro R, et al. A population-based study of the incidence and prognosis of lacunar stroke. *Neurology.* 2006;66(9):1335–1338.
3. Fisher C. The arterial lesions underlying lacunes. *Acta Neuropathol.* 1969;12(1):1–15.
4. White CL, Szychowski JM, Roldan A, et al. Clinical features and racial/ethnic differences among the 3020 participants in the secondary prevention of small subcortical strokes (SPS3) trial. *J Stroke Cerebrovasc Dis.* 2013;22(6):764–774.
5. Jackson C, Sudlow C. Are lacunar strokes really different? A systematic review of differences in risk factor profiles between lacunar and nonlacunar infarcts. *Stroke.* 2005;36(4): 891–901.
6. Mead G, Lewis S, Wardlaw J, et al. Severe ipsilateral carotid stenosis and middle cerebral artery disease in lacunar ischaemic stroke: Innocent bystanders? *J Neurol.* 2002;249(3): 266–271.

7. Jackson CA, Hutchison A, Dennis MS, et al. Differences between ischemic stroke sub-types in vascular outcomes support a distinct lacunar ischemic stroke arteriopathy: a prospective, hospital-based study. *Stroke.* 2009;40(12):3679–3684.

8. Khan U, Porteous L, Hassan A, Markus HS. Risk factor profile of cerebral small vessel disease and its subtypes. *J Neurol Neurosurg Psych.* 2007;78(7):702–706.

9. Choi JC. Genetics of cerebral small vessel disease. *J Stroke.* 2015;17(1):7–16.

10. Zhang Z, Xu G, Liu D, et al. Angiotensin-converting enzyme insertion/deletion polymorphism contributes to ischemic stroke risk: a meta-analysis of 50 case-control studies. *PLoS ONE.* 2012;7(10):e46495.

11. Paternoster L, Chen W, Sudlow CL. Genetic determinants of white matter hyperintensities on brain scans: a systematic assessment of 19 candidate gene polymorphisms in 46 studies in 19,000 subjects. *Stroke.* 2009;40(6):2020–2026.

12. Caplan LR. Lacunar infarction and small vessel disease: pathology and pathophysiology. *J Stroke.* 2015;17(1):2–6.

13. Fisher CM. Lacunes: small, deep cerebral infarcts. *Neurology.* 1998;50(4):841–841a.

14. Fisher CM. Capsular infarcts: The underlying vascular lesions. *Arch Neurol.* 1979;36(2):65–73.

15. Fisher CM. Cerebral miliary aneurysms in hypertension. *Am J Pathol.* 1972;66(2):313–330.

16. Pantoni L, Gorelick PB, eds. *Cerebral Small Vessel Disease.* United Kingdom: Cambridge University Press; 2014.

17. Rosenblum WI. Fibrinoid necrosis of small brain arteries and arterioles and miliary aneurysms as causes of hypertensive hemorrhage: a critical reappraisal. *Acta Neuropathol.* 2008;116(4):361–369.

18. Chung J, Kim BJ, Sohn CH, et al. Branch atheromatous plaque: a major cause of lacunar infarction (high-resolution MRI study). *Cerebrovasc Dis Extra.* 2012;2(1):36.

19. Caplan LR. Intracranial branch atheromatous disease: a neglected, understudied, and underused concept. *Neurology.* 1989;39(9):1246–1250.

20. Weiller C, Ringelstein EB, Reiche W, et al. The large striatocapsular infarct: a clinical and pathophysiological entity. *Arch Neurol.* 1990;47(10):1085–1091.

21. Donnan GA, Bladin PF, Berkovic SF, et al. The stroke syndrome of striatocapsular infarction. *Brain.* 1991;114(Pt 1A)(Pt 1A):51–70.

22. Bailey EL, Smith C, Sudlow CL, Wardlaw JM. Pathology of lacunar ischemic stroke in humans—a systematic review. *Brain Path.* 2012;22(5):583–591.

23. Ogata J. The arterial lesions underlying cerebral infarction. *Neuropathology.* 1999;19(1):112–118.

24. Challa, VR, Bell, MA, Moody, DM. A combined hematoxylin-eosin, alkaline phosphatase and high-resolution microradiographic study of lacunes. *Clin Neuropathol.* 1990;9(4):196–204

25. De Reuck J. The human periventricular arterial blood supply and the anatomy of cerebral infarctions. *Eur Neurol.* 1971;5(6):3213–34.

26. Folsom AR, Yatsuya H, Mosley TH, et al. Risk of intraparenchymal hemorrhage with magnetic resonance imaging—defined leukoaraiosis and brain infarcts. *Ann Neurol.* 2012;71(4):552–559.

27. Fernando MS, Simpson JE, Matthews F, et al. White matter lesions in an unselected cohort of the elderly: molecular pathology suggests origin from chronic hypoperfusion injury. *Stroke.* 2006;37(6):1391–1398.

28. Pantoni L, Garcia JH, Gutierrez JA. Cerebral white matter is highly vulnerable to ischemia. *Stroke.* 1996;27(9):1641–1647.

29. Nezu T, Yokota C, Uehara T, et al. Preserved acetazolamide reactivity in lacunar patients with severe white-matter lesions: 15O-labeled gas and H2O positron emission tomography studies. *J Cereb Blood Flow Metab.* 2012;32(5):844–850.

30. Wardlaw JM, Smith C, Dichgans M. Mechanisms of sporadic cerebral small vessel disease: Insights from neuroimaging. *Lancet Neurol.* 2013;12(5):483–497.

31. Wardlaw JM, Doubal F, Armitage P, et al. Lacunar stroke is associated with diffuse blood–brain barrier dysfunction. *Ann Neuro.l* 2009;65(2):194–202.

32. Wardlaw JM, Sandercock PA, Dennis MS, Starr J. Is breakdown of the blood-brain barrier responsible for lacunar stroke, leukoaraiosis, and dementia? *Stroke.* 2003;34(3): 806–812.

33. Grinberg LT, Thal DR. Vascular pathology in the aged human brain. *Acta Neuropathol.* 2010;119(3):277–290.

34. Igase M, Tabara Y, Igase K, et al. Asymptomatic cerebral microbleeds seen in healthy subjects have a strong association with asymptomatic lacunar infarction. *Circ J.* 2009;73(3):530–533.

35. Poels MM, Vernooij MW, Ikram MA, et al. Prevalence and risk factors of cerebral microbleeds: An update of the rotterdam scan study. *Stroke.* 2010;41(10 Suppl):S103-S106.

36. Akoudad S, Darweesh SK, Leening MJ, et al. Use of coumarin anticoagulants and cerebral microbleeds in the general population. *Stroke.* 2014;45(11):3436–3439.

37. Darweesh SK, Leening MJ, Akoudad S, et al. Clopidogrel use is associated with an increased prevalence of cerebral microbleeds in a stroke-free population: the Rotterdam study. *J Am Heart Assoc.* 2013;2(5):e000359.

38. Vernooij MW, Haag MD, van der Lugt A, et al. Use of antithrombotic drugs and the presence of cerebral microbleeds: the Rotterdam scan study. *Arch Neurol.* 2009;66(6): 714–720.

39. Greenberg SM, Vernooij MW, Cordonnier C, et al. Cerebral microbleeds: a guide to detection and interpretation. *Lancet Neurol.* 2009;8(2):165–174.

40. Yates PA, Villemagne VL, Ellis KA, et al. Cerebral microbleeds: a review of clinical, genetic, and neuroimaging associations. *Front Neurol.* 2013;4:205.

41. Qureshi AI, Tuhrim S, Broderick JP, et al. Spontaneous intracerebral hemorrhage. *N Eng J Med.* 2001;344(19):1450–1460.

42. Roob G, Lechner A, Schmidt R, et al. Frequency and location of microbleeds in patients with primary intracerebral hemorrhage. *Stroke.* 2000;31(11):2665266–9.

43. Charidimou A, Kakar P, Fox Z, Werring DJ. Cerebral microbleeds and recurrent stroke risk: systematic review and meta-analysis of prospective ischemic stroke and transient ischemic attack cohorts. *Stroke.* 2013;44(4):995–1001.

44. Salamon N. Neuroimaging of cerebral small vessel disease. *Brain Path.* 2014;24(5):519–524.

45. Kang CK, Park CA, Lee H, et al. Hypertension correlates with lenticulostriate arteries visualized by 7T magnetic resonance angiography. *Hypertension.* 2009;54(5):1050.

46. Kang CK, Park CW, Han JY, et al. Imaging and analysis of lenticulostriate arteries using 7.0—Tesla magnetic resonance angiography. *Magnetic Reson Med.* 2009;61(1):136.

47. Zwanenburg JJ, Hendrikse J, Takahara T, et al. MR angiography of the cerebral perforating arteries with magnetization prepared anatomical reference at 7T: comparison with time of flight. *J Magnetic Reson Imag.* 2008;28(6):1519.

48. Bae KT, Park SH, Moon CH, et al. Dual echo arteriovenography imaging with 7T MRI. *J Magnetic Reson Imag.* 2010;31(1):255.

49. Nelson RF, Pullicino P, Kendall BE, Marshall J. Computed tomography in patients presenting with lacunar syndromes. *Stroke.* 1980;11(3):256–261.

50. Donnan GA, Tress BM, Bladin PF. A prospective study of lacunar infarction using computerized tomography. *Neurology.* 1982;32(1):49–56.

51. Chamorro A, Sacco RL, Mohr JP, et al. Clinical-computed tomographic correlations of lacunar infarction in the stroke data bank. *Stroke.* 1991;22(2):175–181.

52. Wardlaw JM, Smith EE, Biessels GJ, et al. Neuroimaging standards for research into small vessel disease and its contribution to ageing and neurodegeneration. *Lancet Neurol.* 2013; 12(8):822–838.

53. Loos CM, Staals J, Wardlaw JM, van Oostenbrugge RJ. Cavitation of deep lacunar infarcts in patients with first-ever lacunar stroke: a 2-year follow-up study with MR. *Stroke.* 2012;43(8):2245–2247.

54. Moreau F, Patel S, Lauzon ML, et al. Cavitation after acute symptomatic lacunar stroke depends on time, location, and MRI sequence. *Stroke.* 2012;43(7):1837–1842.

55. Potter GM, Doubal FN, Jackson CA, et al. Counting cavitating lacunes underestimates the burden of lacunar infarction. *Stroke.* 2010;41(2):267–272.

56. Gerraty RP, Parsons MW, Barber PA, et al. Examining the lacunar hypothesis with diffusion and perfusion magnetic resonance imaging. *Stroke.* 2002;33(8):2019.

57. Franke CL, van Swieten JC, van Gijn J. Residual lesions on computed tomography after intracerebral hemorrhage. *Stroke.* 1991;22(12):1530–1533.

58. Hamedani AG, Rose KM, Peterlin BL, et al. Migraine and white matter hyperintensities: the ARIC MRI study. *Neurology.* 2013;81(15):1308–1313.

59. Dinia L, Bonzano L, Albano B, et al. White matter lesions progression in migraine with aura: a clinical and MRI longitudinal study. *J Neuroimag.* 2013;23(1):47–52.

60. Fisher CM. Lacunar strokes and infarcts: a review. *Neurology.* 1982;32(8):871–876.

61. Schonewille WJ, Tuhrim S, Singer MB, Atlas SW. Diffusion-weighted MRI in acute lacunar syndromes: a clinical-radiological correlation study. *Stroke.* 1999;30(10):2066.

62. Altmann M, Thommessen B, Rønning OM, et al. Diagnostic accuracy and risk factors of the different lacunar syndromes. *J Stroke Cerebrovasc Dis.* 2014;23(8):2085–2090.

63. Gan R, Sacco RL, Kargman DE, et al. Testing the validity of the lacunar hypothesis: the northern Manhattan stroke study experience. *Neurology.* 1997;48(5):1204–1211.

64. Donnan GA, O'Malley HM, Quang L, et al. The capsular warning syndrome pathogenesis and clinical features. *Neurology.* 1993;43(5):957.

65. Paul NL, Simoni M, Chandratheva A, Rothwell PM. Population-based study of capsular warning syndrome and prognosis after early recurrent TIA. *Neurology.* 2012;79(13): 1356–1362.

66. Arauz A, Patino-Rodriguez HM, Vargas-Gonzalez JC, et al. Clinical spectrum of artery of Percheron infarct: clinical-radiological correlations. *J Stroke Cerebrovasc Dis.* 2014;23(5):1083–1088. doi: 10.1016/j.jstrokecerebrovasdis.2013.09.011. Epub October 19, 2013.

67. Gorelick PB, Scuteri A, Black SE, et al. Vascular contributions to cognitive impairment and dementia: a statement for healthcare professionals from the American Heart Association/American Stroke Association. *Stroke.* 2011;42(9):2672–2713.

68. Jellinger KA. Pathology and pathogenesis of vascular cognitive impairment—a critical update. *Frontiers in Aging Neurosci.* 2013;5.

69. Caplan LR, Schoene WC. Clinical features of subcortical arteriosclerotic encephalopathy (Binswanger disease). *Neurology.* 1978;28(12):1206.

70. Babikian V, Ropper AH. Binswanger's disease: a review. *Stroke.* 1987;18(1):2–12.

71. Akiguchi I, Budka H, Shirakashi Y, et al. MRI features of Binswanger's disease predict prognosis and associated pathology. *Ann Clin Transl Neurol.* 2014;1(10):813–821.

72. Jauch EC, Saver JL, Adams HP Jr, et al. Guidelines for the early management of patients with acute ischemic stroke. *Stroke.* 2013;44(3):870–947.

73. Hacke W, Kaste M, Bluhmki E, et al. Thrombolysis with alteplase 3 to 4.5 hours after acute ischemic stroke. *N Engl J Med.* 2008;359(13):1317–1329.

74. National Institute of Neurological Disorders and Stroke r-tPA Stroke Study Group. Tissue plasminogen activator for acute ischemic stroke. *N Engl J Med.* 1995;333:1581–1587.

75. Hsia AW, Sachdev HS, Tomlinson J, et al. Efficacy of IV tissue plasminogen activator in acute stroke: does stroke subtype really matter? *Neurology.* 2003;61(1):71–75.

76. Melkas S, Putaala J, Oksala NK, et al. Small-vessel disease relates to poor poststroke survival in a 12-year follow-up. *Neurology.* 2011;76(8):734–739.

77. Jacova C, Pearce LA, Costello R, et al. Cognitive impairment in lacunar strokes: the SPS3 trial. *Ann Neurol.* 2012;72(3):351–362.

78. O'Brien TJ, Erkinjuntti T, Reisberg B, et al. Vascular cognitive impairment. *Lancet Neurol.* 2003;2(2):89–98.

79. Benavente OR, White CL, Pearce L, et al. The secondary prevention of small subcortical strokes (SPS3) study. *Int J Stroke.* 2011;6(2):164–175.

80. Kernan WN, Ovbiagele B, Black HR, et al. Guidelines for the prevention of stroke in patients with stroke and transient ischemic attack. *Stroke.* 2014;45(7):2160–2236.

81. Kwok CS, Shoamanesh A, Copley HC, et al. Efficacy of antiplatelet therapy in secondary prevention following lacunar stroke: pooled analysis of randomized trials. *Stroke.* 2015;46(4):1014–1023.

82. Benavente OR, Hart RG, SPS3 Investigators, et al. Effects of clopidogrel added to aspirin in patients with recent lacunar stroke. *N Engl J Med.* 2012;367(9):817–825.

83. Wang Y, Wang Y, Zhao X, et al. Clopidogrel with aspirin in acute minor stroke or transient ischemic attack. *N Engl J Med.* 2013;369:11–19.

84. Johnston SC, Easton JD, Farrant M, et al. Platelet-oriented inhibition in new TIA and minor ischemic stroke (POINT) trial: rationale and design. *Int J Stroke.* 2013;8(6): 479–483.

85. Stone NJ, et al. 2013 ACC/AHA guideline on the treatment of blood cholesterol to reduce atherosclerotic cardiovascular risk in adults. *Circulation.* 2013: https://doi.org/10.1161/01 .cir.0000437738.63853.7a.

86. Amarenco P, Labreuche J. Lipid management in the prevention of stroke: review and updated meta-analysis of statins for stroke prevention. *Lancet Neurol.* 2009;8(5):453–463.

87. Amarenco P, Goldstein LB, Szarek M, et al. Effects of intense low-density lipoprotein cholesterol reduction in patients with stroke or transient ischemic attack the stroke prevention by aggressive reduction in cholesterol levels (SPARCL) trial. *Stroke.* 2007;38(12):3198–3204.

88. Amarenco P, Benavente O, Goldstein LB, et al. Results of the stroke prevention by aggressive reduction in cholesterol levels (SPARCL) trial by stroke subtypes. *Stroke.* 2009;40(4): 1405–1409.

89. PROGRESS Collaborative Group. Randomised trial of a perindopril-based blood-pressure-lowering regimen among 6105 individuals with previous stroke or transient ischaemic attack. *Lancet Neurol.* 2001;358(9287):1033.

90. Diener HC, Sacco RL, Yusuf S, et al. Effects of aspirin plus extended-release dipyridamole versus clopidogrel and telmisartan on disability and cognitive function after recurrent stroke in patients with ischaemic stroke in the Prevention Regimen for Effectively Avoiding Second Strokes (PRoFESS) trial: a double-blind, active and placebo-controlled study. *Lancet Neurol.* 2008;7(10):875–884.

91. SPS3 Study Group. Blood-pressure targets in patients with recent lacunar stroke: the SPS3 randomised trial. *Lancet.* 2013;382(9891):507–515.

92. Hankey GJ. An optimum blood pressure target after lacunar stroke? *Lancet*. 2013; 382(9891):482–484.

93. Smith EE, Rosand J, Knudsen KA, et al. Leukoaraiosis is associated with warfarin-related hemorrhage following ischemic stroke. *Neurology*. 2002;59(2):193–197.

94. Neumann-Haefelin T, Hoelig S, Berkefeld J, et al. Leukoaraiosis is a risk factor for symptomatic intracerebral hemorrhage after thrombolysis for acute stroke. *Stroke*. 2006;37(10): 2463–2466.

95. Palumbo V, Boulanger JM, Hill MD, et al. Leukoaraiosis and intracerebral hemorrhage after thrombolysis in acute stroke. *Neurology*. 2007;68(13):1020–1024.

96. Demchuk AM, Khan F, Hill MD, et al. Importance of leukoaraiosis on CT for tissue plasminogen activator decision making: evaluation of the NINDS rt-PA stroke study. *Cerebrovasc Dis*. 2008;26(2):120–125.

97. Shoamanesh A, Kwok CS, Lim PA, Benavente OR. Postthrombolysis intracranial hemorrhage risk of cerebral microbleeds in acute stroke patients: a systematic review and meta-analysis. *Int J Stroke*. 2013;8(5):348–356.

98. Gregoire SM, Jager HR, Yousry TA, et al. Brain microbleeds as a potential risk factor for antiplatelet-related intracerebral haemorrhage: hospital-based, case-control study. *J Neurol Neurosurg Psychiatry*. 2010;81(6):679–684.

99. Lovelock CE, Cordonnier C, Naka H, et al. Antithrombotic drug use, cerebral microbleeds, and intracerebral hemorrhage: a systematic review of published and unpublished studies. *Stroke*. 2010;41(6):1222–1228.

Cryptogenic Stroke 15

James E. Siegler and Sheryl Martin-Schild

INTRODUCTION

Cryptogenic stroke is, at the same time, one of the most infuriating and most intriguing stroke etiologies encountered in the clinical and research setting. Although many definitions exist, for reasons of simplicity we will define *cryptogenic stroke* as an embolic cerebral infarction of unknown etiology that is larger than 1.5 cm at its widest dimension on neuroimaging.

To be classified as a cryptogenic stroke, each of the major etiologies of stroke must be evaluated for and excluded. A complete evaluation for stroke is recommended for any incident stroke, whether it be acute (less than 24 hours from symptom onset) or remote (greater than 2 weeks from symptom onset or unknown time of onset). By definition, the underlying pathogenesis of cryptogenic stroke remains unclear. That being said, in this chapter we explore the plausible mechanisms by which these strokes occur, recommendations for clinical evaluation, and the current management strategies. Some of the etiologies described here might more aptly be characterized as "other" as opposed to "cryptogenic." However, we have decided to include these etiologies in our discussion because they are sometimes missed or remain unclear during the initial evaluation for stroke.

The identification of cryptogenic stroke appears to be limited by two major forces: insufficient evaluation by the primary provider (e.g., abbreviated evaluation) and transient nature of the occult etiology, which prohibits detection (e.g., paroxysmal atrial fibrillation). Because the underlying etiology is not always identified, this raises a number of concerns for both the patient and the provider. There is no truly standardized guideline for evaluation. And there are no standardized treatments for cryptogenic stroke in which the etiology remains unclear. Therefore, patients and providers may be less compliant with aggressive management for this condition, which is otherwise associated with high rates of stroke recurrence and mortality.

EPIDEMIOLOGY

Cryptogenic stroke accounts for 30% of all strokes and is more common in younger patients. According to data from the Northern Manhattan study, more than half of stroke patients younger than 45 years experienced a cryptogenic infarct (55% vs. 42% in patients >45 years).[1] Data from this same group and others also show a higher predilection of cryptogenic strokes among blacks and Hispanics when compared to whites, although this finding is hardly conclusive because strokes of all subtypes are more common among these ethnic groups.[2,3] To date, there appears to be no gender predominance.[4] Compared to lacunar infarctions, cryptogenic strokes have been known to recur more frequently. As many as 3% of patients with cryptogenic stroke will experience a subsequent stroke within 30 days.[5] At 1 year, the risk of recurrent stroke rises to 30% for cryptogenic stroke patients as compared to 16% due to large-vessel disease, 15% due to cardioembolic disease, and 2% due to small-vessel disease, according to one cohort.[6] More recent data indicate the annual recurrence rate for cryptogenic stroke is lower than prior estimates, on the order of 3% to 6%.[7] From these data, it is reasonable to infer that, the mechanism of stroke being unknown, the secondary prevention of the underlying etiology is not sufficiently targeted by current medical management strategies. An underlying malignancy may persist for months after an initial cerebrovascular insult, and a patient with paroxysmal atrial fibrillation (PAF) could experience a second stroke years later if not appropriately anticoagulated. Therefore, it is critical to attempt a thorough evaluation of these patients for the occult, but often identifiable, etiologies of primary stroke.

EVALUATION AND TREATMENT

Initial Evaluation

Recommended evaluation for acute stroke is discussed in other chapters but the salient elements are repeated here.[8] Cardiogenic causes of stroke (e.g., atrial fibrillation, mural thrombus, myocardial infarction) should be ruled out by laboratory testing for troponin and/or CKMB with an initial electrocardiogram (EKG), in-hospital telemetry for a minimum of 24 hours, and a transthoracic echocardiogram (TTE). If a cardiogenic source is suspected in spite of negative testing using the preceding modalities, a transesophageal echocardiogram (TEE) should be performed. With this study, one has the option to intravenously infuse agitated saline ("bubble" study) and/or intravenous contrast to increase the sensitivity for detecting an apical thrombus. The use of a TEE is superior to TTE alone for detecting a possible right–to–left shunt, as in the case of a patent foramen ovale (PFO) or atrial septal defect or in the case of a small thrombus of the left atrium due to anatomic proximity of this chamber to the esophagus. It should be noted that the presence of microbubbles in the left atrium or ventricle after agitated saline injection does not always indicate the presence of an intracardiac shunt because pulmonary arteriovenous malformations may also produce this phenomenon. After the acute hospitalization, selected patients may be further evaluated for cardioembolic causes of their cryptogenic stroke. Prospective trials have demonstrated a high prevalence of PAF,[9] and outpatient telemetry is increasingly used to detect these clinically significant events.

Large-vessel disease is typically excluded using ultrasonic imaging with carotid Doppler (specifically for anterior circulation infarctions) and transcranial Doppler (better for posterior circulation infarctions) or with computed tomographic angiography (CTA) or magnetic resonance angiography (MRA) of the head and neck. Both CTA and MRA have sufficient sensitivity and specificity when compared to the gold standard of cerebral angiography for large- and small-vessel cerebrovascular disease.[10] CTA may be more rapidly acquired in the emergency room than MRA; however, it comes with multiple risks, including radiation exposure and acute kidney injury. The provider must certainly consider the patient's allergy status (especially an allergy to iodine) and renal function when deciding between these latter two modalities, particularly given the higher risk of acute kidney injury and chronic kidney disease witnessed among stroke patients. This risk is not shared by MRA when contrast (gadolinium) is avoided. However, in the presence of severe renal insufficiency, intravenous gadolinium may precipitate a rare reaction called nephrogenic systemic fibrosis—a fibroblastic proliferation with resultant deposition of collagen and connective tissue within the heart, lungs, liver, and skin.

Parent vessel disease of small vessel infarction is evaluated with the use of CTA, MRA, or conventional cerebral angiography. More commonly, patients with small-vessel strokes present with a history of hypertension, diabetes, dyslipidemia, or tobacco use. For this reason, hemoglobin A1c and a lipid panel should be checked. In obese patients or patients with appropriate clinical history, a polysomnogram should be performed in order to evaluate for obstructive sleep apnea, which also carries a high risk of small-vessel ischemic disease. Tobacco cessation counseling should also be provided where appropriate.

One challenge encountered by physicians during stroke evaluation is the identification of small degrees of stenosis or mild plaque formation.[11] Because these vascular changes are detected *after* the ischemic event, these seemingly inconsequential elements may represent *prior* plaque burden or instability and could easily have caused the stroke during an episode of plaque disruption. Unfortunately, there is no way of knowing this unless previous vessel imaging (before the index event) was obtained.

Once cardioembolic, large-vessel atherothrombotic disease and small-vessel ischemia are sufficiently excluded, the remaining 30% of stroke patients are classified as having experienced cryptogenic strokes. At this point, the patient and family medical and social histories, laboratory data, and advanced neuroimaging rise in importance. See Figure 15.1 for a summary of the most common risk factors associated with cryptogenic stroke.

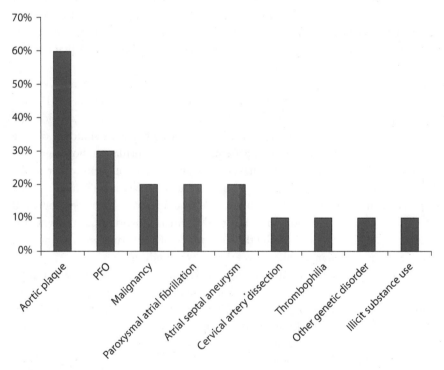

FIGURE 15.1 Estimated prevalence of cryptogenic stroke risk factors among all stroke patients

Paroxysmal Atrial Fibrillation

Possibly representing the most common etiology of cryptogenic stroke, paroxysmal atrial fibrillation may account for up to 20% of cryptogenic sources of embolism. Indeed, PAF is known to be more common than *persistent* atrial fibrillation; however, both have been associated with cerebral embolism. The identification of PAF is one of the principal reasons for performing inpatient telemetry monitoring for all patients who suffer from stroke. Many centers also pursue outpatient telemetry monitoring using portable devices, such as the Holter monitor, which may detect PAF in 10% to 15% of patients with cryptogenic stroke. As can be expected, there is a logarithmic relationship between PAF detection and duration of outpatient monitoring. Unfortunately, compliance with portable devices remains suboptimal, with up to one-third of total days with the device going unmonitored and one in four patients being fully noncompliant with these devices. For these reasons, a number of centers are diverting their outpatient monitoring practices toward implantable devices, which are more sensitive for detecting PAF 6 to 12 months after the initial ischemic event. The rate of detecting PAF continues to increase between 6 and 12 months (from 8.9% to 12.4% according to the CRYSTAL AF study group),[12] which argues for the use of such devices; however, this may not be economically feasible for most patients, and the cost-effectiveness of this practice has not been investigated.

The detection of PAF during outpatient telemetry monitoring warrants therapeutic anticoagulation and rhythm control using Class Ia, Ic, or III antiarrhythmic agents, with or without the use of atrioventricular nodal blocking agents.[13] Vitamin K antagonists (VKAs) have long been the standard of care for therapeutic anticoagulation in patients with atrial fibrillation; however, they require routine monitoring and have numerous interactions with other medications.[8] Newer anticoagulant classes such as the direct factor Xa inhibitors (e.g., apixaban) and direct thrombin inhibitors (e.g., dabigatran) have been approved for use in patients with non-valvular atrial fibrillation who suffer stroke. Clinical trial data have demonstrated the superiority of apixaban[14] and dabigatran[15] to VKAs in secondary stroke prevention for this indication.

According to recent data by Granger et al, apixaban has been shown to have superior efficacy for preventing recurrent ischemic events in non-valvular atrial fibrillation (hazard ratio [HR] 0.79, 95% confidence interval [CI] 0.66–0.95, $p < 0.001$ for noninferiority, $p = 0.01$ for superiority), while also associated with lower risk of major bleeding compared to VKAs (HR 0.69, 95% CI 0.60 to 0.80, $p < 0.001$).[14] One benefit of these newer oral anticoagulants is that there is no need for level monitoring. However, unlike VKAs, there is no known reversal agent for apixaban. (Dabigatran can now be effectively reversed using the monoclonal antibody, idaracizumab.) And with the exception of rivar-oxaban, which is dosed once daily with the largest meal, both apixaban and dabigatran are dosed twice daily. Intravenous or subcutaneous therapies are currently not recommended for routine outpatient use in non-valvular atrial fibrillation.

Among patients who are unable to tolerate anticoagulation therapy for non-valvular atrial fibrillation, left atrial appendage closure using the WATCHMAN device can be considered.[16]

Hypercoagulable State

A hypercoagulable state should be suspected in young patients with stroke, and in patients who have a family history of deep vein thrombosis; early stroke or myocardial infarction; pulmonary embolism; chronic thromboembolic pulmonary arterial hypertension; or, in the case of females, miscarriage or infertility. Hypercoagulable states can be divided into those that can be inherited or acquired. The known heritable hypercoagulable states can be assessed serologically. Antiphospholipid antibody syndrome (APLAS) is identified by the presence of antibodies to cardiolipin, beta2 glycoprotein, phosphatidylserine, or an elevated dilute russell viper venom assay. Mutations in factor V Leiden, prothrombin gene, MTHFR gene, as well as deficient protein C or S levels and elevated factor VIII activity also carry an increased risk of thromboembolic events, including stroke (Figure 15.2).[17]

The acquired hypercoagulable states, for the most part, include pregnancy (particularly third trimester) and malignancy. The risk of stroke appears greatest during the postpartum period,[18–20] but there may also be significant risk during the third trimester, with up to 26 per 100,000 deliveries complicated by cerebrovascular disease.[20–23] In epidemiologic series, malignancy has been identified as a causative agent in approximately 1 of every 1,000 ischemic strokes, with some data suggesting as many as one in five cryptogenic stroke patients have an underlying malignancy.[24] Unfortunately, as the lifespan of the world population continues to rise, the incidence of strokes and malignancy are likely to increase. Cancer is associated with ischemic stroke for two major reasons: (a) the intrinsic factors inherent to the cancer themselves and (b) the treatment of these cancers. Certain malignancies—namely, those of adenocarcinomatous origin—are infamous for producing procoagulant substances such as mucin and tissue factor. These products have been demonstrated to activate factors VII and X of the coagulation cascade, thereby inducing embolic events.[25] Two sensitive measures in the evaluation of cryptogenic malignancies include the serum D-dimer level and a multi-infarct pattern on neuroimaging.[24,26] Other tumor markers (e.g., carcinoembryonic antigen, CA 19-9) may also be tested, but there is no

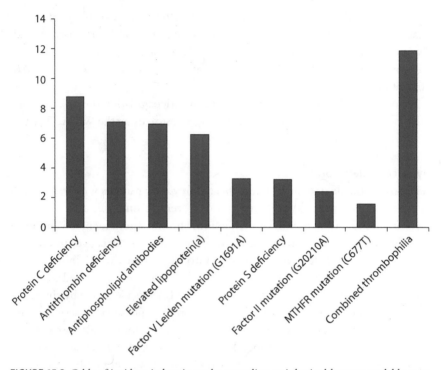

FIGURE 15.2 Odds of incident ischemic stroke according to inherited hypercoagulable state in children

Source: Data adapted from Reference 17.

recommended biomarker panel for the evaluation of suspected malignancy in cryptogenic stroke.[8] Typically, the provider will proceed with full-body imaging, either via positron emission tomography (PET) or computed tomographic (CT) imaging of the chest, abdomen, and pelvis.[24]

In patients actively undergoing chemotherapy, the risk of stroke increases depending on the pharmacologic regimen. In one study of 10,963 patients by Li et al, platinum-based regimens carried the highest risk of chemotherapy-associated stroke.[27] However, it is unclear whether these strokes were due to the malignancy itself or the treatment. One can also imagine the side effects of the chemotherapeutic to have directly toxic effects on the cardiovascular system and, therefore, produce a stroke in such manner. For instance, anthracycline-derived regimens produce a dose-related cardiomyopathy, which can produce embolic events via atrial fibrillation or impaired atrial or ventricular contraction.

Cancer thought to be in remission is highly problematic to the clinician. This is aggravated by cases in which the patient may also have undergone whole-brain radiation for prior intracranial metastases, which can produce a vasculopathy with a high risk of subsequent stroke.[28] It is not always clear whether the new cryptogenic event is related to a hypercoagulable state in the setting of an indolent primary cancer, a hypercoagulable state in the setting of a secondary malignancy, or it is related to prior chemotherapy-associated cardio- and cerebrovascular changes. Low-molecular weight heparin, dosed twice daily, is the preferred treatment modality for secondary prevention of malignancy-associated ischemic stroke[29] and may be an appropriate secondary prevention strategy in selected pregnant patients if no other causative process is identified.

Cervical Artery Dissection

In patients who present with concurrent neck pain or have recently sustained neck manipulation or injury, the diagnosis of cervical artery dissection (CAD) should be suspected. CAD is a relatively rare condition, occurring among 2.6 per 100,000 people, and is more common in younger patients with stroke (mean age 45 years).[30] Despite its low overall incidence in the total stroke population, CAD accounts for as many as one in four strokes among younger patients.[31] Risk factors for CAD include extrinsic factors such as recent infection, aortic root dilation, migraine, and hyperhomocystinemia, as well as genetic factors such as Ehlers-Danlos syndrome, Marfan syndrome, fibromuscular dysplasia, and mutation in the 5,10-methyltetrahydrofolate reductase gene (MTHFR 677TT genotype).[30, 32] From a pathophysiologic perspective, CAD occurs when traumatic forces disrupt the arterial wall intima and media, allowing arterial blood to fill the newly created intra-luminal space. It takes place more frequently in the carotid artery, usually within 2 cm of the internal carotid artery bifurcation, although vertebral dissections also occur. Stroke may ensue in as few as several minutes or up to weeks later via thrombus formation within the intra-luminal space. Pathophysiologically, the blood that fills this space eventually stagnates, and the exposed subendothelial factors promote platelet adhesion and thrombus formation.

Carotid and vertebral artery dissection can be identified using head and neck CTA or MRA with a T_1-weighted axial fat-saturation sequence. MRA of the head and neck is often considered a superior imaging modality to CTA because the fat-saturation sequence permits optimal characterization of the vessel wall compared to CTA, which is largely limited to depicting intraluminal pathology. In contrast, a CTA should be used in patients with suspected vessel calcification and plaque disruption, which is hyperintense on CT imaging and less well characterized on MRA. CTA is also preferred in some cases where vertebral disease is suspected because it has higher resolution than MRA when evaluating these smaller posterior vessels.[33] Finally, in cases where the patient is agitated or delirious and cannot remain stationary, CTA may be superior to MRA due to its more rapid completion time. Clearly, each has its own advantages, and it is up to the judgment of the clinician to determine the appropriate imaging modality. If imaged using MRA or CTA within the first few days of the dissection, one should see the characteristic hyperintense "crescent sign" reflecting the false lumen of the cervical vessel.[33] Carotid duplex ultrasonography may also be performed, but it carries a lower sensitivity for detecting CAD than the aforementioned modalities.

Regarding CAD management, no consensus has been reached by expert opinion regarding the use of anticoagulation or antiplatelet therapy during the acute or chronic phase of the illness.[30] Current data from nonrandomized trials suggest no difference in death or disability between patients who receive either treatment, and the most recent phase II feasibility trial (Cervical Artery Dissection in Stroke Study) failed to detect a clinically meaningful benefit of anticoagulation over antiplatelet therapy for secondary stroke prevention.[34] Regarding alternative interventions, endovascular therapy is not routinely recommended for CAD but may be considered in cases of CAD recurrence. In my experience when treating patients with idiopathic or traumatic CAD, we typically use antiplatelet therapy the acute setting (less than 1–2 weeks) to prevent stroke progression or recurrence. This can be followed by a short course of therapeutic anticoagulation (less than 3 months) once the stroke has completed and the risk of subsequent intracranial hemorrhage is sufficiently low. Antiplatelet therapy is resumed indefinitely thereafter, pending no contraindications (e.g., recent gastrointestinal bleed, thrombocytopenia, etc.). Again, this course of treatment may be appropriate for idiopathic or traumatic CAD that is complicated by cerebral ischemia, but it certainly is not recommended for routine management of all patients with CAD and stroke.

Patent Foramen Ovale

The concept that a patent foramen ovale (PFO) may contribute to ischemic cerebral events has gained much attention in recent years. PFO is certainly not uncommon in the general population and has been reported in up to one in four healthy persons.[35] Theoretically, two mechanisms for associated stroke are possible with a PFO. First, it can be thought that thrombotic debris from a deep vein thrombosis embolizes from a distal extremity to the right atrium where it is diverted across an interatrial shunt (often a PFO) into the systemic arterial circulation to produce an ischemic infarction. This is supported by observational data demonstrating a high prevalence of deep vein thrombosis in stroke patients with PFO.[36] Second, a PFO may create a small nidus for clot formation on the left side of the heart that also has the potential to systemically embolize.

One meta-analysis has demonstrated a nearly two times greater risk of PFO in stroke patients when compared to healthy controls. This risk was greater among patients with cryptogenic infarctions (Odds ratio [OR] 3.16, 95% CI 2.30–4.35) and younger patients with stroke (OR 6.00, 95% CI 3.72–9.68).[37] In this meta-analysis, the prevalence of PFO among stroke patients was double that of the non-stroke controls (32% vs. 16%).

Until recently, PFO closure was not found to reduce the likelihood of a recurrent ischemic stroke in patients without an alternative source of embolism. Three major trials published in the *New England Journal of Medicine* in 2013 demonstrated no reduction in recurrent stroke risk or 30-day mortality after PFO closure when compared to standard medical management.[38–40] This was followed by three clinical trials whose results were published in 2017 demonstrating superiority of PFO closure in secondary stroke prevention.[41–43] In the RESPECT trial (Randomized Evaluation of Recurrent Stroke Comparing PFO Closure to Established Current Standard of Care Treatment), PFO closure with the Amplatzer Occluder followed by short-term (6 months) antiplatelet therapy was superior to medical management alone for secondary stroke prevention (HR 0.55, 95% CI 0.31–0.999, p = 0.04).[42] Similarly, the Gore REDUCE demonstrated a significant reduction in clinical and radiographic infarctions among patients whose PFOs were closed using the Helex Septal Occluder or Cardioform Septal Occluder when compared to those whose PFOs were not. Both groups received antiplatelet therapy.[43] Finally, the CLOSE investigators (Patent Foramen Ovale Closure or Anticoagulants versus Antiplatelet Therapy to Prevent Stroke Recurrence) also found a lower rate of recurrent ischemic strokes in patients who underwent closure using any approved device (HR 0.03, 95% CI 0.00–0.26, P < 0.001).[41] Importantly, patients in these trials were specifically selected for enrollment if no alternative etiology of stroke was identified. Therefore, PFO closure would not be recommended in the routine care of stroke patients when an alternative mechanism is suspected.

Cardiac Wall Motion Abnormalities

The fact that structural changes in the heart contribute to embolic strokes is not unusual. Besides atrial fibrillation and PFO, we also know that apical wall hypokinesis is particularly thrombogenic and may benefit from therapeutic anticoagulation for secondary stroke prevention.[44]

Recently, data have suggested specific anatomical abnormalities in the left atrium may contribute to cryptogenic stroke. Left atrial size and morphology have been demonstrated to correlate with PAF and stroke or transient ischemic attack (TIA) independently of other cardiovascular risk factors.[45,46] Certain morphologic variants of the left atrium are found in higher frequency in patients with cryptogenic stroke (e.g., cauliflower, windsock, and cactus variants more so than the chicken wing variant).[47] Atrial septal aneurysm, found in as many as 15% to 20% of patients with stroke who undergo TEE,[48,49] also confers eight-fold higher odds of thromboembolic stroke and should be treated with anticoagulation.[50]

Atrial cardiopathy[51] is also being specifically evaluated in the ongoing ARCADIA randomized clinical trial (Atrial Cardiopathy and Antithrombotic Drugs in Prevention after Cryptogenic Stroke, NCT03192215). To meet criteria for inclusion in this multi-center double-blind, double-dummy trial— among other criteria—the patient must demonstrate evidence of atrial cardiopathy defined as a serum N-terminal brain natriuretic peptide level >250 pg/mL, left atrial size >3 cm/mL^2, or a p-wave terminal force >5000 μV*ms on electrocardiography. Any of these metrics are presumably related to atrial systolic dysfunction and could be potentially thrombogenic even in the absence of atrial fibrillation.

Atheromatous Aortic Disease

Atherosclerotic disease of the aortic arch is associated with a high risk of ischemic stroke. This risk increases with plaque sizes >1 mm in diameter and is greatest after 4 mm[52] and with ulcerative morphology.[53] According to one clinical trial, ulcerated plaques are far more frequently seen among patients with an unclear etiology of stroke when compared to patients with a known stroke etiology (61% vs. 22%, $p < 0.001$).[54] Transesophageal echocardiogram remains the preferred imaging modality for detection of this abnormality. Unfortunately, due to the high prevalence of aortic arch atheromatous disease, it is unclear whether the stroke is due to an ulcerated or thromboembolic plaque or if the stroke is due to yet another underlying cryptogenic etiology. It remains technically challenging to causally relate aortic arch disease with ischemic stroke.

HMG-coA reductase inhibitors ("statins") promote plaque stabilization and regression in patients with aortic atheromas.[55] In combination with antiplatelet therapy for secondary prevention, statins remain the gold standard of treatment for patients with stroke likely related to aortic atherosclerotic disease. Although some investigators have identified a relationship between larger aortic plaques and hypercoaguability[56] and early data suggested benefit of oral anticoagulation in secondary stroke prevention,[57,58] recent trials have failed to show superiority of VKA over aspirin.[53] Furthermore, guidelines do not recommend the routine surgical removal of aortic plaque or stenting,[8] although this may be considered in young patients without aortic calcification or in extreme cases.[59]

Substance Abuse

Besides tobacco and alcohol use, other substances are associated with a greater risk of stroke. As many as 10% of strokes may be related in part to illicit substance use.[60] Published data have demonstrated a six-fold greater risk of stroke among drug abusers, even after adjusting for known stroke risk factors. Furthermore, this risk increases to nearly 50-fold for patients whose symptoms began within 6 hours of drug use.[61] A urine toxin screen should be performed on patients suspected of substance abuse as well as any young patient with cryptogenic stroke.

Cocaine is the most common of the illicit substances associated with ischemic stroke. It may produce stroke in a myriad of ways, ranging from intracranial vasculitis to thromboembolism secondary to cocaine-associated cardiomyopathy. From a pathophysiologic perspective, there appears to be a dose-dependent cerebral vasoconstriction response to cocaine administration, and these effects are known to accumulate over time.[62] In one epidemiologic series of more than 3 million patients, cocaine was associated with a two-fold risk of both ischemic and hemorrhagic infarctions, with a high rate of mortality.[63] Traditionally, it is thought that acute cocaine use may cause a rapid escalation in blood pressure and vasospasm due to its short half-life; however, cocaine metabolites may continue to produce cerebrovascular effects for several days after use.[64]

Amphetamines are also associated with ischemic stroke and intracranial hemorrhage,[65,66] although some studies have been unable to replicate the association with stroke.[63] The sequelae of ischemic stroke may be due to amphetamine-related hypertension, vasoconstriction, and/or vasculitis, as in the case of cocaine abuse.[65,66] Other recreational stimulants, such as ephedrine and phencyclidine, may also contribute to similar pathophysiologic changes and result in stroke.

The direct effect of opioids has not been related to ischemic stroke. However, the intravenous administration of opioids has been causally related to the development of infectious endocarditis and subsequent cerebral embolism.[60] Opioid effects on respiratory drive have been increasingly implicated result in profound systemic hypoxia, with or without cardiac arrest, and anoxic brain injury.

Marijuana use has been associated with a nearly two-fold risk of ischemic stroke after adjusting for other stroke risk factors,[61] although its mechanism remains unclear.[65] Lysergic acid diethylamide (LSD) is a known vasoconstrictor that has been related to strokes secondary to carotid vasoconstriction.[67,68] However, stroke due to LSD is exquisitely uncommon. Performance-enhancers may also be suspected in certain cryptogenic stroke populations, but this is also rare.[65]

Other Genetic Disorders

Given appropriate past medical and family history, certain genetic causes other than hypercoagulability should be considered. Sickle-cell disease remains the number-one cause of stroke in children. One in four patients with homozygous mutation for hemoglobin S will experience stroke by the age of 45 (1 in 10 for heterozygotes).[69] Sickle-cell disease is known for producing a variety of stroke syndromes ranging from large- and small-vessel strokes, to moyamoya syndrome, to silent infarcts.[70] Screening for patients at high risk of stroke can be performed using transcranial Doppler. In patients with sickle cell, stroke is best prevented and treated with exchange transfusions[71] although many patients will go on to experience recurrent strokes. For patients with moyamoya syndrome, recurrent stroke may be prevented via pial synangiosis.[72]

Cerebral autosomal dominant arteriopathy with subcortical infarcts and leukoencephalopathy (CADASIL) is a rare, autosomal dominant cause of small-vessel stroke in the young.[73] It should be considered in young- to middle-aged patients who have a history of migraines, prior small-vessel strokes, and widespread leukoaraiosis on neuroimaging. CADASIL has no proven treatment.

Fabry disease, an X-linked lysosomal storage disorder, is an uncommon cause of stroke among young patients. In one large series, 4.9% of men and 2.5% of women younger than 55 with cryptogenic stroke carried the mutation.[74] The mean age of stroke onset was between 38 and 40 years. Because of its relatively high prevalence (authors estimate 1.2% of young stroke patients), it should be screened for in young patients with cerebral infarction and multi-organ dysfunction, especially cardiomyopathy and proteinuria.[74] Fabry disease is successfully treated with enzyme replacement therapy. Secondary stroke prevention is dependent on the etiology of stroke (e.g., cardioembolic due to cardiomyopathy vs. small-vessel vasculopathy).

Homocystinuria is a syndrome consisting of many autosomal recessive enzyme deficiencies. Stroke occurs not uncommonly in children with these conditions, and it should be excluded in any child with stroke, static encephalopathy, and Marfanoid skeletal composition.[70] Half of patients improve with pyridoxine supplementation, but this does not independently correlate with neurologic prognosis.[75]

Mitochondrial myopathy, encephalopathy, lactic acidosis, and stroke-like episodes (MELAS) is a maternally inherited disorder characterized by developmental delay, sensorineural hearing loss, short stature, seizures, migraines, and cognitive decline secondary to stroke-like lesions in the central nervous system. It should be suspected in any young patient with strokes, particularly if the strokes are distributed cortically and if they change in size over time.

MELAS can be diagnosed by muscle biopsy or mitochondrial mutation analysis.[70]

Connective tissue disorders such as Marfan's syndrome and Ehlers–Danlos type IV can cause ischemic stroke via arterial dissection, but this is likely to be detected on intra- and extracranial vessel imaging. These syndromes should be suspected in stroke patients with pectus carinatum or excavatum, scoliosis, or aortic dissection and easy bruising or joint flexibility, respectively.[70] Marfan's syndrome is transmitted in an autosomal dominant pattern between parents and offspring due to mutation in the fibrillin 1 protein, and cerebral ischemia is traditionally the sequelae of prosthetic heart valves, mitral valve prolapse, and atrial fibrillation, rather than aortic dissection.[76] Ehlers-Danlos is similarly transmitted in autosomal dominant fashion, but it describes the phenotype associated with a defect in collagen III. In contrast to Marfan's, stroke in Ehlers-Danlos syndrome occurs in the setting of arterial dissection, but intracranial hemorrhage may also occur following ruptured cerebral aneurysms or large vessels.[77,78] Other heritable connective tissue disorders that have been associated with ischemic stroke include osteogenesis imperfecta and pseudoxanthoma elasticum.[70,78] These deserve evaluation in the appropriate clinical context.

FUTURE DIRECTIONS

The future of cryptogenic stroke lies more in etiologic determination than in treatment randomization. Several ongoing trials are investigating the efficacy of long-term cardiac event monitoring (clinical trials NCT02216370, NCT01025947).[79,80] The EMBRACE (Event Monitor Belt for Recording Atrial Fibrillation after a Cerebral Ischemic Event) investigators have described a doubled rate of anticoagulation initiation in patients with long-term cardiac rhythm monitoring, with presumable improvement in clinical outcomes.[81] In the search for PAF, the SECRETO (Searching for Explanations for Cryptogenic Stroke in the Young: Revealing the Etiology, Triggers, and Outcome) study consortium is a Finnish study group performing a 10-year observational case-control study of young cryptogenic stroke patients aged 18 to 49 years. Their primary outcome measures include composite thrombotic event and new-onset atrial fibrillation (NCT01934725). In spite of these trials, there are no trials to the authors' knowledge that intend to evaluate the optimum duration of outpatient cardiac monitoring. According to results of the SURPRISE trial, Christensen et al describe a mean of 109 days (SD ± 48) before the first episode of PAF is detected,[82] findings similar to the REVEAL AF study (median time to PAF detection 123 days using implantable monitor).[83] Therefore, to capture at least 95% of PAF events in cryptogenic patients, monitoring should persist for more than 200 days. At present, short-term outpatient cardiac event monitoring appears to be cost effective,[84] but 200 days of either an external or implantable event monitor has not been assessed in a cost-benefit analysis.

The Biomarkers of Acute Stroke Etiology (BASE) collaboration is sequencing serum RNA samples from the peripheral blood of patients with stroke in order to identify associated genetic biomarkers with stroke etiology (NCT02014896). It is expected that some of these markers may be more indicative of cardioembolic sources of stroke because they may relate to left atrial strain and thrombus formation—potentially less invasive and more sensitive than left atrial dilation, which remains a poor clinical marker suggestive of cardioembolic disease.[9]

Anticoagulation for secondary stroke prevention in patients with cryptogenic stroke has not been shown to be superior to antiplatelet therapy at this time, although clinical trials are ongoing. The recently concluded prospective, randomized, multi-center NAVIGATE-ESUS trial (New Approach riVaroxaban Inhibition of Factor Xa in a Global trial versus Aspirin to prevenT Embolism in Embolic Stroke of Undetermined Source), comparing standard dose rivaroxaban versus aspirin, failed to prove superiority of anticoagulation over aspirin. (Unpublished data) The ongoing RE-SPECT-ESUS (Randomized, Double-Blind, Evaluation in Secondary Stroke Prevention Comparing the EfficaCy and Safety of Oral Thrombin Inhibitor Dabigatran Etexilate Versus Acetylsalicylic Acid, NCT02239120) and ARCADIA trials (previously described) should provide us with additional insight into the possible benefit of anticoagulation for secondary stroke prevention in this at-risk population.

CONCLUSIONS

Cryptogenic stroke accounts for up to one-third of all stroke etiologies. At present, there are no evidence-based guidelines for the evaluation of cryptogenic stroke, leaving these decisions to the judgment of the treating clinician. Often, the etiology of stroke remains unclear due to incomplete evaluation or due to the transient nature of its pathogenesis. However, in many instances, the etiology of cryptogenic stroke can be determined after integration of a thorough medical history with laboratory and imaging studies, as well as protracted outpatient cardiac monitoring. The author's recommendations are seen in Figure 15.3. Patients with cryptogenic stroke have a non-trivial rate of recurrence when compared to other major stroke etiologies. Furthermore, possibly due to a higher likelihood of inadequate secondary stroke prevention, these patients may be at greater risk of poorer outcomes when compared to patients with other stroke mechanisms.[85,86]

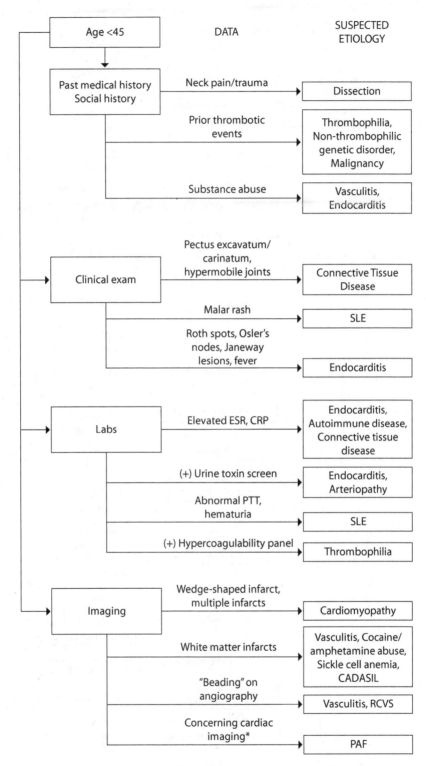

FIGURE 15.3 Recommendations for diagnostic evaluation of cryptogenic stroke

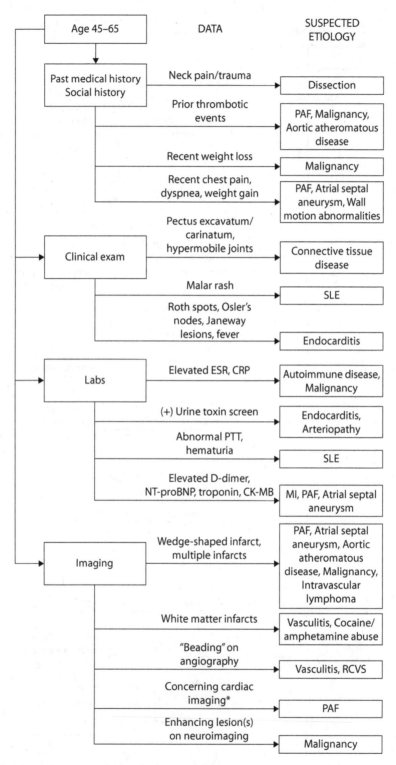

FIGURE 15.3 Recommendations for diagnostic evaluation of cryptogenic stroke (*continued*)

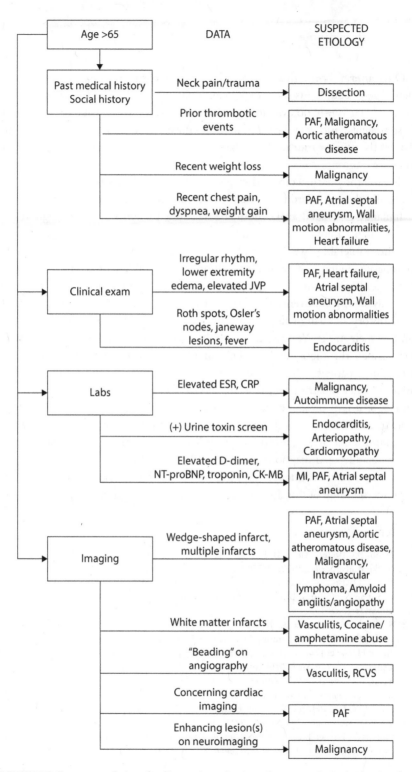

FIGURE 15.3 Recommendations for diagnostic evaluation of cryptogenic stroke (*continued*)

RCVS, reversible cerebral vasoconstriction syndrome; *Concerning cardiac imaging includes left atrial enlargement,[86] left ventricular wall thickness,[86] *p*-wave maximum (height),[87] and *p*-wave dispersion (width).[88]

Only after a thorough evaluation has been performed to exclude the afore-mentioned occult causes of stroke can a patient be classified as cryptogenic. There are currently no available guidelines for secondary stroke prevention in these patients, and data have not proven efficacy of anticoagulation over anti-platelet therapy for routine secondary prevention. Additional phase III clinical trials are ongoing.

Because the pharmacologic therapies used in secondary stroke prevention can drastically change according to the identification of an occult cause of stroke (e.g., malignancy-associated stroke should be treated with low-molecular weight hepa-rin, and non-valvular PAF should be optimally treated with a novel oral antico-agulant, if tolerable), we have made several recommendations here regarding an appropriate sequence of evaluation techniques. Patients at a moderate risk of PAF should undergo extended outpatient telemetry to identify these infrequent but clinically significant events. Older patients or those with a strong family or per-sonal history of malignancy should be appropriately evaluated for cancer as a cause of their stroke. Young patients or those with a personal or family history of unexplained thromboembolic events should be screened for hypercoagulable state. Those patients who fit phenotypic profiles for autoimmune, collagen vas-cular, or other inflammatory diseases should also undergo additional evaluation because many of these are treated dramatically differently (e.g., prednisone for acute giant cell arteritis or disease-modifying therapeutics for systemic lupus ery-thematosus). Ultimately, it is up to the judgment of the treating clinician to pur-sue these additional diagnostic tests. Trials investigating the optimal diagnostic and therapeutic modalities for cryptogenic stroke should continue to illuminate our understanding of this diverse and perplexing patient population.

References

1. Jacobs BS, Boden-Albala B, Lin IF, et al. Stroke in the young in the northern manhattan stroke study. *Stroke*. 2002;33:2789–2793.
2. White H, Boden-Albala B, Wang C, Elkind MS, et al. Ischemic stroke subtype inci-dence among whites, blacks, and hispanics: The northern manhattan study. *Circulation*. 2005;111:1327–1331.
3. Schneider AT, Kissela B, Woo D, et al. Ischemic stroke subtypes: a population-based study of incidence rates among blacks and whites. *Stroke*. 2004;35:1552–1556.
4. Amin H, Greer DM. Cryptogenic stroke-the appropriate diagnostic evaluation. *Cur Treat Options Cardiovasc Med*. 2014;16:280.
5. Sacco RL, Foulkes MA, Mohr JP, et al. Determinants of early recurrence of cerebral infarction. The stroke data bank. *Stroke*. 1989;20:983–989.
6. Bang OY, Lee PH, Joo SY, et al. Frequency and mechanisms of stroke recurrence after cryptogenic stroke. *Ann Neurol*. 2003;54:227–234.
7. Hart RG, Diener HC, Coutts SB, et al. Embolic strokes of undetermined source: the case for a new clinical construct. *Lancet. Neurol*. 2014;13:429–438.

8. Jauch EC, Saver JL, Adams HP, Jr., et al. Guidelines for the early management of patients with acute ischemic stroke: a guideline for healthcare professionals from the American Heart Association/American Stroke Association. *Stroke.* 2013;44:870–947.

9. Tayal AH, Tian M, Kelly KM, et al. Atrial fibrillation detected by mobile cardiac outpatient telemetry in cryptogenic tia or stroke. *Neurology.* 2008;71:1696–1701.

10. Latchaw RE, Alberts MJ, Lev MH, et al. Recommendations for imaging of acute ischemic stroke: A scientific statement from the American Heart Association. *Stroke.* 2009; 40:3646–3678.

11. Coutinho JM, Derkatch S, Potvin AR, et al. Nonstenotic carotid plaque on ct angiography in patients with cryptogenic stroke. *Neurology.* 2016;87:665–672.

12. Sanna T, Diener HC, Passman RS, et al. Cryptogenic stroke and underlying atrial fibrillation. *New Engl J Med.* 2014;370:2478–2486.

13. Tsadok MA, Jackevicius CA, Essebag V, et al. Rhythm versus rate control therapy and subsequent stroke or transient ischemic attack in patients with atrial fibrillation. *Circulation.* 2012;126:2680–2687.

14. Granger CB, Alexander JH, McMurray JJ, et al. Apixaban versus warfarin in patients with atrial fibrillation. *New Engl J Med.* 2011;365:981–992.

15. Connolly SJ, Ezekowitz MD, Yusuf S, et al. Dabigatran versus warfarin in patients with atrial fibrillation. *New Engl J Med.* 2009;361:1139–1151.

16. Holmes DR, Reddy VY, Turi ZG, t al. Percutaneous closure of the left atrial appendage versus warfarin therapy for prevention of stroke in patients with atrial fibrillation: a randomised non-inferiority trial. *Lancet.* 2009;374:534–542.

17. Kenet G, Lutkhoff LK, Albisetti M, et al. Impact of thrombophilia on risk of arterial ischemic stroke or cerebral sinovenous thrombosis in neonates and children: a systematic review and meta-analysis of observational studies. *Circulation.* 2010;121:1838–1847.

18. Kittner SJ, Stern BJ, Feeser BR, et al. Pregnancy and the risk of stroke. *New Engl J Med.* 1996;335:768–774.

19. James AH, Bushnell CD, Jamison MG, et al. Incidence and risk factors for stroke in pregnancy and the puerperium. *ObstetGynecol.* 2005;106:509–516.

20. Lamy C, Hamon JB, Coste J, et al. Ischemic stroke in young women: risk of recurrence during subsequent pregnancies. French study group on stroke in pregnancy. *Neurology.* 2000;55:269–274.

21. Jaigobin C, Silver FL. Stroke and pregnancy. *Stroke.* 2000;31:2948–2951.

22. Lanska DJ, Kryscio RJ. Risk factors for peripartum and postpartum stroke and intracranial venous thrombosis. *Stroke.* 2000;31:1274–1282.

23. Davie CA, O'Brien P. Stroke and pregnancy. *J Neurol Neurosurg Psychiatry.* 2008;79: 240–245.

24. Kim SJ, Park JH, Lee MJ, et al. Clues to occult cancer in patients with ischemic stroke. *PloS ONE.* 2012;7:e44959.

25. Bick RL. Cancer-associated thrombosis. *New Engl J Med..* 2003;349:109–111.

26. Kim SG, Hong JM, Kim HY, et al. Ischemic stroke in cancer patients with and without conventional mechanisms: a multicenter study in korea. *Stroke.* 2010;41:798–801.

27. Li SH, Chen WH, Tang Y, et al. Incidence of ischemic stroke post-chemotherapy: a retrospective review of 10,963 patients. *Clin Neurol Neurosurg.* 2006;108:150–156.

28. Campen CJ, Kranick SM, Kasner SE, et al. Cranial irradiation increases risk of stroke in pediatric brain tumor survivors. *Stroke.* 2012;43:3035–3040.

29. Lee AY, Levine MN, Baker RI, et al. Low-molecular-weight heparin versus a coumarin for the prevention of recurrent venous thromboembolism in patients with cancer. *New Engl J Med.* 2003;349:146–153.

30. Debette S, Leys D. Cervical-artery dissections: predisposing factors, diagnosis, and out-come. *Lancet Neurol.* 2009;8:668–678.

31. Schievink WI. Spontaneous dissection of the carotid and vertebral arteries. *New Engl J Med.* 2001;344:898–906.

32. Gdynia HJ, Kuhnlein P, Ludolph AC, et al. Connective tissue disorders in dissections of the carotid or vertebral arteries. *Journal Clin Neurosci.* 2008;15:489–494.

33. Levy C, Laissy JP, Raveau V, et al. Carotid and vertebral artery dissections: three-dimensional time-of-flight mr angiography and mr imaging versus conventional angi-ography. *Radiology.* 1994;190:97–103.

34. investigators Ct, Markus HS, Hayter E, Levi C, Feldman A, et al. Antiplatelet treatment compared with anticoagulation treatment for cervical artery dissection (cadiss): a ran-domised trial. *Lancet Neurol.* 2015;14:361–367.

35. Meissner I, Khandheria BK, Heit JA, et al. Patent foramen ovale: innocent or guilty? Evidence from a prospective population-based study. *J Am Coll Cardiol.* 2006;47: 440–445.

36. Stollberger C, Slany J, Schuster I, et al. The prevalence of deep venous thrombosis in patients with suspected paradoxical embolism. *Ann Intern Med.* 1993;119:461–465.

37. Overell JR, Bone I, Lees KR. Interatrial septal abnormalities and stroke: a meta-analysis of case-control studies. *Neurology.* 2000;55:1172–1179.

38. Furlan AJ, Reisman M, Massaro J, et al. Closure or medical therapy for cryptogenic stroke with patent foramen ovale. *New Engl J Med.* 2012;366:991–999.

39. Carroll JD, Saver JL, Thaler DE, Smalling RW, Berry S, MacDonald LA, et al. Closure of patent foramen ovale versus medical therapy after cryptogenic stroke. *New Engl J Med..* 2013;368:1092–1100.

40. Meier B, Kalesan B, Mattle HP, et al. Percutaneous closure of patent foramen ovale in cryptogenic embolism. *New Engl J Med.e.* 2013;368:1083–1091.

41. Mas JL, Derumeaux G, Guillon B, et al. Patent foramen ovale closure or anticoagulation vs. Antiplatelets after stroke. *New Engl J Med.* 2017;377:1011–1021.

42. Saver JL, Carroll JD, Thaler DE, et al. Long-term outcomes of patent foramen ovale clo-sure or medical therapy after stroke. *New Engl J Med.* 2017;377:1022–1032.

43. Sondergaard L, Kasner SE, Rhodes JF, et al. Patent foramen ovale closure or antiplatelet therapy for cryptogenic stroke. *New England J Med.* 2017;377:1033–1042.

44. Visser CA, Kan G, Meltzer RS, et al. Embolic potential of left ventricular thrombus after myocardial infarction: a two-dimensional echocardiographic study of 119 patients. *J Am Coll Cardiol.* 1985;5:1276–1280.

45. Taina M, Sipola P, Muuronen A, et al. Determinants of left atrial appendage volume in stroke patients without chronic atrial fibrillation. *PloS ONE.* 2014;9:e90903.

46. Taina M, Vanninen R, Hedman M, et al. Left atrial appendage volume increased in more than half of patients with cryptogenic stroke. *PloS ONE.* 2013;8:e79519.

47. Di Biase L, Santangeli P, Anselmino M, et al. Does the left atrial appendage morphology correlate with the risk of stroke in patients with atrial fibrillation? Results from a multi-center study. *J Am Coll Cardiol.* 2012;60:531–538.

48. Pearson AC, Nagelhout D, Castello R, et al. Atrial septal aneurysm and stroke: a trans-esophageal echocardiographic study. *J Am CollCardiol.* 1991;18:1223–1229.

49. Belkin RN, Kisslo J. Atrial septal aneurysm: recognition and clinical relevance. *AmHeart J.* 1990;120:948–957.

50. Cabanes L, Mas JL, Cohen A, et al. Atrial septal aneurysm and patent foramen ovale as risk factors for cryptogenic stroke in patients less than 55 years of age. A study using trans-esophageal echocardiography. *Stroke.* 1993;24:1865–1873.

51. Kamel H, Bartz TM, Elkind MSV, et al. Atrial cardiopathy and the risk of ischemic stroke in the CHS (Cardiovascular Health Study). *Stroke.* 2018;49:980–986.

52. Amarenco P, Cohen A, Tzourio C, et al. Atherosclerotic disease of the aortic arch and the risk of ischemic stroke. *New Engl J Med.* 1994;331:1474–1479.

53. Di Tullio MR, Russo C, Jin Z, et al. Aortic arch plaques and risk of recurrent stroke and death. *Circulation.* 2009;119:2376–2382.

54. Amarenco P, Duyckaerts C, Tzourio C, et al. The prevalence of ulcerated plaques in the aortic arch in patients with stroke. *New Engl J Med.* 1992;326:221–225.

55. Lima JA, Desai MY, Steen H, et al. Statin-induced cholesterol lowering and plaque regression after 6 months of magnetic resonance imaging-monitored therapy. *Circulation.* 2004;110:2336–2341.

56. Di Tullio MR, Homma S, Jin Z, et al. Aortic atherosclerosis, hypercoagulability, and stroke the APRIS (Aortic Plaque and Risk of Ischemic Stroke) study. *J AmColl Cardiol.* 2008;52:855–861.

57. Dressler FA, Craig WR, Castello R, et al. Mobile aortic atheroma and systemic emboli: efficacy of anticoagulation and influence of plaque morphology on recurrent stroke. *J Am Coll Cardiol.* 1998;31:134–138.

58. Ferrari E, Vidal R, Chevallier T, et al. Atherosclerosis of the thoracic aorta and aortic debris as a marker of poor prognosis: benefit of oral anticoagulants. *J AmColl Cardiol.* 1999;33:1317–1322.

59. Sen S. Aortic arch plaque in stroke. *Curr CardiolRep.* 2009;11:28–35.

60. Barbieux M, Veran O, Detante O. [Ischemic strokes in young adults and illegal drugs]. *Rev Med Interne.* 2012;33:35–40.

61. Kaku DA, Lowenstein DH. Emergence of recreational drug abuse as a major risk factor for stroke in young adults. *Ann Intern Med.* 1990;113:821–827.

62. Kaufman MJ, Levin JM, Ross MH, et al. Cocaine-induced cerebral vasoconstriction detected in humans with magnetic resonance angiography. *JAMA.* 1998;279:376–380.

63. Westover AN, McBride S, Haley RW. Stroke in young adults who abuse amphetamines or cocaine: a population-based study of hospitalized patients. *Arch Gen Psychiatry.* 2007;64:495–502.

64. Saez CG, Olivares P, Pallavicini J, et al. Increased number of circulating endothelial cells and plasma markers of endothelial damage in chronic cocaine users. *ThrombRes.* 2011;128:e18–23.

65. Fonseca AC, Ferro JM. Drug abuse and stroke. *Curr Neurol Neurosci Rep.* 2013;13:325

66. Salanova V, Taubner R. Intracerebral haemorrhage and vasculitis secondary to amphetamine use. *Postgrad Med J..* 1984;60:429–430.

67. Lieberman AN, Bloom W, Kishore PS, et al. Carotid artery occlusion following ingestion of LSD. *Stroke.* 1974;5:213–215.

68. Sobel J, Espinas OE, Friedman SA. Carotid artery obstruction following LSD capsule ingestion. *Arch Intern Med.* 1971;127:290–291.

69. Ohene-Frempong K, Weiner SJ, Sleeper LA, et al. Cerebrovascular accidents in sickle cell disease: rates and risk factors. *Blood.* 1998;91:288–294.

70. Dichgans M. Genetics of ischaemic stroke. *Lancet Neurol.* 2007;6:149–161.

71. Switzer JA, Hess DC, Nichols FT, et al. Pathophysiology and treatment of stroke in sickle-cell disease: present and future. *Lancet Neurol.* 2006;5:501–512.

72. Scott RM, Smith JL, Robertson RL, et al. Long-term outcome in children with moyamoya syndrome after cranial revascularization by pial synangiosis. *J Neurosurg.* 2004; 100:142–149.

73. Chabriat H, Joutel A, Dichgans M, et al. CADASIL. *The Lancet. Neurology.* 2009; 8:643–653.

74. Rolfs A, Bottcher T, Zschiesche M, et al. Prevalence of fabry disease in patients with cryptogenic stroke: a prospective study. *Lancet.* 2005;366:1794–1796.

75. Yap S, Boers GH, Wilcken B, et al. Vascular outcome in patients with homocystinuria due to cystathionine beta-synthase deficiency treated chronically: a multicenter observational study. *Arterioscler Thromb Vasc Biol.* 2001;21:2080–2085.

76. Wityk RJ, Zanferrari C, Oppenheimer S. Neurovascular complications of marfan syndrome: a retrospective, hospital-based study. *Stroke.* 2002;33:680–684.

77. North KN, Whiteman DA, Pepin MG, et al. Cerebrovascular complications in ehlers-danlos syndrome type IV. *Ann Neurol.* 1995;38:960–964.

78. Schievink WI, Michels VV, Piepgras DG. Neurovascular manifestations of heritable connective tissue disorders. a review. *Stroke.* 1994;25:889–903.

79. Wachter R, Weber-Kruger M, Seegers J, et al. Age-dependent yield of screening for undetected atrial fibrillation in stroke patients: the Find-AF Study. *J Neurol.* 2013;260: 2042–2045.

80. Weber-Kruger M, Gelbrich G, Stahrenberg R, et al. Finding atrial fibrillation in stroke patients: randomized evaluation of enhanced and prolonged Holter monitoring—find-AF (RANDOMISED)—rationale and design. *Am Heart J.* 2014;168:438–445 e431.

81. Gladstone DJ, Spring M, Dorian P, et al. Atrial fibrillation in patients with cryptogenic stroke. *New Engl J Med.* 2014;370:2467–2477.

82. Christensen LM, Krieger DW, Hojberg S, et al. Paroxysmal atrial fibrillation occurs often in cryptogenic ischaemic stroke. Final results from the SURPRISE Study. *Eur J Neurol.* 2014;21:884–889.

83. Reiffel JA, Verma A, Kowey PR, et al. Incidence of previously undiagnosed atrial fibrillation using insertable cardiac monitors in a high-risk population: the REVEAL AF study. *JAMA Cardiol.* 2017;2:1120–1127.

84. Kamel H, Hegde M, Johnson DR, et al. Cost-effectiveness of outpatient cardiac monitoring to detect atrial fibrillation after ischemic stroke. *Stroke.* 2010;41:1514–1520.

85. Murat Sumer M, Erturk O. Ischemic stroke subtypes: risk factors, functional outcome and recurrence. *Neurol Sci.* 2002;22:449–454.

86. Petty GW, Brown RD, Jr., Whisnant JP, et al. Ischemic stroke subtypes : a population-based study of functional outcome, survival, and recurrence. *Stroke.* 2000;31:1062–1068.

87. Vaziri SM, Larson MG, Benjamin EJ, et al. Echocardiographic predictors of nonrheumatic atrial fibrillation. The Framingham Heart Study. *Circulation.* 1994;89:724–730.

88. Dilaveris PE, Gialafos EJ, Sideris SK, et al. Simple electrocardiographic markers for the prediction of paroxysmal idiopathic atrial fibrillation. *Am Heart J.* 1998;135:733–738.

INDEX

Page numbers in *italics* represent tables and figures.